Pediatric Thoracic Surgery

CURRENT TOPICS IN GENERAL THORACIC SURGERY
AN INTERNATIONAL SERIES

Series Editors
Richard M. Peters, MD
I. Vogt-Moykopf, MD
Watts R. Webb, MD
Earle W. Wilkins, Jr., MD

Pediatric Thoracic Surgery
James C. Fallis, MD, FRCS(C)
Robert M. Filler, MD, FRCS(C)
Georges Lemoine, MD

Pediatric Thoracic Surgery

Edited by

James C. Fallis, MD, FRCS(C)

Assistant Professor
Departments of Pediatrics and Surgery
University of Toronto Faculty of Medicine

Emergency Services
The Hospital for Sick Children
Toronto, Ontario, Canada

Robert M. Filler, MD, FRCS(C)

Professor
Department of Surgery
University of Toronto Faculty of Medicine

Surgeon-in-Chief
The Hospital for Sick Children
Toronto, Ontario, Canada

Georges Lemoine, MD

Associate Professor
Department of Thoracic and Cardiovascular Surgery
Pediatric Unit
Centre Medico-Chirurgical de la Porte de Choisy, Paris, France

Elsevier
New York • Amsterdam • London • Tokyo

Elsevier Science Publishing Co., Inc.
655 Avenue of the Americas, New York, New York, 10010

© 1991 by Elsevier Science Publishing Co., Inc.

Library of Congress Cataloging in Publication Data

Pediatric thoracic surgery / edited by James C. Fallis, Robert M. Filler,
    Georges Lemoine.
        p. cm. – (Current topics in general thoracic surgery)
        Includes index.
        ISBN 0-444-01605-8 (hard cover : alk. paper)
        1. Chest – Surgery. 2. Children – Surgery. I. Fallis, James C.
    II. Filler, Robert M. III. Lemoine, Georges. IV. Series.
        [DNLM: 1. Thoracic Surgery – in infancy & childhood. WF 980 P371]
    RD536.P44   1991
    617.9'8 – dc20
    DNLM/DLC   91-28185
    for Library of Congress   CIP

Current printing (last digit):
10 9 8 7 6 5 4 3 2 1

Manufactured in the United States of America

Contents

Part I
Special Problems / 1

Chapter 1
Imaging of Pediatric Surgical Disease of the Chest / 3
Philip Stanley, MD
Discussion / 13
Philippe Baudain, MD, Chartal Durand, MD, Jean-Francois Dyon, MD and Patrice Francois, MD

Chapter 2
Pediatric Anesthesia: Special Requirements for Intrathoracic Procedures / 23
Derek Blackstock, MB, FFARCSI, FRCP(C) and David J. Steward, MB, FRCP(C)
Discussion / 32
Gary G. Johnson, MD

Chapter 3
Intensive Airway and Respiratory Techniques / 35
David S. Jardine, MD and Robert K. Crone, MD
Discussion / 44
Didier Moulin, MD

Foreword to the Series

CURRENT TOPICS IN GENERAL THORACIC SURGERY: AN INTERNATIONAL SE-RIES is the successor to INTERNATIONAL TRENDS IN GENERAL THORACIC SUR-GERY; the latter is six years and eight volumes old. This volume represents the passing of the series into new hands, new series editors, and a new publisher, Elsevier Science Publishing Company, Inc.

The world has been made progressively smaller by our technological advances in travel. The jumbo jet assures that any physician may have a patient with disease acquired in any part of the world and patients of any race, nationality, and language. Compendiums of medical knowledge have an international readership and, we believe, should include the views of the international medical community. The electronic communications revolution is giving us new exciting tools for dissemination of knowledge and communication between individuals. These improved communications methods may speed discourse between editors and authors but the task of assembling medical knowledge from an international group of medical experts (even with the FAX) still requires arduous work by devoted and underpaid editors and authors. This series exists because dedicated editors and authors believe this task is part of their obligation as medical experts.

In the foreword to the first volume of the International Trends in General Thoracic Surgery series, Drs. Norman Delarue and Henry Eschapasse indicated that "A void exists in the sphere of information transfer within the specialty of general thoracic surgery." This void persists and there remains "an obvious need to fill the resultant vacuum." The developers of the INTERNATIONAL TRENDS IN GENERAL THORACIC SURGERY series wanted to reach a wide international audience. Recognizing that most individuals with English as a native language are unilingual, they chose English as the language for the series. "In order to foster international dialogue" they established the format that "the contributions from one medical culture" have been, and will continue to be, discussed "by representatives . . . from another part of the world."

This first volume to be published within the CURRENT TOPICS IN GENERAL THORACIC SURGERY: AN INTERNATIONAL SERIES series was conceived by the INTERNATIONAL TRENDS IN GENERAL THORACIC SURGERY Series Editors and guided to publication by their careful and diplomatic supervision. They stimulated the volume editors to gather an outstanding group of contributors and gave invaluable aid to the new Series Editors and the publisher in bringing this volume to publication.

Co-editors from North America and Europe are responsible for the contents of this volume. We hope in the future to include more contributors from Russia, Eastern Europe, the Southern Hemisphere, and Asia to catalyze a broader authorship and leadership.

The Current Topics in General Thoracic Surgery Series Editors know we have a challenge to meet the standards set by Drs. Norman Delarue and Henry Eschapasse. With their continued counsel and the excellent help of the staff at Elsevier we hope to be able to continue to provide a high quality series.

Richard M. Peters, MD

Preface

Any series presenting world-wide trends in general thoracic surgery would be incomplete without at least one volume describing advances in the management of surgical chest disease in infancy and childhood. Most pediatric general thoracic surgery continues to be carried out by pediatric general surgeons who have developed specialized interest in certain aspects of surgery of the chest and—in conjunction with pediatric colleagues from a number of disciplines such as anesthesia, neonatology, and respirology—supervise important research studies out of which major clinical progress flows and will continue to flow.

This volume is an attempt to survey this broad field for the reader. There is relevant information for all who treat infants and children with thoracic disease, whether pediatric surgeons, anesthesiologists, medical specialists, or adult thoracic surgeons who have occasion to manage chest disease in children from time to time. The contributors, all acknowledged as specialists with international reputation, have put great effort into producing readable and informative chapters. As a manifestation of the international authorship it will be apparent to the reader that English is not the mother tongue for some of the contributors, although all attempts have been made to make the translations easily understood.

The first section hinges on the almost unbelievable technological progress of the last two decades. Advances in imaging capacities now permit preoperative studies hardly anticipated a decade ago. The ability to add artificial oxygenation to artificial circulation presents the potential for extending therapeutic horizons to limits never before envisioned. Technological advances have probably had their most evident application in the services provided by the anesthesiologist and by the pediatric intensivist. These are all detailed for the general benefit of the surgeon, or for the subspecialist working in his own narrower field.

Intrathoracic congenital anomalies are dealt with in the second section. A comprehensive chapter on the embryological basis for thoracic malformations is followed by contributions on clinical aspects of the lesions themselves.

A discussion of acquired esophageal lesions follows, with emphasis on gastroesophageal reflux and caustic burns of the esophagus. The section on tracheobronchial obstruction covers the relatively uncommon entities as well as foreign body aspiration which is so relevant to pediatric practitioners of any specialty.

The chapter on congenital diaphragmatic herniation introduces a philosophy of management which contrasts with the traditional but has immediate application. Phrenic nerve palsy and thoracic cage anomalies cause heated discussion among pediatric surgeons and the international approach to these topics puts the points of disagreement into perspective. This is followed by a section on tumors of chest wall, lung, and mediastinum. A discussion of chest injuries in children has immediate relevance in view of the alarming incidence of major thoracic trauma occurring either alone or in combination with other serious injuries.

Although pulmonary infections and their complications no longer occur with their former frequency, unusual infections now require unusual methods for diagnosis and treatment, as is described in the chapter on lung biopsy and bronchoalveolar lavage. Current management of empyema, bronchiectasis and lung abscess is also included.

The final section on future challenges is appropriate for medical and surgical specialists alike, and sets the stage for pediatric thoracic surgical care in the 90s. It focuses on the two most controversial areas, that of fetal surgery and of lung, heart, and heart-lung transplantation, and on ethical considerations of these topics.

In this volume, as in the series, the chapters are followed by invited comments from individuals half a world away; it is hoped that this international format will stimulate and instruct.

The editors are grateful to the chapter contributors and those providing comments on the chapters, for their enthusiasm and the quality of their submissions.We are also most appreciative of the guidance provided by Drs. Delarue and Eschapasse, the Editors Emeritus of the series.

James C. Fallis, MD, FRCS(C)

Robert M. Filler, MD, FRCS(C)

Georges Lemoine, MD

Contributors

Wolfgang R. Ade, MD
Adjunct Staff, Juro Wada Commemorative Heart and Lung Institute; Yuden Clinic and Akasaka Hospital Medical Center, Denki Building N.10F, 1-7-1 Yuraku-Cho, Chiyoda-Ku, Tokyo 100, Japan

Jean-Pierre Alibeu, MD
Department of Anesthesiology, University Hospital, CHU de Grenoble, BP 217, 38043 Grenoble Cedex 9, France

Kathryn D. Anderson, MD
Vice-Chairman, Department of Surgery, Children's National Medical Center, 111 Michigan Avenue Northwest, Washington, DC 20010-2970

Francisco Asensi, MD
Associate Professor of Pediatrics and Consultant of the Infectious Diseases Section, La Fe University Children's Hospital, Avda. Campanar 21, 46009 Valencia, Spain

Phillip G. Ashmore, MD, FRCS(C)
Head and Chairman, Division of Cardiovascular and Thoracic Surgery, Section of Surgery, British Columbia Children's Hospital, Rm 1L7, 4480 Oak Street, Vancouver, British Columbia V6H 3V4

Robert J. Attorri, MD
Chief Resident of Pediatric Surgery, Department of Surgery, Children's National Medical Center, 111 Michigan Avenue N.W., Washington, DC 20010-2970

Robert H. Bartlett, MD
Professor, Department of Surgery, University of Michigan Medical Center, 1500 East Medical Center Drive, Ann Arbor, Michigan 48109-0331

Philippe Baudain, MD
Professor, Department of Pediatric Radiology, University Joseph Fourier, CHU de Grenoble, 38043 Grenoble Cedex, France

Jean-Paul Binet, MD
Hopital Marie Lannelongue, 133 Avenue de la Resistance, 92350 Le Plessis Robinson, France

Derek Blackstock, MB, FFARCSI, FRCP(C)

Clinical Assistant Professor, Department of Anesthesia, University of British Columbia Faculty of Medicine; Staff Anesthetist British Columbia Children's Hospital, 4480 Oak Street, Vancouver, British Columbia V6H 3V4

Desmond Bohn, MB, BCh, FRCP(C)

Assistant Professor of Anesthesia, University of Toronto Faculty of Medicine; Assistant Director, Department of Critical Care, Hospital for Sick Children, Room 2211, 555 University Avenue, Toronto, Ontario M5G 1X8, Canada

J. Boix-Ochoa, MD

Chairman and Professor, Department of Pediatric Surgery, Hospital Materno-Infantil Vall d'Hebron, 08035 Barcelona, Spain

Albert P. Bos, MD

Pediatric Consultant, Department of Pediatric Surgery, Sophia Children's University Hospital, P.O. Box 70029, 3000 LL Rotterdam, the Netherlands

D. Branscheid, MD

Assistant Head of Surgery, Thoracic Surgery Clinic, Rohrbach Hospital, Amalienstrasse 5, 6900 Heidelberg I, Germany

François C. Bremont, MD

Pediatrician, CHU Purpan-Place du Docteur Baylac, 310059 Toulouse, France

J. M. Casasa, MD

Chief of Surgical Gastroenterology, Department of Pediatric Surgery, Hospital Materno-Infantil, Vall d'Hebron 08035, Barcelona, Spain

Jean Paul Chappuis, MD

Professor, Department of Pediatric Surgery, Hopital Edouard Herriot, Place d'Arsonval, 69003 Lyon Cedex 03, France

Yves P. M. Chavrier, MD

Professor and Chief of Pediatric Surgery, Hopital Nord, Albert Raimond Avenue, 42277 Saint Priest en Jarez, Saint-Etienne, France

Jean-Yves Chevalier, MD

Intensive Care Unit, Hopital Trousseau, 26 Au du Dr. A. Netter, 75012 Paris, France

Arnold G. Coran, MD

Professor and Head, Department of Pediatric Surgery, The University of Michigan Medical Center; Surgeon-in-Chief, C. S. Mott Children's Hospital, Box 0245, Ann Arbor, Michigan 48109-0245

Robert K. Crone, MD

Professor of Anesthesiology and Pediatrics, University of Washington School of Medicine; Director of Anesthesiology, Children's Hospital and Medical Center, 4800 Sand Point Way Northeast, Seattle, Washington 98105

Claire Danel, MD
Associated Professor, Department of Pathology, University Rene Descartes; Department of Anatomy and Pathology, CHU Necker Enfants Malades, 149 rue de Sevres, 75743 Paris Cedex 15, France

Juan C. de Agustin, MD, PhD
Surgeon, Department of Pediatric Surgery, Universidad Autónoma de Madrid; Hospital Infantil del Niño Jesús, Poza de la Sal 15, 28031 Madrid, Spain

M. Jaubert de Beaujeu, MD
Professor of Childrens Pediatrics, Universite Claude Bernard, Cliousclat 26270 Lyon, France

Jean-Louis de Brux, MD
Department of Cardiovascular and Thoracic Surgery, Centre Hospitalier Regional Et Universitaire, CHRU, 49033 Angers Cedex, France

Michel Deneuville, MD
Chief Resident, Thoracic and Cardiovascular Surgery, Pediatric Unit, CMC Porte de Choisy 6, Place de Port au Prince 75013, Paris, France

Jean de Ville de Goyet, MD
Department of Pediatric Surgery and Intensive Care, University of Louvain Medical School, Cliniques Saint-Luc, Avenue Hippocrate 10, 1200 Brussels, Belgium

Chartal Durand, MD
Radiologist, Department of Pediatric Radiology, University Joseph Fourier, CHU de Grenoble, BP 27, 38043 Grenoble Cedex, France

Yves Durandy, MD
Department of Cardiac Surgery, C.R.P Clinique de la Residence du Parc, 13362 Marseille, Cedex 10, France

Guy J. Dutau, MD
Professor of Pediatrics, Unité des Maladies Respiratoires et Allergiques de l'Enfant et de l'Adolescent, CHU Purpan-Place du Docteur Baylac, 310059 Toulouse, France

Jean-Francois Dyon, MD
Professor of Pediatric Surgery, Department of Pediatric Surgery, University Hospital, University Joseph Fourier, Grenoble I, B.P. 217, 38043, Grenoble Cedex 9, France

Martin R. Eichelberger, MD
Director, Emergency Trauma Services, Children's Hospital National Medical Center, 111 Michigan Avenue N.W., Washington, District of Columbia 20010-5000

James C. Fallis, MD, FRCS(C)
Assistant Professor, Departments of Pediatrics and Surgery, University of Toronto Faculty of Medicine; Emergency Service, The Hospital for Sick Children, 555 University Avenue, Toronto, Ontario, M5G 1X8 Canada

Robert M. Filler, MD, FRCS(C)

Professor, Department of Surgery, University of Toronto Faculty of Medicine; Surgeon-in-Chief, Department of Surgery, The Hospital for Sick Children, 555 University Avenue, Toronto, Ontario, M5G 1X8 Canada

Patrice Francois, MD

Department of Pediatrics, CHU de Grenoble, BP 217X, 38043 Grenoble, France

Daniel A. Gillis, MD, BSc, MS, FRCS(C), FACS

Head of Department of Surgery, Dalhousie University; Chief of Surgery, I.W.K. Children's Hospital, P.O. Box 3070, 5850 University Avenue, Halifax, Nova Scotia B3J 3G9, Canada

Stephen W. Gray, PhD

Professor Emeritus of Anatomy and Associate Director, The Thalia and Michael Carlos Center for Surgical Anatomy and Technique and The Alfred A. Davis Research Center for Surgical Anatomy and Technique, Emory University School of Medicine, 1462 Clifton Road Northeast, Suite 303, Atlanta, Georgia 30322

A. Grimfeld, MD

Hopital Trousseau, 26 Au du Dr. A. Netter, Paris, France

Jay L. Grosfeld, MD

Lafayette F. Page Professor and Chairman, Department of Surgery, Indiana University School of Medicine; Surgeon-in-Chief, J. W. Riley Hospital for Children, 702 Barnhill Drive (K-21), Indianapolis, Indiana 46202

J. Alex Haller, Jr., MD

Children's Surgeon-in-Charge, Department of Pediatric Surgery, The Johns Hopkins Hospital, 601 North Broadway, Baltimore, Maryland 21205

Daniel M. Hays, MD

Professor of Surgery and Pediatrics, University of Southern California School of Medicine; Children Hospital of Los Angeles, P.O. Box 54700, Mailstop 70, Los Angeles, California 90054-0700

Frans W. J. Hazebroek, MD, PhD

Department of Pediatric Surgery, Sophia Children's University Hospital, P.O. Box 70029, 3000 LL Rotterdam, the Netherlands

Gerald B. Healy, MD

Otolaryngologist-in-Chief, Department of Otolaryngology and Communication Disorders, The Children's Hospital, 300 Longwood Avenue, Boston, Massachusetts 02115

Thomas M. Holder, MD

Chief, Department of Thoracic and Cardiovascular Surgery, Clinical Professor of Surgery, Department of Surgery, The Children's Mercy Hospital, 2401 Gillham Road, Kansas City, Missouri 64108

Ulrik Hvass, MD

Professor of Thoracic and Cardiovascular Surgery, Xavier Bichat Medical University; Cardiovascular Surgeon, Hopital Bichat 46, rue Henri Huchard, 75018 Paris, France

David S. Jardine, MD
Assistant Professor of Anesthesiology and Pediatrics, Department of Anesthesiology, Children's Hospital and Medical Center, 4800 Sand Point Way Northeast, Box C5371, Seattle, Washington 98105

Francis Jaubert, MD
Professor, Department of Anatomy and Pathology, Hopital Necker Enfants Malades, 149 rue de Sevres, 75743 Paris Cedex 15, France

Dale G. Johnson, MD
Professor of Surgery and Pediatrics, University of Utah School of Medicine; Surgeon-in-Chief, Primary Children's Medical Center, 100 North Medical Drive, Suite 2600, Salt Lake City, Utah 84113-1100

Gary G. Johnson, BA, MD, FRCP(C)
Associate Professor, Department of Anesthesia, University of Ottawa; Chief, Department of Anesthesia, University of Ottawa; Chief, Department of Anesthesiology, Children's Hospital of Eastern Ontario, 401 Smyth Road, Ottawa, Ontario K1H 8L1, Canada

Ann M. Kosloske, MD
Clinical Professor of Surgery and Pediatrics, University of New Mexico School of Medicine; Director of Pediatric Surgery, The Children's Hospital of New Mexico, Albuquerque, New Mexico 87106

S. Krysa, MD
Thoracic Surgery Clinic, Rohrbach Hospital, Amalienstrasse 5, 6900 Heidelberg I, Germany

Leon K. Lacquet, MD, FRCS(C)
Professor and Head, Department of Thoracic and Cardiac Surgery, University Hospital St. Radboud, Postbus 9101, 6500 HB Nijmegen, The Netherlands

Jacob C. Langer, MD, FRCS(C)
Assistant Professor, Department of Surgery and Pediatrics, McMaster University, 1200 Main Street West, Room 4E-2, Hamilton, Ontario L8N 3Z5, Canada

Jean Langlois, MD
Professor in Cardio-vascular Surgery and Chief, Department of Cardiac Surgery, Hopital Bichat 46, rue Henri Huchard, 75018 Paris, France

Georges Lemoine, MD
Associate Professor, Department of Thoracic and Cardiovascular Surgery, Pediatric Unit, Centre Medico-Chirurgical de la Porte de Choisy 6, Place De Port Au Prince, 75013 Paris, France

Abbyann Lynch, PhD
Associate Professor, Department of Pediatrics, University of Toronto; Director, Department of Bioethics, Hospital for Sick Children, 555 University Avenue, Toronto, Ontario, Canada M5G 1X8

David P. Mitchell, MD, FRCS(C)
Department of Otolaryngology, The Hospital for Sick Children, 555 University Avenue, Toronto, Ontario M5G 1X8, Canada

Christopher R. Moir, MD
Senior Associate Consultant in Pediatric Surgery, Assistant Professor of Surgery, Mayo Foundation, 200 First Street Southwest, Rochester, Minnesota 55905

Jan C. Molenaar, MD, PhD, FAAP
Professor, Department of Pediatric Surgery, Sophia Children's University Hospital, P.O. Box 70029, 3000 LL Rotterdam, the Netherlands

Philippe Montupet, MD
Department of Pediatric Surgery, Universite Paris XII; Hopital de Bicetre, Lemoine Unit, CMC Porte de Choisy 6, Place de Port au Prince 75013, Paris, France

Didier Moulin, MD
Assistant Professor, Department of Pediatric Intensive Care, Clinical University of St. Luc, Avenue Hippocrates 10, 1200 Brussels, Belgium

Kurt D. Newman, MD
Assistant Professor, Department of Pediatric Surgery, George Washington University, Children's National Medical Center, 111 Michigan Avenue N.W., Washington, DC 20010

James A. O'Neill, Jr., MD
C.E. Koop Professor of Pediatric Surgery, University of Pennsylvania School of Medicine; Surgeon-in-Chief, Children's Hospital of Philadelphia, 34th and Civic Center Boulevard, Philadelphia, Pennsylvania 19104

Carmen Otero, MD
Assistant, Infectious Diseases Section, La Fe University Children's Hospital, Avda. Campanar 21, 46009 Valencia, Spain

Jean-Bernard Otte, MD
Professor and Head, Department of Pediatric Surgery, Hospital St Luc, 10 Avenue Hippocrate, B1200 Brussels, Belgium

Francisco Paris, MD
Head of Thoracic Surgery, Titular Professor of Surgery, La Fé University Hospital, Avda. Campanar 21, 46009 Valencia, Spain

G. Alexander Patterson, MD, FRCS(C), FACS
Associate Professor, Department of Surgery, University of Toronto Faculty of Medicine, 200 Elizabeth Street, Eaton Wing-10th Floor, Room 230, Toronto, Ontario M5G 2C4, Canada

Desamparados Perez-Tamarit, MD
Assistant of the Infectious Diseases Section, La Fé University Children's Hospital, Avda. Campanar 21, 46009 Valencia, Spain

Arvin I. Philippart, MD
Professor, Department of Surgery, Wayne State University; Chief of Pediatric General Surgery and Chairman of Surgical Services, Children's Hospital of Michigan, 3901 Beaubien, Detroit, Michigan 48201

Claude Planche, MD
Professor of Thoracic and Cardiovascular Surgery, Bicetre Medical University; Cardiovascular Surgeon, Centre Chirurgical Marie-Lannelongue 133, Avenue de la Resistance, 92350 La Plessis Robinson, France

Kevin C. Pringle, MD, ChB, FRACS
Associate Professor of Pediatric Surgery, Department of Surgery, University of Otago–Wellington School of Medicine, P.O. Box 7343, Wellington, New Zealand

Yann Revillon, MD
Professor, Hopital Enfants Malades 149, rue de Sevres, 75015 Paris, France

Santiago Ruiz-Company, MD
Head, Department of Pediatric Surgery, La Fé Children's Hospital, Avda. Campanar 21, 46010 Valencia, Spain

Annie C. Sengelin, MD
Anesthesiologist, CHU Purpan-Place du Docteur Baylac, 310059 Toulouse, France

Alain Serraf, MD
Chief Resident, Pediatric Cardiac Surgery, Marie Lannelongue Hospital, 133 Avenue de la Resistance, 92350 Le Plessis Robinson, France

Hiroyuki Shimada, MD, DMS
Head of Electron Microsurgery, Department of Pathology and Laboratory Medicine, Children's Hospital of Los Angeles, 4650 Sunset Boulevard, Los Angeles, California 90027

John E. Skandalakis, MD, PhD, FACS
Chris Carlos Distinguished Professor and Director, The Thalia and Michael Carlos Center for Surgical Anatomy and Technique and The Alfred A. Davis Research Center for Surgical Anatomy and Technique, Emory University School of Medicine, 1462 Clifton Road Northeast, Suite 303, Atlanta, Georgia 30322

Philip Stanley, MD
Professor of Radiology, Head, Division of Diagnostic Radiology, Children's Hospital of Los Angeles, 4650 Sunset Boulevard, Los Angeles, California 90027

David J. Steward, MB, FRCP(C)
Professor, Department of Anesthesiology, University of Southern California; Director of Anesthesiology, Children's Hospital of Los Angeles, 4650 Sunset Boulevard, Los Angeles, California 90027

Robert L. Telander, MD
Professor, Department of Surgery, University of North Dakota School of Medicine; Chief of Surgery, Fargo Clinic and St. Lukes Hospital, 737 North Broadway, Fargo, North Dakota 58123

Dick Tibboel, MD, PhD
Consultant, Pediatric Surgery Intensive Care Unit, Department of Pediatric Surgery, Sophia Children's University Hospital, P.O. Box 70029, 3000 LL Rotterdam, the Netherlands

Juan G. Utrilla, MD

Assistant Professor of Pediatric Surgery, Universidad Autonoma de Madrid; Chief, Department of Pediatric Surgery, Hospital Infantil "La Paz", Claudio Coello 90, 28006 Madrid, Spain

Jean-Stephane Valla, MD

Professor of Pediatric Surgery, Hopital Lenval, 57 Avenue de la Californie, 06200 Nice, France

I. Vogt-Moykopf, MD

Professor and Director, Thoracic Surgery Clinic, Rohrbach Hospital, Amalienstrasse 5, 6900 Heidelberg I, Germany

Pascal R. Vouhé, MD

Professor of Cardiac Surgery, Department of Cardiovascular Surgery, Laennec Hospital, 42 Rue de Sevres, 75340 Paris Cedex 07, France

Juro Wada, MD, FACS

Director, J. Wada Commemorative Heart-Lung Institute, Yuden Clinic Medical Center, Denki Building N.10F, 1-7-1 Yuraki-Cho, Chiyoda-Ku, Tokyo 100, Japan

David E. Wesson, MD, FRCS(C)

Associate Professor of Surgery, University of Toronto; Director of Trauma Program, The Hospital for Sick Children, Room 1526, 555 University Avenue, Toronto, Ontario, M5G 1X8, Canada

Special Problems

Chapter 1

Imaging of Pediatric Surgical Disease of the Chest

Philip Stanley, MD

It is not possible to encompass the field of radiological imaging in pediatric surgical chest disease in one chapter. This article highlights recent advances and indications for the new imaging procedures.

CONTRAST AGENTS

Many life-threatening reactions to and the discomfort with the classic contrast agents were attributable to their high osmolality. With the introduction of nonionic agents and their reduced osmolality, there has been a tremendous increase in safety.[1] Whereas barium has remained the contrast medium of choice for most esophageal studies, nonionic agents are used for bronchography to demonstrate esophageal leaks and fistulae (Fig. 1.1). For enhancement with computed tomography and for vascular studies, nonionic agents are used exclusively at my pediatric institution.

The choice among iohexol, iopamidol, and ioversol is up to the individual radiologist. There is little difference clinically, given that their safety and opacification are equal. It should be noted that in catheterization procedures, nonionic agents are slightly more thrombogenic than are the classic agents. In addition, they are considerably more expensive.

MAGNETIC RESONANCE IMAGING

Magnetic resonance imaging (MRI) has introduced a new dimension in thoracic imaging. The ability to visualize in the three standard orthogonal planes (coronal, axial, and sagittal), together with the absence of radiation, reduced need for contrast agents, and improved soft tissue resolution, has made MRI the imaging method of choice for many conditions. The extent of paravertebral masses and possible involvement of the spinal contents can be shown (Fig. 1.2) without the need for intrathecal contrast. Magnetic resonance imaging will demonstrate the extent of mediastinal masses[2,3,4] and show their relationship to adjacent airways and major blood vessels (Fig. 1.3). However, because of long scanning time—a disadvantage of MRI—small intraparenchymal metastatic lesions will be missed because of respiratory motion. These lesions are best detected by computed tomography.

Preoperative and postoperative complex great vessel anomalies will be shown (Fig. 1.4). Aortic arch anomalies and their relationship to the compressed airway will be seen without the need for invasive angiography.[5,6] In cases of conotruncal abnormalities it is essential to demonstrate the pulmonary artery prior to surgery; this is often not demonstrated by angiography and will be shown by MRI.[7] For the follow-up of patients with aortic coarctation or systemic pulmonary shunts, MRI is the imaging method of choice[8] (Fig. 1.5). The arterial blood supply and venous drainage of sequestrations[9] will be shown, often without need for angiography (Fig. 1.6).

COMPUTED TOMOGRAPHY

Computed tomography (CT) of the chest has traditionally been used to demonstrate abnormalities of the mediastinum, lung parenchyma, chest wall, and pleura. Some of these areas, especially in the mediastinum, are now better imaged by magnetic resonance, particularly in a stable child

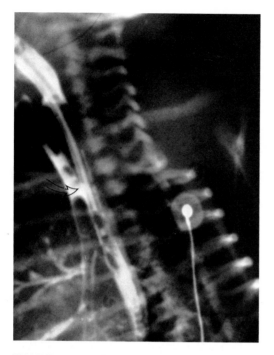

FIGURE 1.1 Esophagram with nonionic contrast showing a tracheoesophageal fistula (arrow). There is contrast in the bronchial tree. The nonionic contrast at a concentration of 200 mg of iodine/ml is approximately normo-osmolar, with minimal irritant affect to the respiratory mucosa.

who can be sedated if necessary. However, CT is usually the method of choice for the demonstration of lung parenchyma (Fig. 1.7), chest wall disease (particularly if bone destruction or periosteal new bone is to be demonstrated), or the mediastinum in a sick, unstable child (Fig. 1.8). With the development of ultrasfast scanning, high-quality dynamic CT of the pediatric airway is possible.[10,11] Computed tomography is the method of choice for providing guidance for biopsies (Fig. 1.9).

BRONCHOGRAPHY

Bronchography is usually performed to demonstrate bronchial and tracheal stenosis, important variants, and bronchiectasis, and to monitor balloon dilatation therapy.[12] It is usually performed immediately after bronchoscopy. Nonionic contrast with 200 mg of iodine/ml is injected through a small polyethylene tube introduced through the side port of an endotracheal tube.

BIOPSY

A needle biopsy under fluoroscopy or with computed tomography is a valuable technique for establishing the nature of mediastinal, lung, or pleural disease. For the diagnosis of lymphoma with the establishment of subtypes, a core of tis-

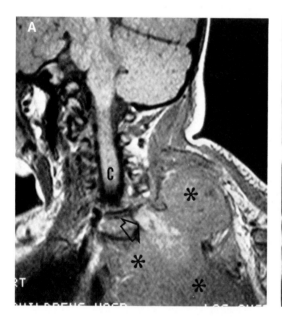
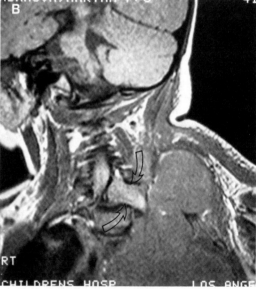

FIGURE 1.2 A. Coronal oblique MRI (short TR, short TE) in a child with intrathoracic lymphoma. There is a large lobulated mass (asterisks) occupying the upper left hemithorax. There is apparent extension (arrow) toward the spinal cord (C). **B.** Section 5 mm posterior to part A demonstrates extension through the intervertebral foramen (arrows), compressing the cord. This cord compression was difficult to visualize in other projections.

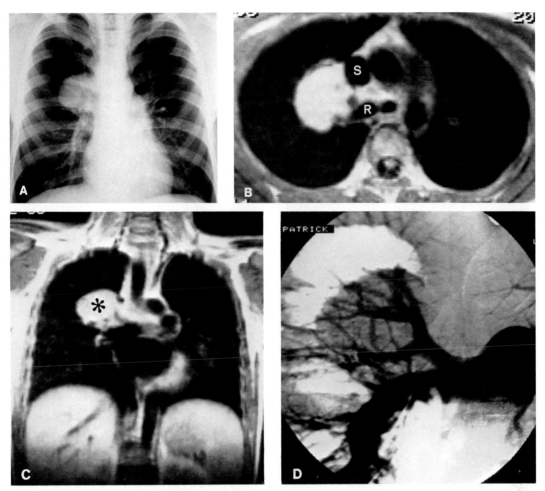

FIGURE 1.3 A. Frontal view of the chest in a 13-year-old boy showing a large perihilar mass. **B.** Axial MRI (short TR, short TE) demonstrating a high signal mass in the superior right hilar region. (R = right main bronchus, S = superior vena cava.) **C.** Coronal MRI (short TR, short TE) revealing high signal mass in the right hilum. The high signal on these sequences is not typical for lymphoma. **D.** Digital subtraction angiogram showing displacement and separation of branches of the right superior pulmonary artery but no aneurysm formation. Histology showed Castleman's disease.

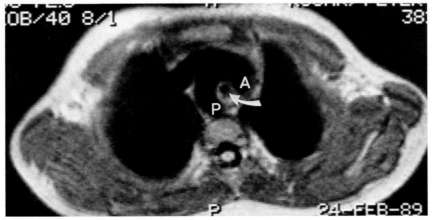

FIGURE 1.4 Axial MRI (gated short TE) in a child with respiratory distress due to a double aortic arch. The anterior (A) and posterior (P) arches encircling the trachea (arrow) are well seen.

sue is required. If the preliminary imaging study demonstrates a large mediastinal mass, a Trucut needle is used, special care being taken to avoid important vascular structures. For patients with a known primary with suspected intrathoracic metastatic disease and for biopsy of the lung, an aspiration biopsy is performed with a small caliber needle. The specimen is sent for cultures as

well as histology. Granulomatous disease can simulate metastases on chest images.

DRAINAGE PROCEDURES

Whereas the majority of empyemata are treated with a combination of antibiotics and surgical drainage, pleural collections and lung abscesses

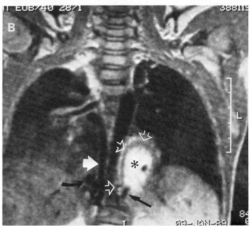

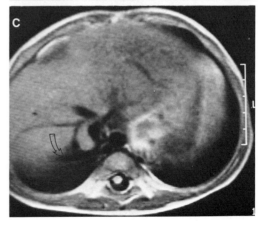

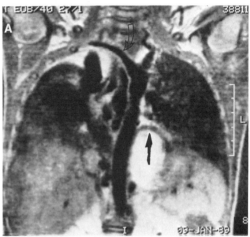

FIGURE 1.5 Postangioplasty MRI (gated short TE) showing residual coarctation (arrow) in this oblique sagittal projection.

→

FIGURE 1.6 Magnetic resonance studies of bilateral sequestrations. **A.** Coronal MRI (gated short TE) at the level of the descending aorta. There is an anomalous right subclavian artery (open arrow) and a sequestered segment at the left base (high signal intensity) with a large nutrient artery (solid black arrow). **B.** Coronal MRI 5 mm anterior to Fig 1.6, A section demonstrating the left basal sequestration (asterisk) with arterial blood supply arising from the aorta (short, white, open arrows). A draining vein (straight, black arrow) is seen emanating from the sequestration. In addition there are abnormal veins (curved black arrow) arising from a smaller sequestration at the right base. The azygous vein is well seen (solid white arrow). **C.** Axial MRI (gated short TE) showing a vein from the base of the right sequestered segment draining into the inferior vena cava (curved open arrows).

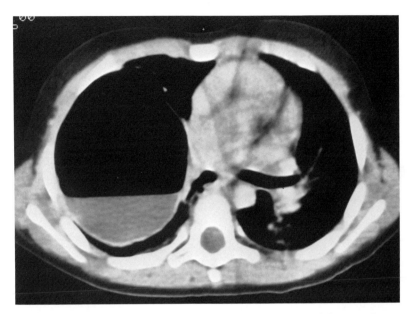

FIGURE 1.7 Axial computed tomography with the patient supine showing a right upper lung cyst with an air fluid level within it.

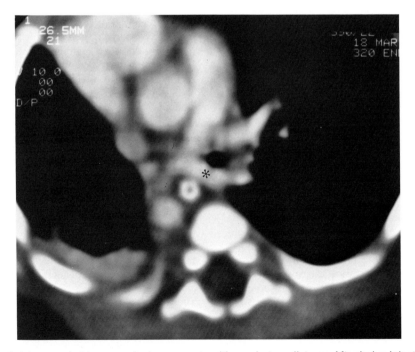

FIGURE 1.8 Axial computed tomography in a neonate with respiratory distress. After bolus injection of contrast, an anomalous left pulmonary artery (asterisk) was shown. There was dextroposition of the heart. The presence of a pulmonary artery sling was confirmed at surgery.

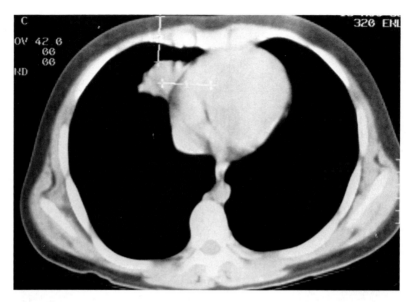

FIGURE 1.9 Axial nonenhanced computed tomography in a patient with treated Hodgkin's disease. It was feared that the right middle lobe mass represented recurrent disease. A thin-needle biopsy showed cocci-diomycosis. Measurements were placed on the scan by cursors as a guide to biopsy.

unresponsive to antibiotics may be drained percutaneously through the chest wall, obviating the need for a thoracotomy with general anesthesia.[13]

ANGIOGRAPHY

Angiography in its broadest sense encompasses arteriography, venography, and lymphangiography.

Arteriography has undergone fundamental changes with the introduction of low osmolality contrast agents and new methods of recording the image. The new methods of image demonstration include use of 100/105 mm cameras and digital subtraction techniques, the latter of which uses a computer to make an initial noncontrast mask and to subtract electronically from subsequent contrast films. With the digital recording, smaller volumes of less-concentrated contrast media may be given and the electronic subtracted image is instantly available, decreasing the time of catheterization; all of these features add to the safety of invasive arteriography.

The initial expectation that good arterial images could be recorded digitally through use of a venous injection has been only partially fulfilled. After central venous injection, it is possible to visualize the major pulmonary arteries (Fig. 1.10) and aorta; this is particularly helpful in sick infants with coarctation or in whom the arterial

access is not available (Fig. 1.11). However, fine arterial detail is not possible with a venous injection. Arteriography of the arch through an arterial catheter is performed at my hospital to demonstrate the effect of trauma, to show bronchial collaterals prior to embolization, to demonstrate blood supply in difficult sequestrations or tumors, and for complex aortic arch anomalies not shown adequately by less invasive techniques (Fig. 1.12). For patients with esophageal atresia, it is essential to demonstrate the side of the descending aorta prior to repair. If there is any doubt on ultrasound studies, the course of the descending aorta can easily be shown by injection through an umbilical catheter. If necessary, this can be performed in the nursery.

Venography and Central Venous Catheters

Many children have central venous catheters, placed through either a subclavian or jugular vein, for measurement of central venous pressure and to provide access for hyperalimentation. These catheters frequently need repositioning using guide wires. In addition, venous occlusions may occur requiring contrast venography to demonstrate the site of the obstruction and show important collaterals, some of which may be suitable for catheterization (Fig. 1.13).

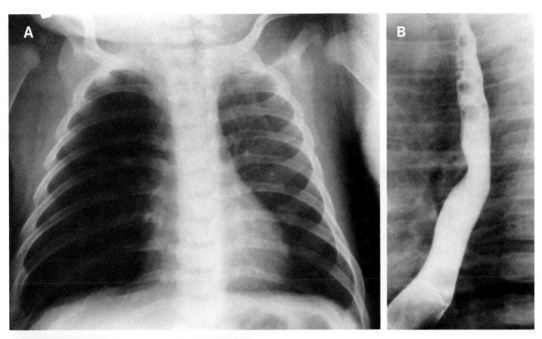

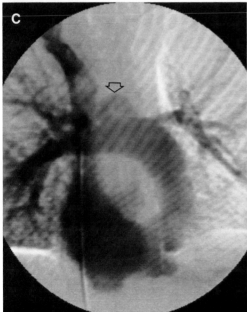

FIGURE 1.10 A. Frontal chest roentgenogram in a 2-month-old child showing overexpansion of the right lung. **B.** Lateral view of barium esophagram demonstrating a rounded mass between the posterior aspect of the trachea and the anterior wall of the esophagus compatible with a pulmonary artery sling. **C.** Digital subtraction angiogram taken by introduction of a small catheter into the femoral vein confirms the presence of an anomalous left pulmonary artery (pulmonary artery sling; arrow).

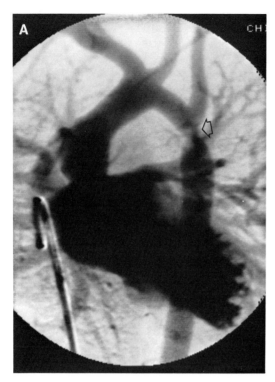

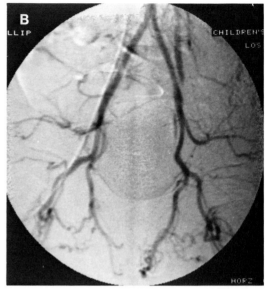

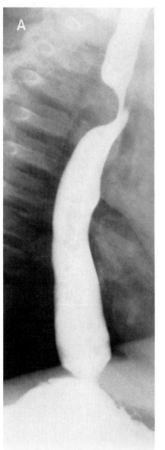

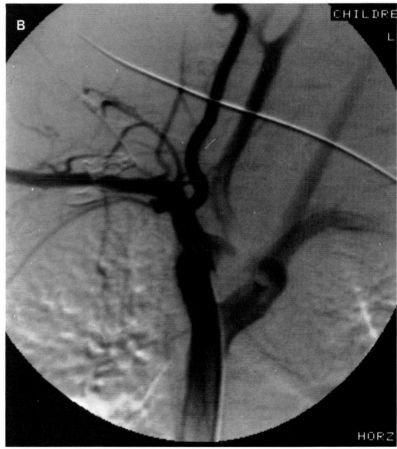

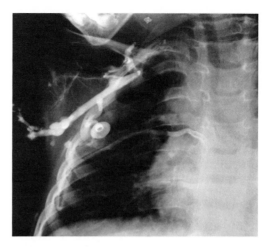

FIGURE 1.13 Right upper extremity venogram demonstrating subclavian obstruction secondary to central venous catheterization. The large intercostal collateral was successfully catheterized to provide access in this patient, who required long-term vascular infusions but had limited venous sites.

FIGURE 1.11 A. Transvenous digital subtraction angiogram showing coarctation of the aorta (arrow). B. There is bilateral femoral artery occlusion secondary to previous angioplasties. Blood supply to the lower extremities is through branches from the internal iliac arteries. This examination was performed as part of an attempted angioplasty and demonstrates why arterial punctures were not successful.

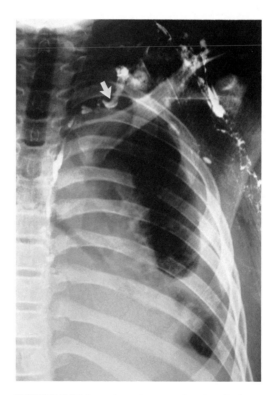

FIGURE 1.14 Lymphangiogram showing leakage from the thoracic duct (arrows) following lymph node biopsy for non-Hodgkin's lymphoma. Contrast is extravasating into a drainage bag covering the open wound.

FIGURE 1.12 A. Esophagram in a 4-month-old child with a wheeze. The large retroesophageal indentation is most probably due to a double aortic arch. B. Aortogram: digital study using an arterial catheter showing a classic double aortic arch. Angiography is undertaken only if MRI is inconclusive.

Lymphangiography

Lymphangiography is an effective radiological technique for demonstrating the internal architecture of lymph nodes. In the chest, it is employed to show ligation or laceration of the thoracic duct (Fig. 1.14). Demonstration of the exact site of obstruction or leakage will determine the correct surgical approach.

SUMMARY

Radiological imaging of the pediatric chest has undergone a revolution with the introduction of new techniques and agents. With these, imaging of the sick or injured child can be accomplished more accurately and with increased safety, enabling the correct therapeutic course to be charted with confidence.

REFERENCES

1. Swanson D: Conventional or low-osmolality: Picking the right contrast media. *Diag Imaging* 1988; 10:191–210.
2. Siegel MJ, Nadel SN, Glazer HS, Sagel SS: Mediastinal lesions in children: Comparison of CT and MR. *Radiology* 1988;160:241–244.
3. Brasch RC, Gooding CA, Lallemand DP, Wesbey GE: Magnetic resonance imaging of the thorax in childhood. *Radiology* 1984;150:463–467.
4. Kangerloo H: Chest MRI in childhood. *Radiol Clin North Am* 1988;26:263–275.
5. Bisset GS, Strife JL, Kirks DR, Bailey WW: Vascular rings: MR imaging. *AJR* 1987;149:251–256.
6. Fletcher BD, Dearborn DG, Mulopulos GP: MR imaging in infants with airway obstruction: Preliminary observations. *Radiology* 1986;160:245–249.
7. Formanek AG, Witcofski RL, D'Souza VJ, et al: MR imaging of the central pulmonary arterial tree in conotruncal malformation. *AJR* 1988;147:1127–1131.
8. Katz ME, Glazer HS, Siegel MJ, et al: Mediastinal vessels: Postoperative evaluation with MR imaging. *Radiology* 1986;161:647–651.
9. Cohen MD, Scales RL, Eigen H, et al: Evaluation of pulmonary parenchymal disease by magnetic resonance imaging. *Br J Radiol* 1987;60:223–230.
10. Frey EE, Sato Y, Smith WL, Franken EA: Cine CT of the mediastinum in pediatric patients. *Radiology* 1987;165:19–23.
11. Brasch RC, Gould RG, Gooding CA, et al: Upper airway obstruction in infants and children: Evaluation with ultrafast CT. *Radiology* 1987;165:459–466.
12. Brown SB, Hedlund GL, Glasier CM, et al: Tracheobronchial stenosis in infants: Successful balloon dilatation therapy. *Radiology* 1987;164:475–478.
13. Silverman SG, Mueller PR, Saini S, et al: Thoracic empyema: Management with image-guided catheter drainage. *Radiology* 1988;169:5–9.

Imaging of Pediatric Surgical Disease of the Chest

Philippe Baudain, MD, Chartal Durand, MD,
Jean-Francois Dyon, MD and Patrice Francois, MD

Radiological examination of the thorax of the child is characterized by (1) the importance of simple examinations, which remain fundamental in positive diagnosis and which influence further investigations; and (2) the introduction of modern techniques, which provide surgeons with the most precise anatomical image for the operation.

The conclusions of the preceding article have been accepted by all; however, this section does diverge in regard to a few points, mainly concerning the indications of radiological examinations and, in particular, the importance of thoracic ultrasound, which was not mentioned.

TECHNIQUES

For plain chest films, filtered x-rays are very useful and rarely fail to show up any mediastinal disorders. The filtered x-ray can be taken at any age, even in the newborn. The position of the aortic arch can be demonstrated without the use of contrast substances.

The esophagus remains the mediastinal plumb line and the esophagogram retains its full importance. In our opinion, it should be performed using barium because a water-soluble contrast agent (even isotonic), if aspirated, may cause congestion of the distal airways. Barium has the advantage of stopping at the large bronchial trunk level and of opacifying any fistula that may have gone unnoticed.

The esophagogram is also useful in clarifying the anatomical type of double aortic arch anomalies without having to resort to angiography or MRI. It also allows specific diagnosis of an esophageal bronchus and is better than MRI in affirming the presence of a duplication embedded in its wall.

Thoracic ultrasound has progressed markedly and often eliminates the need for further ex-

aminations. In infants, it confirms the presence of thymic hypertrophy, the diagnosis of which is made difficult by the volume or unusual topography of the thymus. At all ages, it specifies the liquid, solid, or vascular nature of an anomaly and, most of the time, its topography in relation, for instance, to vascular elements or the diaphragm. Technically speaking, the transducer is placed in specific locations along the chest wall (suprasternal, supraclavicular, intercostal, subxiphoid, or even the transsternal position in babies). Thoracic ultrasound also facilitates the examination of almost all the compartments of the mediastinum, the wall, and even certain parenchymatous anomalies in contact with the wall or diaphragm.

Computed tomography (CT) and magnetic resonance imaging (MRI) are presently competing with one another in the field of thoracic imaging. Each embodies a different approach.

CT has the advantages of quick sections, outstanding spatial definition, and densimetric measurement of anomalies. However, the small size of the child and the absence of fat make interpretation of the images more difficult than with adults. With children younger than 6 years of age, technical difficulties, accentuated at times by the need to inject contrast material, have a considerable effect on the quality of the image.

MRI has the advantages of spontaneous contrast of the vascular structures and perfect mediastinal assessment as a result of cardiac synchronization, which eliminates artifacts caused by heartbeats. Furthermore, sections can be taken in all spatial planes. Spatial definition is mediocre, however, and does not give a clear display of the pulmonary parenchyma. Bone structures and calcifications are not demonstrated as well as with CT.

The choice of methods therefore depends on the age of the child, the availability of equipment, and, especially, on the structure to be examined.

The other techniques are less often used with children. Bronchography is reserved for

© 1991 Elsevier Science Publishing Co., Inc.
655 Avenue of the Americas, New York, NY 10010
Current Topics in General Thoracic Surgery:
An International Series

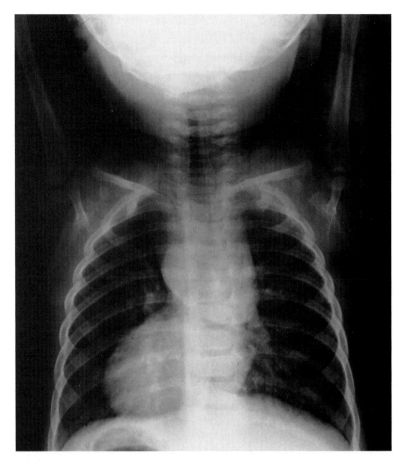

FIGURE D1.1 Frontal filtered image of the mediastinum of a child several months old. Suspected mediastinal opacity.

bronchial stenosing disorders that can be cured by surgery. The indications for angiography, even with digital substraction, are diminishing except in heart diseases and aortic coarctation.

INDICATIONS

It is important to eliminate unnecessary examinations of children, which unfortunately, are too often performed. Certain techniques that are easy to carry out on older children may be of poor quality or may require general anesthesia in younger ones. A supposedly harmless examination like MRI can become aggressive if it requires anesthesia. Age is therefore the first element to be taken into consideration. Further examinations should be proposed depending on radioclinical situations, such as the following.

Discovery of a Mediastinal Anomaly

The first examination to be performed after a plain roentgenogram is the ultrasound. It allows elimination of pseudo-masses which are related to thymic hypertrophy (Figs. D1.1 and D1.2), dilation of the pulmonary artery, eventration, retrocostal xiphoid hernia with hepatic content, or even diaphragmatic hernia with a sac. In the case of a real tumor, the ultrasound specifies the liquid, solid, homogeneous, or heterogeneous nature (Figs. D1.3 and D1.4A) and provides a global picture of the limits and relationships of the mass. It sometimes reveals a pleural or pericardial effusion. A benign or malignant mediastinal tumor almost always justifies the use of sectional imaging. MRI is currently tending to take precedence over CT because of its spontaneous contrast and its ability to reveal extension of the tumor in the three planes (Figs. D1.4B, D1.5, and D1.6). Injection of a contrast substance is reserved for difficult cases (Fig. D1.7). Preference for MRI becomes an obligation in the field of neurogenic tumors, of which extensions into the spinal canal through the intervertebral foramina

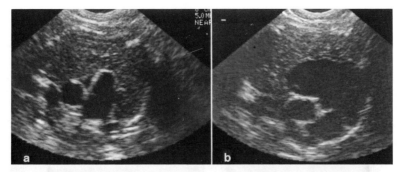

FIGURE D1.2 Same patient; mediastinal ultrasound. **A.** Axial image at the level of the pulmonary artery (P), the aortic arch (A), and the superior vena cava (C). **B.** Sagittal paramedian image. Posterior extension of a structure connecting clearly with the anterior thymic tissue (arrows).

can be especially well displayed on the frontal sections (Fig. D1.5).

Discovery of a Pulmonary Anomaly

The radiological evaluation is based above all on plain roentgenograms. The observation of a lobar or pulmonary emphysema requires the use of bronchoscopy or dynamic bronchography during inspiration-expiration, thus enabling a distinction to be made between acquired and congenital disorders (bronchomalacia or bronchial atresia). CT can be used in several situations: nodules and round opacities, searching for bronchial dilatations or an interstitial syndrome (Fig. D1.8), evaluating pleuropneumopathy with an encysted effusion, identification before needle biopsy, and so on.

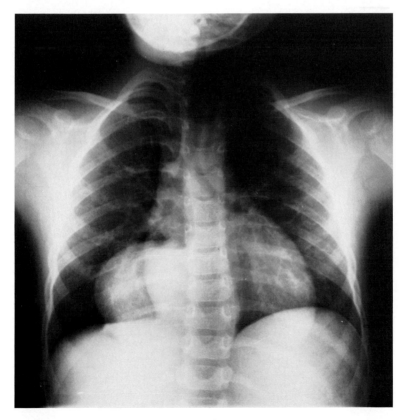

FIGURE D1.3 Frontal filtered image of mediastinum in a 4-year-old child. Lower right posterior mediastinal mass enlarging the last intercostal spaces and causing a curve of the dorsal lumbar column.

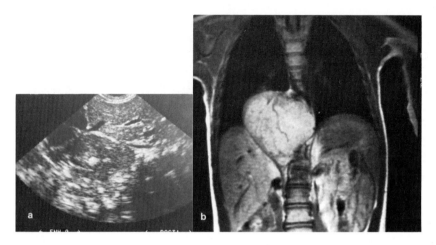

FIGURE D1.4 Same patient as in Fig D1.3: ultrasound and MR image (short TR). **A.** Coronal image showing the echogenic and heterogeneous character of the mass and specifying its topography in the posterior inframediastinal space above the diaphragm and behind its convexity (arrows). **B.** Confrontation with coronal MR image (short TR), which confirms the topography in relation to the diaphragm (arrows) and the heterogeneous character of the mass.

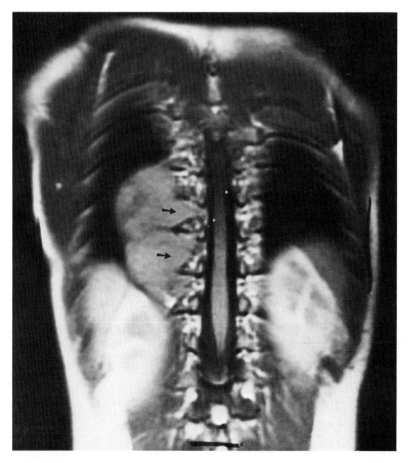

FIGURE D1.5 Frontal MR image (short TR) passing through the spinal canal in the same patient. No compression of the spinal cord but extension of the tumor inside the intervertebral foramina (arrows).

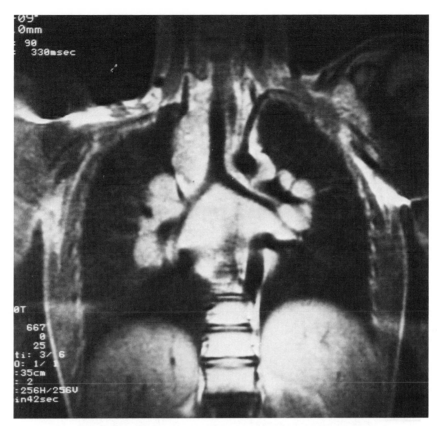

FIGURE D1.6 Sarcoidosis in a 15-year-old patient. Frontal MR image (short TR) passing through the tracheal plane. Numerous voluminous adenopathies.

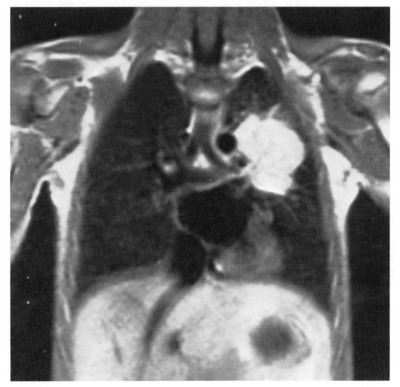

FIGURE D1.7 Frontal MR image (short TR) after injection of contrast material in a 6-year-old patient. Massive take-up of contrast substance affirming the parenchymatous nature of the process. (Inflammatory pseudo-tumor.)

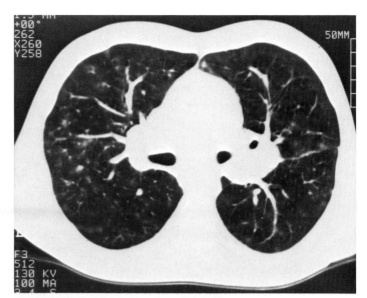

FIGURE D1.8 Same patient as in Figure D1.6: CT scan. Confirmation of adenopathies and, in particular, demonstration of an interstitial syndrome. (These images are visible only on millimetric sections and were not focused on in MRI.)

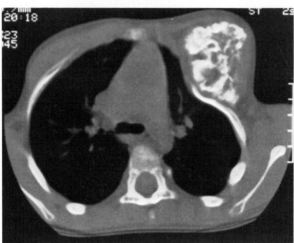

FIGURE D1.9 CT scan of a costal osteochondroma in a 6-year-old patient.

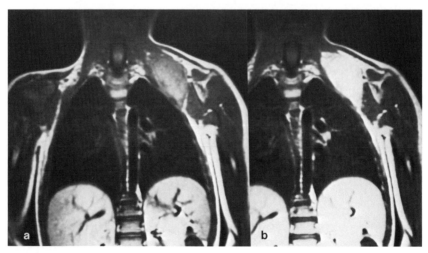

FIGURE D1.10 Tumor of soft parts above left clavicle in a 4-year-old patient. Frontal MR image (short TR) **A** without and **B** with injection of contrast material. Massive take-up of contrasting substance within the lesion, the limits of which become more precise (desmoid tumor).

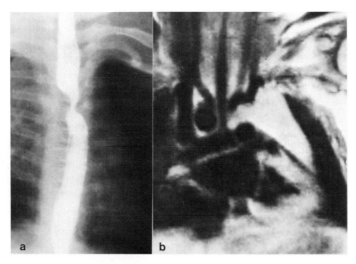

FIGURE D1.11 Combination of an esophagogram and an MR image (short TR) in a 7-year-old patient with an aortic arch anomaly. **A.** Frontal esophagogram showing an aortic arch and a right descending aorta opposite a curved impression with a small radius due to an arterial duct (Neuhauser's anomaly). **B.** Frontal MR image (short TR) passing through the tracheal plane: confirmation of an aortic arch in the right position and tracheal stenosis. However, absence of a view of the arterial duct that had been diagnosed on the esophagogram.

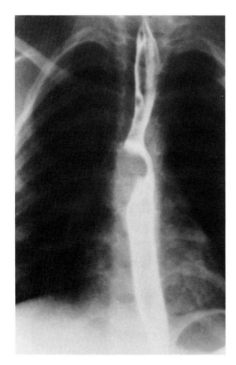

FIGURE D1.12 Frontal esophagogram in a 5-year-old patient. Characteristic appearance of parietal lesion set in the esophageal wall, confirming the diagnosis of esophageal duplication. No other examination is necessary for surgery on this child, and the MRI performed served no purpose.

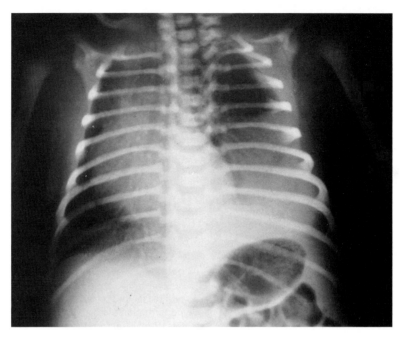

FIGURE D1.13 Frontal chest roentgenogram of an 8-day-old patient. Opacity of the left base partially obscures the lower part of the heart and pushes it to the right.

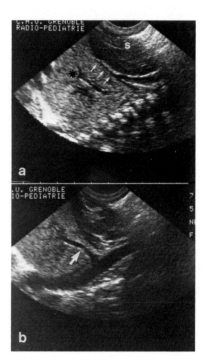

FIGURE D1.14 Same patient as in Fig D1.13: ultrasound sagittal image **A** lateralized to the left and **B** passing through the aortic plane. "Hepatized" mass (*) separated from the spleen (S) by the diaphragm (arrows). Vascular pedicle growing directly from the aorta (arrowhead) enabling the diagnosis of sequestration. (The observation of a venous return in the vena cava allowed the extralobar nature of this sequestration to be confirmed.)

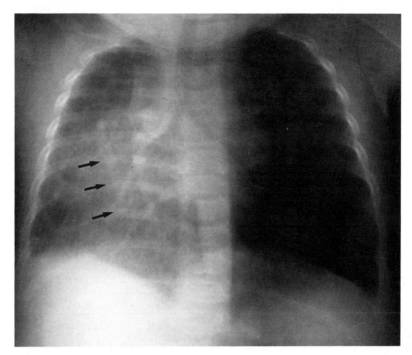

FIGURE D1.15 Filtered radiography of the mediastinum of a 5-month-old patient. Small right lung with extrapleural tissue obscuring the edge of the heart and an abnormal venous pulmonary return of scimitar shadow (arrows).

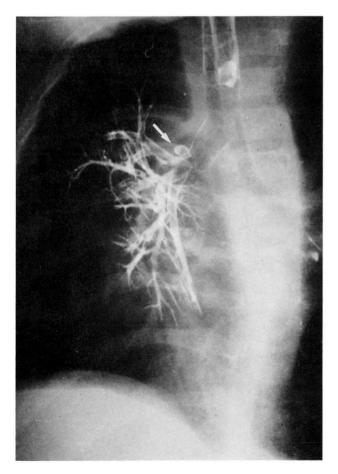

FIGURE D1.16 Same patient as in Figure D1.15: bronchography focusing on the blind pouch characteristic of an aplasia (arrow). This pouch was responsible for a chronic cough, which disappeared after surgery.

Discovery of an Anomaly in the Thoracic Wall

The discovery of an infection or a tumor in the chest wall is, above all, a clinical matter. Investigations begin with plain roentgenograms and an ultrasound study. The choice between CT (Fig. D1.9) and MRI (Fig. D1.10) depends mainly on whether or not there is bone alteration; both methods enable examination of extensions into adjacent soft parts.

Specific Situations

The anatomical assessment of a vascular ring as a double aortic arch justifies the use of simple roentgenograms, a filtered image, and an esophagogram. These examinations are sufficient in specifying the elements of the anomaly that are useful for the surgeon, and there is no need to resort to magnetic resonance imaging or angiography, which for the most part do not provide any additional information (Fig. D1.11). The same reasoning can be applied to the diagnosis of esophageal duplication (Fig. D1.12).

Sequestration can appear in two forms. One form, referred to as *solid,* is asymptomatic and simulates a posterior mediastinum tumor: the other form is air-containing and develops after repeated pneumonias. In the former, diagnosis by ultrasound can focus upon the existence of a vascular pedicle originating from the aorta (Figs. D1.13 and D1.14). In the latter, recurring pneumonias should suggest sequestration, and aggressive examinations would not appear to be necessary if indications for surgery are clear and the surgeon is notified.

Finally, the congenital absence of growth of a lobe, which may or may not be related to an abnormal venous return, often leads to unnecessary investigations. Angiocatheterization should be performed only for cardiac symptomatology. With chronic coughing, bronchography is suggested (Figs. D1.15 and D1.16) and may differentiate between aplasia (with its blind pouch) and real agenesia.

CONCLUSION

Other situations occur in which radiosurgical discussion is essential in order to decide which additional examinations are required and are sufficient for the surgery. Imaging for imaging's sake is to be discouraged where children are concerned.

Chapter 2

Pediatric Anesthesia: Special Requirements for Intrathoracic Procedures

*Derek Blackstock, MB, FFARCSI, FRCP(C) and
David J. Steward, MB, FRCP(C)*

Anesthetic management of the child having a thoracic surgery must be based on a knowledge of the physiology of infancy and childhood, the pathophysiology of the surgical lesion that is present, and the anticipated effects of the surgery and the anesthetic drugs and procedures the patient is to have. Infants having intrathoracic surgery require very careful management to prevent unnecessary physiological stresses, and for these special considerations the reader is directed to a general text of current pediatric anesthesia practice.[1]

GENERAL CONSIDERATIONS

The patient must be fully assessed to determine his or her current status and to confirm that it has been brought to the most optimal state possible prior to the planned procedure. A complete review of the history, physical examination, radiological studies, biochemistry, and pulmonary function tests (if available) must be completed. Acute infection and other disease must be improved whenever possible before surgery. Hypoxemia and intraoperative respiratory complications are increased following upper respiratory tract infection.[2,3] An increased incidence is reported of postoperative pulmonary complications after major surgery performed within 2 to 3 weeks of an upper respiratory tract infection (URI), possibly due to altered respiratory tract reactivity and predisposition to bacterial infections following a viral URI.[4,5] Hence major thoracic surgery should be delayed, if possible, until 3 or 4 weeks have elapsed after such a URI.

© 1991 Elsevier Science Publishing Co., Inc.
655 Avenue of the Americas, New York, NY 10010
Current Topics in General Thoracic Surgery:
An International Series

Intrathoracic surgery may result in major blood losses; the anesthesiologist should confirm that adequate blood and blood products have been ordered and will be available to the operating room during the operation. As there are now increased concerns regarding transfusion of donor blood, alternatives should be considered. Discussions with the parents should detail the risks and benefits of blood transfusion and its alternatives for each child. It is usually considered that below a hemoglobin level of 80 to 90 g/L, oxygen transport to the tissues may become compromised, especially in the presence of cardiorespiratory disease. The decision to transfuse blood must be based on an evaluation of all the factors present in each patient.[6]

Older children having thoracic surgery are often very apprehensive and require special reassurance concerning the planned procedures. Postoperative care and plans for pain management should be carefully discussed. If there is any likelihood that prolonged mechanical ventilation may be required, this should be explained in detail. Preoperative medication may be ordered, but drugs that may cause marked respiratory depression should be avoided. If the anesthesiologist can establish good rapport with the patient and explain all the procedures that will be performed, heavy sedation is usually not required. For those few patients who require sedation, either an oral benzodiazapine (eg, diazepam) or a combination of a barbiturate and narcotic analgesic drug is suitable (eg, pentobarbital 2 mg/kg P.O. 1-½ hours preoperatively and 0.1 mg/kg morphine I.M. 45 minutes preoperatively). Experience with patients who have congenital heart disease indicates that the latter regimen will result in little change in arterial oxygen saturation.[7]

Intraoperatively, pulmonary function may be significantly further compromised, as a result of both anesthesia with controlled ventilation and the intrathoracic surgical manipulations. It is essential that the patient be monitored to continuously assess the adequacy of gas exchange; the use of pulse oximetry and end-expired gas sampling is recommended. In infants and small children surgical retraction within the chest may compress the lungs excessively, kink major airways, and/or restrict the filling of the heart. Such effects must be anticipated at all times during surgery and the surgeon immediately warned if these occur. A decrease in oxygen saturation or bradycardia occurring at any time must be treated by removal of all retractors and ventilation with oxygen. Atropine (10 to 20 $\mu g/kg$) is indicated to block vagal stimuli associated with mediastinal manipulation if bradycardia persists once full oxygenation has been achieved.

MONITORING

The use of a stethoscope—esophageal or precordial, as appropriate—a blood pressure cuff, a pulse oximeter, an electrocardiogram, and a thermometer is essential for all patients. Measurement of end-tidal carbon dioxide and anesthetic gases and vapors is indicated where possible but requires special considerations in infants and children and those with respiratory diseases (to be discussed). Invasive hemodynamic monitoring is required for those having major intrathoracic procedures.

Pulse oximetry confirms adequate oxygenation and improves the anesthetist's response to hypoxia in the operating room.[8] Continuous monitoring of arterial saturation is an essential precaution during thoracic anesthesia when desaturation due to major changes in cardiopulmonary function may occur extremely rapidly. In preterm infants, when hyperoxia must be avoided, the saturation sensor should be placed in a preductal position (eg, on the right hand) and the FIO_2 and ventilation adjusted to maintain a saturation between 90% and 95%[9]; this will ensure a safe arterial oxygen tension. During thoracic surgery, when conditions may change very rapidly, it may sometimes be necessary to err on the side of safety. The reliability of pulse oximetry is improved if all extraneous light is excluded from the sensor—eg, by covering it with foil.[10] The limb on which the sensor is placed should be protected by a rigid cover from the weight of the surgical drapes or any other external pressures. End-tidal carbon dioxide measurement ($PetCO_2$) in infants under 8 kg body weight being ventilated with partial rebreathing (T-piece sys-

tems) will provide meaningful results only if a sampling catheter is placed at the distal tip of the endotracheal tube.[11] In older children and those being ventilated with a nonrebreathing circuit (eg, Siemen's ventilator) sampling at the endotracheal connector provides acceptable values. During thoracotomy and lung retraction in infants and children, the end-tidal CO_2 remains a reliable estimate of the arterial pCO_2, but with pulmonary artery clamping the blood-end-tidal difference increases significantly, rendering end-tidal monitoring unreliable.[12] $PetCO_2$ measurements underestimate the $PaCO_2$ in children with cyanotic congenital heart disease but provide a reliable estimate of $PaCO_2$ in those with acyanotic heart disease.[13] $EtCO_2$ may not correlate well with the arterial pCO_2 in the newborn period or in those with cardiopulmonary disease, but it does permit rapid assessment of pulmonary blood flow and ventilation when there is surgical traction on the lung or heart.[14,15]

Invasive blood pressure monitoring is indicated for major intrathoracic surgery, which may result in rapid changes in cardiopulmonary function with or without significant blood losses. An arterial line is commonly placed in the radial artery, but in infants it may be placed in the femoral artery without an increased incidence of serious complications. Cannulation of the femoral artery should not be performed in the neonate (younger than 1 mo) as there is an increased risk of perfusion-related complications.[16] In infants and young children the systemic blood pressure is a reliable guide to the adequacy of intravascular volume replacement. In older children or when cardiac function may be compromised, central venous pressure (CVP) monitoring should be employed to guide fluid and blood resuscitation in the event of hemorrhage. A CVP catheter may be inserted in the external jugular vein, in which case the use of a 3-mm radius J wire is advised.[17] Alternatively the internal jugular route may be chosen; this has a higher success rate for central passage of the catheter but has a higher complication rate.[18] Measurement of pulmonary capillary wedge pressure and/or cardiac output using a Swan-Ganz catheter is rarely performed in the pediatric patient. If monitoring of left atrial pressure is indicated, a left atrial catheter is inserted by the surgeon in the operating room—eg, after correction of complex congenital cardiac lesions.

CHOICE OF ANESTHETIC TECHNIQUE

The technique for induction of anesthesia may be dictated by the nature of the patient's disease, but the following general principles apply. Preoxygenation, if it can be performed without distressing the child, and manual ventilation of the lungs with oxygen prior to intubation reduce the incidence of hypoxia during induction.[19] A rapid sequence induction with intravenous pentothal and succinylcholine, and endotracheal intubation with cricoid pressure, allows early control of the airway in the patient with abnormal lung compliance or in those at risk of aspiration of gastric contents. Inhalation induction maintains oxygen saturation better than the rapid sequence technique in healthy infants and children, but in some patients rapid control of the airway may be of equal importance. Arterial desaturation and respiratory complications are more frequent during inhalation induction with isoflurane than with halothane.[20] Accurate placement of the tip of the endotracheal tube is very important. When a high inspired concentration of oxygen is used, monitoring the arterial saturation may not immediately detect endobronchial intubation. Auscultation of the chest may also be difficult to interpret in very small infants. Careful inspection of both hemithoraces for equal expansion with ventilation, auscultation of both axillae, and continued monitoring of SaO_2 is necessary to detect endobronchial intubation. The use of the fiberoptic bronchoscope will rapidly confirm the position of the endotracheal tube in difficult cases.[21] The position of the endotracheal tube must always be confirmed again after repositioning the patient for surgery. Double lumen tubes are not commonly used for pediatric patients; such tubes are not commercially available in small sizes, and to place them accurately and securely into a small airway might be difficult.

When isolation of one lung is required, it has been achieved by selective endobronchial intubation combined with the use of a Fogarty catheter as a bronchial blocker, if required.[22,23] Selective endobronchial intubation in children may be achieved by placing the bevel of the endotracheal tube facing away from the side to be intubated as the tube is advanced in the trachea.[24] The endotracheal tube connections should be easily accessible in case suctioning is required intraoperatively.

MAINTENANCE OF ANESTHESIA

A balanced technique using a volatile anesthetic agent, muscle relaxant, and low-dose narcotic analgesic permits extubation of the trachea immediately after the anesthetic. The use of high doses of narcotics (eg, fentanyl 25 μg/kg) reduces the metabolic response to surgery[25] and the stress responses of the reactive pulmonary vasculature,[26] but respiratory failure and the need for ventilatory support in the postoperative period is common. Clearance of fentanyl is unpredictable in the neonate (especially the preterm)[27] and blood levels of the drug may rebound with accompanying ventilatory depression. Hence any infant who has received other than minimal doses of fentanyl (≤ 2 μg/kg) should be very closely observed postoperatively.

Halothane has been considered the drug of choice for patients with obstructive lung disease[28] as this drug is a bronchodilator and improves dynamic lung compliance.[29] Isoflurane may have an action essentially similar to that of halothane on the lungs but causes less myocardial depression[30]; isoflurane is often favored for small infants undergoing thoracic surgery.

The anesthesia circuit that is usually preferred for infants and small children is the T-piece, which is lightweight, convenient, readily humidified and scavenged, and easily attached to a ventilator. An additional advantage of the T-piece system is that by limiting the fresh gas flow rate, excessive effective alveolar ventilation and consequent hypocapnia can be avoided. Formulas have been recommended to determine the fresh gas flow necessary to produce desired $PaCO_2$,[31] but the availability of end-tidal CO_2 monitoring will permit a much closer control of carbon dioxide levels during anesthesia.[32]

It is suggested that during thoracic surgery the arterial carbon dioxide should be maintained at near-normal levels, unless there is a specific indication of hyperventilation (eg, to modify changes in pulmonary vascular resistance). This can be achieved by setting a fresh gas flow rate into the T-piece based on the following formula and using end-tidal CO_2 monitoring to adjust the level as required.

Fresh gas flow requirements[31] for T-piece systems during controlled ventilation to predict $pCO_2 = \pm 37$:

Patients 10 to 30 kg $\rightarrow$ 1000 ml + 100 ml/kg

Patients over 30 Kg $\rightarrow$ 2000 ml + 50 ml/kg.

The delivered minute volume must equal 1.5 times this fresh gas flow.[31]

The use of heated and humidified inspired gases maintains body temperature and decreases postoperative atelectasis.[33] Passing the fresh gases from the anesthesia machine through a heated humidifier with a heated gas delivery hose (Fisher and Paykel Model #MR 620) and monitoring the inspired gas temperature at the patient will achieve this goal.

Hypoxemia may occur during transfer to the recovery room even in healthy pediatric patients,[34,35] but this can be prevented by oxygen administration.[36] It is therefore most important to ensure that postthoracotomy patients, who may have significantly impaired gas exchange, are provided with oxygen during transportation.

POSTOPERATIVE CARE

Many patients may be extubated at the end of the procedure, provided that they demonstrate adequate ventilatory function. Otherwise, a nasotracheal tube should be inserted and mechanical ventilation continued.

Relief of pain in the postoperative period improves patient comfort and reduces the psychological impact of the hospital experience.[37] Adequate analgesia can also be expected to minimize oxygen demands[38] and reduce the incidence of postoperative complications.[39]

There are now many methods to ameliorate postoperative pain, and all may be applied to pediatric patients; in many cases a combination of methods may be appropriate—eg, regional analgesia combined with systemic analgesic drugs.

Regional analgesic techniques are advantageous in that they provide very good pain relief and may improve ventilation with no central nervous system depression and none of the side effects of narcotic drugs. In addition, the incidence of postoperative lung complications may be reduced.[40] After thoracic surgery intercostal nerve blocks (using local analgesic drugs or cryoanalgesia), intrapleural block, or epidural block have been used.

Intercostal nerve blocks in infants and small children may be performed by the surgeon while the chest is open or percutaneously by the anesthesiologist. Bupivacaine is the usual drug of choice, and its duration of action may be extended by the addition of an equal volume of low-molecular-weight dextran to the solution.[41] If the percutaneous route is chosen the risk of pneumothorax in small children may be reduced by inserting the needle almost parallel to—rather than vertical to—the rib.[42] Given that systemic absorption of drugs from the intercostal space is very rapid, the total dose should be carefully measured and not exceed 2 to 3 mg/kg of bupivacaine. The injection should be made as far lateral to the spine as possible to minimize the risk of intrathecal spread of the local analgesic agent and resultant total spinal block.[43]

Cryopexy to the intercostal nerves can be performed while the chest is open and is reported to relieve pain for 2 to 3 weeks in adult patients. Each intercostal nerve to be blocked must be identified, exposed, isolated, and mobilized and a cryoprobe tip applied. Two 30-second freeze cycles with an intervening 5-second thaw interval

have been recommended.[44] Cryopexy may be particularly advantageous when the risk of postoperative complications is high and the need for physiotherapy great, for example, in the patient with cystic fibrosis.[45]

Intrapleural block using a continuous infusion of bupivacaine through an intrapleural catheter has been demonstrated to be effective in children.[46] A 20-gauge epidural catheter is passed into the pleural space with a Tuohy needle before chest closure. The interior tip is loosely sutured at the posterior aspect of the incision. A chest drain was inserted in the usual fashion. Bupivacaine 0.25% with 1:200,000 epinephrine was infused at a maximum rate of 0.5 ml/kg/h. However, at this rate of infusion, serum bupivacaine concentrations may approach toxic levels and caution is required.

Epidural morphine may be used to provide analgesia following thoracic surgery in children and has been introduced through the lumbar,[47] caudal,[48] or thoracic route.[49] Epidural narcotic analgesia may give very good pain relief and facilitate early ambulation and effective physiotherapy. The common side effects are pruritus and nausea and vomiting. A dose of 0.05 mg/kg preservative-free morphine administered through the lumbar route did not affect respiratory rate, tidal volume, minute ventilation, or end-tidal CO_2 but did reduce the ventilatory response to carbon dioxide for 22 hours. The use of epidural morphine 0.075 mg/kg by the caudal route did not provide complete analgesia, but it markedly reduced the need for systemic narcotic drugs and was not accompanied by significant respiratory depression. However, delayed respiratory depression has been reported following the use of caudal morphine.[50] Patients treated with epidural opiates must be carefully observed for signs of impending respiratory depression for at least 24 hours after the last dose is administered.

Systemic narcotic analgesics following thoracic surgery should be given by continuous intravenous infusion; in older children their administration may be patient controlled. A continuous infusion of 10 to 30 µg/kg/h of morphine provides good relief of pain and minimal respiratory depression following cardiac surgery.[51] This infusion may be preceded by one or more bolus loading doses of 0.1 mg/kg morphine as required to establish analgesia.

Patient-controlled analgesia (PCA) regimens have been used in children as young as 5 years.[52,53] The pump may be programmed to provide a basal infusion rate (15 µg/kg/h), which is supplemented by on-demand doses of 10 to 30 µg/kg every 10 to 15 minutes. Children can easily be taught to push the PCA button when they feel pain and may achieve excellent analgesia by this means. Parents should be reassured that excessive doses are prevented by the lock-out procedure that is programmed into the apparatus but should be cautioned not to press the button for the child.

ANESTHETIC IMPLICATIONS FOR SOME PROCEDURES

Endoscopy

Laryngoscopy and Bronchoscopy

Young infants and children may require laryngoscopy to define clearly any lesions obstructing the airway or to remove a foreign body. When airway obstruction is life-threatening, awake laryngoscopy following oxygenation and the application of topical lidocaine may be the safest technique. When the degree of respiratory distress is less, mask induction with halothane in oxygen provides a safety margin should the airway suddenly become obstructed. Induction may be carried out with the child held in the parent's or assistant's arms, and as sleep occurs monitoring equipment should be gently applied. The level of anesthesia is deepened with 2% to 4% halothane in oxygen. At this stage ventilation may be gently assisted. Paradoxical breathing has been noted at end-tidal concentrations of 1% halothane, and this increases as the concentration increases. In addition, ventilation is depressed at 1.5% halothane when compared with 0.5% and 1% end-tidal concentrations. In infants younger than 6 months of age a greater depression of ventilation is seen.[54,55]

When an adequate depth of anesthesia has been reached laryngoscopy should be performed and topical anesthesia of the larynx, trachea, and bronchi established with lidocaine. A total dose should not exceed 5 mg/kg, and the maximum dose of 1.5 mg/kg should be used when sprayed directly into the trachea. Should the vocal cords move or the patient cough, anesthesia should be further deepened; coughing with the rigid bronchoscope in place may cause injury. Spontaneous ventilation should be maintained throughout unless the patient becomes hypoxic or seriously hypercarbic and/or arrhythmias occur. In this case very gentle positive pressure ventilation may be given in order to assist the patient's own spontaneous respirations. The maintenance of spontaneous respiration is essential to obtain accurate assessment of dynamic airway obstruction due to collapse or compression. Spontaneous ventilation during foreign body removal may also

add a margin of safety should difficulties arise. The possibility of sudden development of a pneumothorax should constantly be considered during pediatric bronchoscopy.[56,57] The use of the Storz pediatric bronchoscope permits good visualization of even the smallest infant's airway, but when using the 2.5, 3, and 3.5 mm internal diameter bronchoscopes significant hypercarbia may occur.[58,59] Inadequate ventilation is related to increased resistance to airflow resulting within small bronchoscopes when the telescope is in place. Although resistance to inspiration can be easily overcome by a ventilator or hand ventilation, the passive elastic recoil of the chest wall and lung may be inadequate to expel gas during the usual time for expiration. The end result can be increased trapping of gas in the lung with an ever-increasing lung volume. In such circumstances it is necessary to remove the telescope to allow the lung to deflate. With the size 2.5 bronchoscope both inspiration and expiration are severely limited while the telescope is in place, and the endoscopist should remove the telescope regularly to allow adequate ventilation; otherwise serious hypoxia and hypercarbia will result. The common practice of attaching a flexible extension to the Jackson-Rees T-piece to ventilate through a bronchoscope markedly increases the circuit dead space. Attaching the T-piece directly to the side arm of the bronchoscope eliminates this dead space but requires that the anesthetist gently support the equipment. If the bronchoscope is advanced into a main stem bronchus there may be inadequate ventilation of the controlateral lung and consequent desaturation. Constant monitoring of the pulse oximeter will detect this.

Removal of a foreign body from the trachea or a main stem bronchus requires close cooperation between the endoscopist and the anesthetist. Inadequate ventilation may require the endoscopist to readjust the position of the bronchoscope. Impaction or fragmentation of a foreign body with debris in either or both the main stem bronchi may result in an immediate life-threatening situation. The removal of these foreign bodies is absolutely essential, and efforts to do this take precedence over all other maneuvers. Throughout anesthesia when a foreign body is present in the airway the surgeon must be readily available to perform a bronchoscopy or emergency tracheostomy or cricothyrotomy should the airway become completely obstructed. If a foreign body lodges in the trachea and causes total obstruction but cannot be rapidly extracted, it should be pushed down into a main bronchus to permit ventilation of the contralateral lung. Emergency thoracotomy and bronchotomy has been described but has failed to prevent a fatal cardiac arrest.[60]

Esophagoscopy

Esophagoscopy of pediatric patients generally requires general anesthesia. When there are obstructing lesions of the esophagus and/or gastroesophageal reflux it is important to recognize the risk of pulmonary aspiration during induction of anesthesia. Preoperatively H_2 histamine blocking agents[61] and/or metoclopramide[62] should be given to reduce the volume and acidity of the gastric contents. Anesthesia should be induced using a rapid sequence technique and cricoid pressure applied until the endotracheal tube is safely in place. It is important that the child does not cough or strain during the procedure as this will increase the risk of perforation of the esophagus; hence adequate anesthesia must be ensured. In small infants it should be recognized that the passage of the esophagoscope may compress the airways distal to the endotracheal tube and compromise ventilation. Accordingly ventilation and oxygen saturation must be constantly monitored during the examination.

Anesthesia for Surgery of Intrapulmonary Lesions

Intrapulmonary lesions and malformations of the lung may cause significant respiratory compromise. Increased inspired concentrations of oxygen are often required to prevent serious hypoxia associated with manipulation of the mediastinum and lung tissue. The administration of nitrous oxide should be avoided in patients with pneumothorax, gas-containing cysts, or lobar emphysema. Bronchogenic cysts do not usually communicate with the tracheobronchial tree but may compress major airways. Lung cysts may communicate with the airway and may increase in size and lead to tension pneumothorax. Lobar emphysema in the infant may be due to endobronchial obstruction, bronchomalacia, or extrinsic bronchial compression; in each case air trapping may occur and may be increased by positive pressure ventilation.[63] Hence excessive positive pressure ventilation must be avoided until the thorax is open and the remaining normal lung tissue is decompressed.

Tracheoesophageal Fistula

Infants with tracheoesophageal fistula (TEF) require special care during anesthesia. Many affected infants also have other congenital anomalies,[64] which may complicate their care and add to morbidity and mortality. In most cases (90%) the proximal esophagus ends blindly and a fistula is present between the distal esophagus and the trachea. Regurgitation of gastric contents through the fistula and aspiration from the blind esophageal pouch can result in a severe pneumonia. This will usually not improve until the fistula is ligated. Infants who also have respiratory distress syndrome and poorly compliant lungs requiring ventilation at high pressures are at grave risk of developing a large leak through the fistula.[65] This may compromise ventilation, either as a result of the leak through a gastrostomy or subsequent to gastric distension; in extreme cases rupture of the stomach and pneumoperitoneum may occur. Control of the leak may be achieved by placing a fogarty catheter in the lower esophagus through the gastrostomy.[66] It has also been suggested that a Fogarty catheter may be positioned into the fistula itself with the aid of a small fiberoptic flexible bronchoscope.[67] Alternatively an emergency thoracotomy to control the fistula may be lifesaving.

Endotracheal intubation must be very carefully performed in the patient with TEF, as there is a danger of intubating the fistula. Awake intubation is still preferred by many authorities for infants with TEF. Optimally the tip of the tube should be placed distal to the fistula but proximal to the carina. Sometimes, however, the fistula is very close to the carina, making such placement very difficult. Various maneuvers have been suggested to correctly place the tip of the tube. Intubation with the bevel facing posteriorly is considered advisable to minimize the risk of intubating the fistula. It has been suggested that observing the cessation of escape of gases bubbled underwater through a gastrostomy tube may aid in placement of the tip below the fistula.[68] A refinement of this technique is to sample gases passing from the gastrostomy tube using a capnograph or anesthesia gas analyzer.[69] When the sampled gases contain no carbon dioxide or anesthetic agents it is assumed that the tip lies below the fistula. In practice many prefer to position the tip by advancing the tube until one-lung ventilation occurs and then withdrawing the tube slightly until bilateral breath sounds are heard. It is then assumed that the tip is positioned ideally just above the carina. After intubation, tracheobronchial suctioning should be performed and ventilation gently assisted until the chest is open and the fistula secured. Breath sounds and oxygen saturation should be closely monitored, as there is a danger that major airways may become kinked as the fistula is approached.

Tracheal Stenosis

Tracheal stenosis may occur as an isolated lesion or may accompany other defects (eg, tracheoesophageal fistula).[70] Ventilation of the patient during resection of the stenotic lesion may be maintained by using sterile endotracheal or endobronchial tubes inserted by the surgical team[71] or by means of jet ventilation.[72] Once the stenosed segment has been resected and the posterior wall of the trachea repaired, an endotracheal tube can be advanced past the anastomosis and the repair of the anterior wall completed.

Congenital Diaphragmatic Hernia

The management of patients with congenital diaphragmatic hernia has evolved as more has been learned of the pathophysiology of this condition. The rush to emergency surgery of former years has been replaced by an extended period of preoperative resuscitation and stabilization; the wisdom of this approach has been confirmed by the finding that surgical correction of the lesion may tend to compromise pulmonary function rather than improve it.[73] Preoperative management may include neuromuscular blockade and controlled ventilation, sedation with large doses of fentanyl, correction of metabolic acidosis, and other measures to minimize pulmonary vasoconstriction. In some patients preoperative extracorporeal membrane oxygenation (ECMO) may be indicated. An operation should be performed only when the pulmonary status is improved and stable. Anesthesia management should be designed to maintain optimal ventilatory care intraoperatively and avoid any further damage to the lungs.

Mediastinal Tumors

Children with mediastinal masses require very careful preoperative assessment and anesthetic care, as life-threatening airway obstruction or cardiovascular collapse secondary to cardiac compression may occur after induction of general anesthesia.[74,75] Chest radiography and the degree of symptomatology may not give a reliable indication of the potential for airway obstruction after induction, but a history of orthopnea should be considered prognostic for possible major problems.[76,77] Computed tomography scan is a reliable method to identify the extent of airway compression. Pulmonary function tests can identify both intrathoracic and extrathoracic obstruction in asymptomatic patients.[78]

Echocardiography will help in assessing myocardial contractility. Encasement of the heart or major vessels may seriously impede venous return and the fixed cardiac output may be further depressed by the general anesthetic agents, the supine position, and loss of spontaneous respiration.[79]

Children with a greater than 33% decrease in luminal area are at increased risk of airway obstruction during general anesthesia. Where there is involvement of the pericardium or obstruction of the great vessels the risk of general anesthesia is prohibitive and a tissue diagnosis by needle biopsy under local anesthesia is advisable. If surgical resection is required, femoral-femoral bypass should be available before anesthesia is induced.

REFERENCES

1. Steward DJ: *Manual of pediatric anesthesia.* 3rd ed. New York: Churchill Livingstone, 1989.
2. Desoto H, Patel RI, Soliman IE, Hannallah RS: Changes in oxygen saturation following general anesthesia in children with upper respiratory infection signs and symptoms undergoing otolaryngological procedures. *Anesthesiology* 1988;68:276–279.
3. Tait R, Knight PR. Intraoperative respiratory complications in patients with upper respiratory tract infections. *Can J Anesth* 1987;34:3300–3303.
4. Tait AR, Ketcham TR, Klein MJ, Knight PR: Perioperative respiratory complications in patients with upper respiratory tract infections. *Anesthesiology* 1983;59:A433.
5. McGill WA, Coveler LA, Epstein BS: Subacute respiratory infection in small children. *Anesth Analg* 1979;58:331–333.
6. Consensus conference: Perioperative red blood cell transfusion. *JAMA* 1988;260:2700–2703.
7. De Bock TL, Petrilli RL, Davis PJ, Motoyama EK: Effect of premedication on preoperative arterial oxygen saturation in children with congenital heart disease. *Anesthesiology* 1987;67:A492.
8. Cote CJ, Goldstein EA, Cote MA, Hoaglin DC, et al: A single blind study of pulse oximetry in children. *Anesthesiology* 1988;68:184–188.
9. Deckhart R, Steward DJ: Noninvasive arterial hemoglobin oxygen saturation versus transcutaneous oxygen tension monitoring in the preterm infant. *Crit Care Med* 1984;12:935–939.
10. Siegel MN, Gravenstein N: Preventing ambient light from affecting pulse oximetry. *Anesthesiology* 1987;67:280.
11. Badgwell JM, Heavner JE, May WS, et al: End-tidal PCO_2 monitoring in infants and children ventilated with either a partial rebreathing or a non-rebreathing circuit. *Anesthesiology* 1987;66:405–410.
12. Heneghan CPH, Scallan MJH, Branthwaite MA: End tidal carbon dioxide during thoracotomy: Its relation to blood levels in adults and children. *Anaesthesia* 1981;36:1017–1021.
13. Burrows FA: Physiologic dead space, venous admixture, and the arterial to end-tidal carbon dioxide difference in infants and children undergoing cardiac surgery. *Anesthesiology* 1989;70:215–219.
14. Watkins AM, Weinding AM: Monitoring of end tidal CO_2 in neonatal intensive care. *Arch Dis Child* August 1987;62(8):837–839.
15. Schuller JL, Bovill JG, Nijvild A: End-tidal carbon dioxide concentration as an indicator of pulmonary blood flow during closed heart surgery in children: A report of two cases. *Br J Anesth* 1985;57(12):1257–1259.
16. Glenski JA, Beynen FM, Brady J: A prospective evaluation of femoral artery monitoring in pediatric patients. *Anesthesiology* 1987;66:227–229.

17. Nordstrom L, Fletcher R: Comparison of two different J-wires for central venous cannulation via the external jugular vein. *Anesth Analg* 1983;62:365.

18. Belani KG, Buckley JJ, Gordon JR, Cataneda W: Percutaneous cervical central venous line placement: A comparison of the internal and external jugular routes. *Anesth Analg* 1980;59:40–44.

19. Laycock GJA, McNicol LR: Forum-hypoxemia during induction of anesthesia—An audit of children who underwent general anesthesia for routine elective surgery. *Anaesthesia* 1988;43:981–984.

20. Phillips AJ, Brimacombe JR, Simpson DL: Anesthetic induction with isoflurane or halothane. *Anaesthesia* 1988;43:927–929.

21. Deitrich KA, Atrauss RH, Cabalka AK, et al: Use of flexible fiberoptic endoscopy for determination of endotracheal tube position in the pediatric patient. *Crit Care Med* 1988;16(9):884–887.

22. Vale R: Selective bronchial blocking in a small child. *Br J Anesth* 1969;41:453.

23. Rao CC, Krishna G, Grosfeld JL, Weber TR: One lung pediatric anesthesia. *Anesth Analg* 1981;60(6):450–452.

24. Baraka A, Akel S, Muallem M, et al. Bronchial intubation in children: Does the tube bevel determine the side of intubation? *Anesthesiology* 1987;67:869–870.

25. Sofianos E, Alevizou F, Zissis N, et al: Hormonal response to thoracic surgery: Effects of high-dose fentanyl anesthesia, compared with halotane anesthesia. *Acta Anesth Belgica* 1985;36(2):89–96.

26. Hickey PR, Hansen DD, Wessel DL, et al: Blunting of stress responses in the pulmonary circulation of infants by fentanyl. *Anesth Analg* 1985;64:1137–1142.

27. Koehntop DE, Rodman JH, Brundage DM, et al: Pharmacokinetics of fentanyl in neonates. *Anesth Analg* 1986;65:227–232.

28. Gold MI: Anesthesia for the asthmatic patient. *Anesth Analg* 1970;49:881.

29. Colgan FJ: Performance of the lungs and bronchi during inhalation anesthesia. *Anesthesiology* 1965;26:778.

30. Wolf WJ, Neal MB, Peterson MD: The hemodynamic and cardiovascular effects of isoflurane and halothane anesthesia in children. *Anesthesiology* 1986;64:328–333.

31. Rose DK, Froese AB: The regulation of $PaCO_2$ during controlled ventilation of children with a T piece. *Can Anesth Soc J* 1979;26:102–113.

32. Badgwell JM, McEvedy BAB, Lerman J: Fresh gas formulae do not accurately predict end-tidal PCO_2 in paediatric patients. *Can J Anesth* 1988;35:581–586.

33. Fonkalsrud EW, Calmes S, Barcliffe LT, Barrett CT: Reduction of operative heat loss and pulmonary secretions in neonates by use of heated and humidified Anesthetic gases. *J Thorac Cardiovasc Surg* 1980;80(5):718–723.

34. Pullerits J, Burrows FA, Roy WL: Arterial desaturation in healthy children during transfer to the recovery room. *Can J Anesth* 1987;34(5):470–473.

35. Bideshwar KK, Harnik EV, Mitchard R, et al: Postoperative arterial oxygen saturation in the pediatric population during transportation. *Anesth Analg* 1988;67:280–282.

36. Patel R, Norden J, Hannallah RS: Oxygen administration prevents hypoxemia during post-anesthetic transport in children. *Anesthesiology* 1988;69:616–618.

37. Vernon DTA, Schulman JL, Foley JM: Changes in children's behavior after hospitalization. *Am J Dis Child* 1966;111:581.

38. Evelyn R, Steward DJ: Oxygen consumption in the early postoperative period: Effect of analgesic therapy and subsequent activity. *Can J Anesth* 1987;34:595–596.

39. Pflug AE, Bonica JJ: Physiopathology and control of postoperative pain. *Arch Surg* 1977;112:773–781.

40. Wiklund L: Regional blockade versus analgesic therapy. *Acta Anesth Scand* 1982;74:(suppl)169–172.

41. Kaplan JA, Miller ED, Gallagher EG: Postoperative analgesia for thoracotomy patients. *Anesth Analg* 1975;54:773–777.

42. Shelly MP, Park GR: Intercostal nerve blockade for children. *Anaesthesia* 1987;42:541–544.

43. Benumof J, Semenza J: Total spinal following intrathoracic intercostal nerve blocks. *Anesthesiology* 1975;43:124–125.

44. Katz J, Nelson W, Forest R, Bruce DL: Cryoanalgesia for post-thoracotomy pain. *Lancet* 1980;1:512–514.

45. Robinson DA, Branthwaite MA: Pleural surgery in patients with cystic fibrosis. *Anaesthesia* 1984;39:655–659.

46. McIlvaine WB, Knox RF, Fennessey PV, Goldstein M: Continuous infusion of bupivacaine via intrapleural catheter for analgesia after thoracotomy in children. *Anesthesiology* 1988;60:261–264.

47. Attia J, Ecoffey C, Sandouk P, et al: Epidural morphine in children: Pharmacokinetics and CO_2 sensitivity. *Anesthesiology* 1986;65:590–594.

48. Rosen KR, Rosen DA: Caudal epidural morphine for control of pain following open heart surgery in children. *Anesthesiology* 1989;70:418–421.

49. Shapiro LA, Jedaikin RJ, Shalev D, Hoffman S: Epidural morphine analgesia in children. *Anesthesiology* 1984;61:210–212.

50. Krane EJ: Delayed respiratory depression in a child after caudal epidural morphine. *Anesth Analg* 1988;67:79–82.

51. Lynn AM, Opheim KE, Tyler DC: Morphine infusion after pediatric cardiac surgery. *Crit Care Med* 1984;12:863–866.

52. Means LJ, Allen HM, Lookabill RN, Krishna G: Recovery room initiation of patient controlled analgesia in pediatric patients. *Anesthesiology* 1988;69:A772.

53. Dodd E, Wang JM, Rauck RL: Patient controlled analgesia for post-surgical patients ages 6–16 years. *Anesthesiology* 1988;69:A372.

54. Lindahl SG, Yates AP, Hatch DJ: Respiratory depression in children at different end-tidal halothane concentrations. *Anaesthesia* 1987;42:1267–1275.

55. Olsson AK, Lindahl SG: Ventilation, dynamic compliance and ventilatory response to CO_2: Effects of age and body weight in infants and children. *Anaesthesia* 1985;40:229–236.

56. Berry FA: Pediatric anesthesia. *Otolaryngol Clin N Am* 1981;14:533.

57. Gallagher MJ, Muller BJ: Tension pneumothorax during pediatric bronchoscopy. *Anesthesiology* 1981;55:685.

58. Rah KH, Salzberg AM, Boyan CP, et al: Respiratory acidosis with the small Storz-Hopkins bronchoscopes: Occurrence and management. *Ann Thorac Surg* 1979;27:197.

59. Wallace CT, Baker JD, Othersen HB: Problems with ventilation during pediatric bronchoscopy. Presented at the Section of Anesthesia Abstracts, American Academy of Pediatricians; April 1977; New Orleans, La.

60. Ward CF, Benumof JL: Anesthesia for airway foreign body extraction in children. *Anesth Rev* 1977;13.

61. Young ET, Goudsouzian NG, Shah BS: Effect of ranitidine on intragastric pH in children. *Anesth Analg* 1986;65:S170.

62. Rao TLK, Madhavareddy S, Chinthagada M, El-Etr AA: Metoclopramide and cimetidine to reduce gastric fluid pH and volume. *Anesthesiology Analg* 1984;63:1014–1016.

63. Cote CJ: Anesthetic management of congenital lobar emphysema. *Anesthesiology* 1974;49:296.

64. German JC, Mahour GH, Woolley MM: Esophageal atresia and associated anomalies. *J Pediatr Surg* 1976;11:299.

65. Templeton JM, Templeton JJ, Schnaufer I, et al: Management of esophageal atresia and tracheoesophageal fistula in the neonate with severe respiratory distress syndrome. *J Pediatr Surg* 1985; 20:394–397.

66. Karl HW: Control of life-threatening air leak after gastrostomy in an infant with respiratory distress syndrome and tracheoesophageal fistula. *Anesthesiology Analg* 1985;62:670–672.

67. Bloch EC, Filston HC: A thin fiberoptic bronchoscope as an aid to occlusion of the fistula in infants with tracheoesophageal fistula. *Anesth Analg* 1988; 67:791–793.

68. Dierdorf SF, Krishna G: Anesthetic management of neonatal surgical emergencies. *Anesth Analg* 1981; 60:204–215.

69. Schwartz N, Eisenkraft JB: Positioning the endotracheal tube in an infant with tracheoesophageal fistula. *Anesthesiology* 1988;69:289–290.

70. Borland LM, Reilly JS, Smith SD: Anesthetic management of tracheoesophageal fistula with distal tracheal stenosis. *Anesthesiology* 1987;67:132–133.

71. Grillo HC, Zannani P: Management of obstructive tracheal disease in children. *J Pediatr Surg* 1984; 19:414.

72. Obara H, Maekawa N, Iwai S, et al: Reconstruction of the trachea in children with tracheal stenosis by using jet ventilation. *Anesthesiology* 1988;68:441–443.

73. Sakai H, Tamura M, Hosokawa Y, et al: Effect of surgical repair on respiratory mechanics in congenital diaphragmatic hernia. *J Pediatr* 1987; 111:432–438.

74. Azizkhan RG, Dudgeon DL, Buck JR, et al: Life-threatening airway obstruction as a complication to the management of mediastinal masses in children. *J Pediatr Surg* 1985;20:816–822.

75. Keon TP: Death on induction of anesthesia for cervical node biopsy. *Anesthesiology* 1981;55:471–472.

76. Piro AH, Weiss DR, Hellman S: Mediastinal Hodgkin's disease: A possible danger for intubation anesthesia. *Int J Radiat Oncol Biol Phys* 1976;1:415–419.

77. Kirks DR, Fram EK, Vock P, et al: Tracheal compression by mediastinal masses in children: CT evaluation. *AJR* 1983;141:647–651.

78. Degraff AC, Bouhuys A: Mechanics of airflow in airway obstruction. *Ann Rev Med* 1973;24:111–134.

79. Neuman GG, Weingarter AE, Abramowitz RM, et al: The anesthetic management of the patient with an anterior mediastinal mass. *Anesthesiology* 1984; 60:144–147.

DISCUSSION

Pediatric Anesthesia: Special Requirements for Intrathoracic Procedures

Gary G. Johnson, MD

Intrathoracic surgery represents a small percentage of all surgery in children if one excludes cardiac surgery. Accordingly, there is a need for an appreciation of the special anesthetic considerations involving thoracic surgical interventions. This chapter by Blackstock and Steward is well referenced for the problems and approaches recommended, and it includes many clinical "pearls" for the successful management of anesthesia.

Endoscopy of the airway and esophagus in children is much more common than intrathoracic surgery, and the anesthetic approaches for endoscopy are crisply presented.

The section on general considerations did not present the adverse effect of the lateral decubitus position (LDP) on the matching of ventilation and perfusion. Given that most intrathoracic surgery is done in the LDP, this is an important consideration, especially in infants, in whom the rib cage is less stable, functional residual capacity is reduced close to residual volume, and airway closure is more likely to occur in the dependent lung. In the LDP, both spontaneously breathing infants and those who are positive pressure ventilated have been shown to distribute more ventilation to the nondependent lung. As in adults, a vertical gravity gradient increases dependent lung blood flow. As a result, infants and children are at risk for ventilation/perfusion mismatch and desaturation during anesthesia for thoracic surgery in the LDP and require careful monitoring.

Monitoring with pulse oximeters and endtidal CO_2 (ETCO$_2$) monitors is a voluntary monitoring standard of both Canadian and American anesthesiology associations for all intubated patients. This standard is now mandated by legislation in some U.S. states (New York, New Jersey). The authors have outlined factors that bear on the accuracy and reliability of these monitors, especially in infants under anesthesia.

A recent study comparing mainstream versus sidestream (aspirating) capnographs demonstrated that a new mainstream CO_2 analyzer (Novametrix 1260) was as accurate as distal endotracheal sampling with a sidestream monitor in patients as small as 4.3 kg. This mainstream unit was also more accurate than the usual proximal endotracheal sidestream sampling, which is generally inaccurate below 12 kg.[1] This is a significant advance for infants in providing a more rapid and accurate ETCO$_2$ measurement and by avoiding the technical problems of distal sidestream sampling and the slow response time of transcutaneous CO_2 monitoring.

Oximetry's importance is clearly demonstrated during one-lung anesthesia, where desaturation may occur and not respond to modest increases in positive end-expiratory pressure applied to the dependent lung. In this circumstance, the oximeter provides beat-to-beat oxygen saturation monitoring that guides the need and timing for clamping the pulmonary artery of the surgical lung in order to decrease venous admixture and avoid hypoxia.

The anesthetic techniques presented by Blackstock and Steward fairly reflect current practice, with some minor institutional preference shown, such as for the Jackson-Rees T-piece anesthesia circuit. Other commonly used and equally acceptable anesthesia circuits for thoracic surgery in children are the Mapleson D, the Bain circuit (a coaxial Mapleson D) and circle systems with low-resistance valves. Circles are not recommended for infants and especially not for neonates in my practice.

655 Avenue of the Americas, New York, NY 10010
*Current Topics in General Thoracic Surgery:
An International Series*

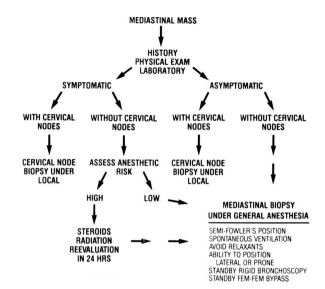

MEDIASTINAL MASS

HISTORY
PHYSICAL EXAM
LABORATORY

SYMPTOMATIC   ASYMPTOMATIC

WITH CERVICAL   WITHOUT CERVICAL   WITH CERVICAL   WITHOUT CERVICAL
NODES   NODES   NODES   NODES

CERVICAL NODE   ASSESS ANESTHETIC   CERVICAL NODE
BIOPSY UNDER   RISK   BIOPSY UNDER
LOCAL   LOCAL

HIGH   LOW

STEROIDS   MEDIASTINAL BIOPSY
RADIATION   UNDER GENERAL ANESTHESIA
REEVALUATION   SEMI-FOWLER'S POSITION
IN 24 HRS   SPONTANEOUS VENTILATION
                        AVOID RELAXANTS
                        ABILITY TO POSITION
                          LATERAL OR PRONE
                        STANDBY RIGID BRONCHOSCOPY
                        STANDBY FEM-FEM BYPASS

FIGURE D2.1 Decision tree for management of a child with anterior mediastinal mass. *Reproduced from Morray and Krane,*[4] *with permission.*

Blackstock and Steward recommend the use of formal airway heaters-humidifiers. There is no mention of the use of heat and moisture exchangers (HMEs or "artificial noses") presumably because of the risk of blood or secretions obstructing the channels of the material used in the HME adapters, thereby increasing airway resistance during thoracic surgery.

The section on postoperative care was devoted almost exclusively to postoperative pain management, an aspect of pediatric care that has been regrettably overlooked in the past. This emphasis is warranted. The options for pain management are presented for use alone or in combinations. The use of cryopexy in children has been limited and should not be considered clearly established, though cryopexy in cystic fibrosis patients postsurgery seems logical, if not ideal. Experience with regional anesthesia techniques in children has lagged behind that in adults, but their use is expanding and their benefit is clearly established. Continuous narcotic infusion is the preferred route for systemic analgesia in my hospital's practice and is the basic approach for major thoracic surgery. The use of patient-controlled analgesia (PCA) devices in school-age children is a natural advancement over continuous narcotic infusions and appears promising. PCAs must be considered and organized preoperatively in order to adequately instruct the patient and parents. In fact, the whole of the pain control strategy should be carefully selected and individually planned as part of the preoperative patient management scheme instead of the all too frequent approach of ordering routine analgesics, on a sliding scale, *pro re na'ta.* The inadequacy of the p.r.n. approach in children is shown by the study of Beyer et al (1983), where 6 of 50 children received no analgesic medication after cardiac surgery in the first 3 days; in addition they received a fraction of the administrations of analgesics and at less than recommended dosages when compared with a group of 50 adults after cardiac surgery.[2]

Many valuable clinical tips are offered in the comments on the anesthetic management of several major thoracic surgical procedures. The discussion on mediastinal masses illustrates the importance of preoperative patient assessment. CT scans, echocardiography, and flow-volume loops are especially valuable in identifying children with anterior mediastinal masses. These children are at risk for acute airway obstruction and/or cardiac collapse during or following induction of anesthesia. Because of this risk, alternatives to open biopsy must be considered, and the surgeon, oncologist, and anesthesiologist should discuss and plan to optimize the patient if anesthesia is contemplated.[3] Should airway obstruction or cardiovascular collapse occur during or after induction, preplanned approaches must be carried out rapidly, including the immediate change of position, from supine (Fowler's) to a lateral or even prone position. If the problem is airway obstruction, rigid instrumentation with a bronchoscope may be required. An emergency sternotomy has been employed to relieve cardiac compression and, to a lesser extent, airway obstruction. A femoral-femoral bypass has also been recommended. These approaches and others require clinical anticipation and prior preparation of equipment and personnel to achieve a favorable outcome. The decision tree outlines an approach to this uncommon but potentially life-threatening problem of the child with an anterior mediastinal mass (Fig. D2.1.)[4]

REFERENCES

1. Ilillier S, Lerman J: Mainstream vs. sidestream capnography in anesthetized infants and children. Abstract presentation. American Society of Anesthesiologists, October 14–18, 1989.
2. Beyer J, DeGood, DE, Ashley LC, Russell GA: Patterns of post-operative analgesic used with adults and children following cardiac surgery. Pain 1983;17:71–81.
3. Pullerits J: Anesthesia for patients with mediastinal masses. Canadian Journal of Anaesthesia 1989; 36:681–688.
4. Morray JP, Krane EJ: Anesthesia for thoracic surgery. In Gregory GA, ed. *Pediatric Anesthesia,* 2nd ed. New York: Churchill Livingstone, 1989.

Chapter 3

Intensive Airway and Respiratory Techniques

David S. Jardine, MD and Robert K. Crone, MD

Respiratory failure is one of the leading reasons for admission to neonatal and pediatric intensive care units. Basic airway management is an important skill for all personnel who work with critically ill infants and children.

Airway management begins with clearing the mouth and oropharynx of secretions. When the child is in the prone position, the tongue and hypopharyngeal structures fall forward, usually clearing the airway of soft tissues. While supine, head positioning and manipulation of the mandible are often necessary to effectively relieve the airway of soft tissue obstruction. In children this is accomplished by moderate extension of the cervical spine and superior displacement of the rami of the mandible. This will usually move the tongue and anterior wall of the hypopharynx enough to clear the airway.[1]

Knowledge of these simple maneuvers is far more important than intubation skills, because clearing the airway and delivering oxygen are most important in supporting respiration in the compromised child. Only in instances where ventilation is impossible due to obstruction of the larynx or trachea is intubation primarily indicated.

Mask ventilation may be facilitated under certain circumstances by the placement of either an oropharyngeal or nasopharyngeal airway. These devices are tolerated only in obtunded or comatose patients. They may induce vomiting, agitation, or laryngospasm in awake or semicomatose children and should be used with caution.

Face masks for manually ventilating children come in a variety of shapes and sizes. Those most commonly used are transparent so that secre-tions can be visualized and so that moisture from exhaled gases may confirm ventilation. Low-profile masks designed to fit a child's face are available in reusable and disposable forms.

It is also important to be familiar with operation of the manual breathing systems for infants and children. Both self-inflating and collapsible systems are available. The self-inflating bags require some form of reservoir to deliver an enriched inspired oxygen concentration above 40%, whereas the collapsible (anesthesia type) bag requires a constant flow of gas and a tight mask fit in order to support positive pressure ventilation. In both types of bags, airway pressure should be monitored when applying positive pressure, because pressure relief valves are unreliable when gas velocity is variable, as is the case during hand ventilation.[2]

In every case of artificial ventilation, the measure of effectiveness is the clinical assessment of chest expansion and the presence of breath sounds. In small infants and children, expansion and distension of the stomach can be mistaken for respiration. Careful assessment of breath sounds is essential in confirming the effectiveness of artificial ventilation. Detection of carbon dioxide by infrared gas analysis or other type of capnometry can confirm the clinical assessment except when pulmonary blood flow is severely impaired.

Endotracheal intubation is indicated whenever prolonged respiratory support will be needed, where protection of the airway from aspiration is necessary, or where proximal airway obstruction can be bypassed. The infant's and young child's larynx is positioned higher in the neck relative to the cervical spine (C3-4) and is funnel shaped. The narrowest portion of the upper airway is at the level of the cricoid cartilage. These anatomical differences make Miller laryngoscope blades (straight) preferable to those that are curved (Macintosh) and favor un-cuffed endotracheal tubes over those with in-flatable cuffs. Endotracheal tubes should be im-plantation tested and the size should be carefully selected. Several formulae are available for de-termining endotracheal tube size[3]; however, the following age-specific guidelines may be helpful:

	I.D. (uncuffed)
Premature infant	2.5–3.0
Full-term infant to 6 months	3.0–3.5
6 months to 1 year	3.5–4.0
1–2 years	4.0–4.5
3–4 years	4.5–5.0
5–6 years	5.0–5.5
6–9 years	5.5–6.0

The correct-size endotracheal tube should produce an audible leak at a constant inflation pressure of approximately 20 cm H_2O or, in the case of abnormal lung compliance, at an inflation pressure just above that required to inflate the lungs.

Endotracheal intubation techniques vary widely and depend upon the indications for in-tubation. An emergency intubation in a comatose child can be accomplished after bag and mask ventilation with oxygen by direct laryngoscopy without the use of anesthetic agents or muscle relaxants. In more controlled circumstances in-travenous or inhalational anesthetics and muscle relaxants such as those in the following list may be appropriate to facilitate endotracheal intu-bation. These drugs should be used only by those familiar with their actions and where precautions to prevent aspiration of stomach contents can be taken.

Commonly used anesthetics to facilitate intuba-tion:

sodium thiopental	2–4 mg/kg
methohexital	1–2 mg/kg
ketamine	1–2 mg/kg

Commonly used muscle relaxants to facilitate in-tubation:

succinylcholine	1–2 mg/kg
vecuronium	0.1 mg/kg
atracurium	0.5 mg/kg
pancuronium	0.1 mg/kg

Oral tracheal intubations are easier to per-form than are nasotracheal intubations and hence should be used in emergency situations. Although nasotracheal intubations can be more difficult to perform, nasally placed tubes are usu-ally better tolerated and more easily secured for long-term management.

After intubation, the position of the tube should be confirmed clinically by bilateral aus-culation of equal breath sounds, by observation of symmetrical chest motion, and by chest roent-genogram. Recently, an electromagnetic locater device has become commercially available to confirm the position of specially designed en-dotracheal tubes for infants and children.[4]

In recent years, endotracheal tubes have been left in place in infants and children for in-creasing periods of time. It is not uncommon to leave a child's trachea intubated for more than 2 weeks and up to 6 weeks without performing a tracheostomy. This approach has been possible because of proper humidification and improved techniques of nursing care, including endotra-cheal suctioning, continuous sedation of chron-ically intubated patients, and careful patient sur-veillance.

TRACHEOSTOMY

Indications

Indications for the placement of a tracheostomy fall into three broad, frequently overlapping cate-gories: airway obstruction, assisted ventilation, and pulmonary toilet.[5] The indications for tra-cheostomy in children differ somewhat from those in adults. On one hand, a small amount of swelling of the tracheal wall obstructs a child's trachea more easily than does a similar amount of swelling in an adult trachea. On the other hand, if the child is able to tolerate the tracheal ob-struction, he or she may eventually outgrow the problem without any medical intervention (un-like the adult).

The small size of the infant's trachea makes airway obstruction particularly dangerous. The normal anterior-posterior diameter of the infant's glottis is 4.5 mm.[6] One millimeter of circumfer-ential tracheal edema reduces the glottic lumen to 30% of normal. This unfavorable situation is compounded by the physics of gas flow. Turbu-lent flow of gas past an obstruction is inversely proportional to the fifth power of the radius of the lumen.[7,8] Gas exchange will be dramatically reduced by minor degrees of impingement on an infant's trachea. For the same reason, a child is unable to tolerate lesions that would not produce symptoms in an adult.

Pediatric anatomic anomalies that may ne-cessitate tracheostomy are most frequently man-ifested in the neonatal period or in infancy, though some may not appear until childhood. The most common abnormalities include vocal cord paralysis (congenital and postbirth injury), subglottic stenosis, tracheal stenosis, cystic hy-groma, tracheal hemangioma, and laryngeal cyst.[9,10] The accurate diagnosis of these problems is frequently made during bronchoscopic examination of the larynx and trachea while the patient is anesthetized. If the obstruction is of sufficient magnitude, consideration should be given to performing a tracheostomy at the time of bronchoscopy.

The tracheostomy is now only infrequently employed in the management of pediatric infectious diseases that result in airway obstruction. A few years ago, diseases such as epiglottitis and laryngotracheobronchitis (croup) were routinely managed with a tracheostomy.[6,11,12] Recent studies have demonstrated the safety and efficacy of managing patients with epiglottitis and croup with nasotracheal intubation rather than with a tracheostomy.[11,13,14] In our institution, a tracheostomy for epiglottitis has not been performed in more than 10 years. In addition, the treatment of croup with racemic epinephrine has dramatically decreased the need for any sort of invasive airway management in the therapy of this illness.[15] Finally, in children, just as in adults, a tracheostomy may be necessary to relieve airway obstruction following facial or cervical trauma.[16,17]

Infants may also require tracheostomy because of the need for assisted ventilation. The advent of neonatal intensive care has enabled small preterm infants to survive despite severe respiratory illness. Many of these patients will require lengthy periods of mechanical ventilation to treat infant respiratory distress syndrome and bronchopulmonary dysplasia. Prolonged nasotracheal intubation may result in acquired subglottic stenosis.[18–21] To reduce the frequency of this complication, a tracheostomy may be performed. The optimal timing of tracheostomy for children who require long-term intubation remains controversial.[22] In many neonatal intensive care units, infants requiring mechanical ventilatory support for longer than 30 to 45 days will undergo tracheostomy. Although the trend for longer periods of nasotracheal intubation has become more common.

The decline of polio in the United States in the 1950s dramatically decreased the number of tracheostomies performed to facilitate mechanical ventilation and pulmonary toilet. Nevertheless, several pediatric diseases predictably result in prolonged neuromuscular failure. The victims of these diseases may receive a tracheostomy for the same indications as the polio victims of three decades ago. Older children with Guillain-Barré syndrome and respiratory failure may require a tracheostomy if a lengthy course of mechanical ventilation is anticipated.[23]

The timing of the tracheostomy will depend upon a number of issues, including the patient's underlying illness and the severity of the condition that makes tracheostomy necessary. If possible, emergency tracheostomy under unfavorable conditions should be avoided as the complications are more likely.[24,25]

Procedure

The surgical technique for pediatric tracheostomy has been well described.[25–27] If possible, the tracheostomy should be performed on a patient receiving general anesthesia through an endotracheal tube or bronchoscope. The neck should be gently extended, with a roll placed under the shoulders. Hyperextension should be avoided, as it could make the procedure more difficult and result in caudad displacement of the stoma when the neck is returned to a more normal position.

Postoperative Nursing Care

Care from attentive, trained nurses is essential for the well-being of the patient with a tracheostomy.[27] Until a tract of granulation tissue has formed in the stoma between the cervical epithelium and the tracheal endothelium, precautions should be taken to prevent the accidental displacement of the tracheostomy tube. Although stay sutures facilitate replacement of the tracheostomy tube it may still be difficult, especially in an emergency situation with a struggling patient. The hastily replaced tube may be incorrectly located in the pretracheal soft tissue[28] resulting in asphyxiation. If positive pressure ventilation is attempted with the tube in this position, subcutaneous and mediastinal emphysema may be followed by a life-threatening tension pneumothorax.[29] Because of these risks, patients at our institution remain in the intensive care unit for several days postoperatively. Smaller children have arm restraints placed to prevent them from pulling at the tracheostomy tube. If necessary, sedation is given until the child grows accustomed to the tracheostomy and the tract matures with the formation of granulation tissue. If accidental displacement of the tracheostomy tube does occur, replacement may be facilitated by gently inserting a lighted #O Miller laryngoscope blade into the stoma and identifying the tracheal lumen before a small endotracheal tube is passed.

In addition to avoiding accidental displacement of the tracheostomy tube, the patient must be monitored for obstruction of the tracheostomy tube. The tube may be obstructed by dried tracheal mucus. In some cases the patient's chin may obstruct the tube. Humidified gas may be administered to prevent drying and inspissation of secretions. Gentle suction applied with a catheter may be necessary to remove tenacious or copious secretions. Many patients will also require chest physical therapy to aid in the removal of thick secretions.[30] The skin must also be monitored for signs of irritation or infection.

Complications

Any surgery upon the airway involves risk. The complication rate following tracheostomy has been reported to be 10% to 30%, with a death rate of 3%.[31,32] Early postoperative complications include air leak, hemorrhage, and aspiration. Air leak is seen much more frequently in children than in adults[28,33] and may be life-threatening.[34] The risk of complications declines with the age of the patient. Some life-threatening complications, such as accidental decannulation or tracheostomy tube obstruction, may occur anytime after the placement of a tracheostomy,[35] so the safety and well-being of patients with a tracheostomy requires constant vigilance.

Swallowing dysfunction after tracheostomy may lead to aspiration of saliva and food.[36] This may be due in part to the anchoring of the trachea to the skin of the neck, preventing the cephalad movement of the trachea during swallowing.[37] Children who have a tracheostomy often have difficulty learning to eat. The high frequency of pneumonia observed after tracheostomy[38] may be in part attributable to the problem of recurrent aspiration. Aerophagia, another form of swallowing dysfunction, occurs with modest frequency in pediatric patients following tracheostomy.[39]

Late complications include granulation tissue formation, tracheal stenosis,[40] infection of the stoma, pneumonia, fused vocal cords, and distal tracheomalacia. An uncommon but particularly dangerous late complication is erosion of the tracheostomy tube into the innominate artery.[41] Although infection of the stoma and distal tracheomalacia may be evident prior to decannulation, granulation formation and fused vocal cords may not be apparent until decannulation is attempted.

Decannulation

As many as 36% of children will experience problems at the time of decannulation.[42] These difficulties are most frequent in patients younger than 1 year of age. Structural abnormalities that result in decannulation problems include subglottic stenosis, tracheomalacia at the tracheostomy site, granuloma tissue obstructing the trachea, and fused vocal cords. If respiratory distress is encountered at the time of decannulation, it should not be attributed to the patient's psychological dependence on the tracheostomy tube. It is important to evaluate the airway with either bronchoscopy or a lateral neck roentgenogram.[43] Psychological factors should not be considered until structural causes of respiratory embarrassment have been eliminated.

BRONCHOSCOPY
Rigid or Flexible Bronchoscopy?

Bronchoscopy may be performed for diagnostic or therapeutic indications. A decision must be made as to whether the problem is best addressed by rigid or flexible bronchoscopy. Rigid bronchoscopy is commonly employed for both diagnostic and therapeutic indications. Compared with fiberoptic bronchoscopy, rigid bronchoscopy has the advantage of superior optics and a much larger lumen through which instruments may be passed or suction may be applied. The inability of this bronchoscope to bend is its major limitation. Fiberoptic bronchoscopy has several advantages over rigid bronchoscopy. It is less traumatic to the patient; in certain instances, it may be performed without general anesthesia. The flexibility of the fiberoptic bronchoscope extends the surgeon's ability to examine the tracheobronchial tree beyond those regions that may be seen through a rigid bronchoscope. These diagnostic advantages come at a price: the fiberoptic bronchoscope has a very small lumen. Many therapeutic procedures exceed the capabilities of the fiberoptic bronchoscope and must be performed with a rigid bronchoscope.

Indications

Infants manifest a variety of airway anomalies during the first few months of life. Many of these anomalies are diagnosed with bronchoscopy. These abnormalities may be classified as disorders of phonation, respiration, or deglutition.[9,10] Inspiratory stridor is a common neonatal problem, the cause of which is most frequently found to be laryngotracheomalacia. During bronchoscopy, the glottic structures appear to collapse into the tracheal lumen when the patient inspires, giving rise to the crowing sound that is audible during the inspiratory phase of crying. Bronchoscopy may also be indicated for the infant who is hoarse or aphonic or has an abnormal cry. Frequently, varying degrees of vocal cord paralysis will be found to be the cause of these anomalies.

Respiratory difficulties in neonates may take a variety of forms. Among these are stridor, inspiratory retractions, cyanosis, cough, and apnea. Although foreign body aspiration may produce these signs in older children, this is an uncommon problem in neonates. Instead, infants usually suffer from anatomic anomalies, of which vocal cord paralysis is the most common cause, but which may also be caused by a tracheo-esophageal fistula, vascular ring, subglottic stenosis (congenital or acquired), tracheal web, cystic hygroma, or tracheal hemangioma.

In recent years a newly recognized disorder—necrotizing tracheobronchitis—has been noted among intubated, mechanically ventilated preterm neonates.[44] This illness is characterized by tracheal obstruction from sloughed, necrotic tracheal mucosa[45] and is an indication for emergency rigid bronchoscopy to remove the obstruction.[46,47] Rigid bronchoscopy is preferred, as the severely ill infant may not tolerate the airway obstruction produced during fiberoptic bronchoscopy.[48]

Disorders of deglutition are often due to anomalies of both the esophagus and trachea. These derangements may be manifested by a poor suck reflex, choking and cyanosis during feeding, excessive oropharyngeal secretions, and vomiting. Some of the abnormalities that may be diagnosed during bronchoscopy include laryngeal cleft, tracheoesophageal fistula, esophageal stricture, and esophageal atresia.

Perhaps the most common therapeutic indication for bronchoscopy in children is the aspiration of foreign material. This problem primarily affects children between 1 and 4 years of age.[49,50] Eighty-one percent of the children who aspirate foreign body are younger than 3 years old. The most common foreign body is vegetable matter,[51] with peanuts being a particularly egregious offender.[49]

Bronchoscopy may also be performed to diagnose opportunistic pulmonary infections in immunosuppressed patients or to remove inspissated secretions that have caused bronchial obstruction in patients with a variety of illnesses. Although fiberoptic bronchoscopy has limited utility in removing tenacious secretions, both rigid and fiberoptic bronchoscopy are useful in the diagnosis of pneumonia in immunosuppressed patients. These specimens may be obtained by bronchial washings or bronchial brushings.

Techniques have been developed in which the fiberoptic bronchoscope is used to aid in endotracheal intubation of patients with airway abnormalities that would preclude intubation by more conventional means.[52,53]

Anesthesia

There is no doubt that both rigid and fiberoptic bronchoscopy may be performed without anesthesia for selected indications,[48,54] but the procedure is easier and less traumatic if the patient is anesthetized.

If the patient is to undergo rigid bronchoscopy, general inhalation anesthesia may be given by mask until he or she is deeply anesthetized and airway reflexes have been ablated. The vocal cords may then be sprayed with a solution of 2% to 4% lidocaine (not to exceed 5 mg/kg total dose) to further diminish the risk of coughing or laryngospasm during the procedure. Neuromuscular relaxation is elective and should not be employed if vocal cord function is to be assessed during the procedure. During the procedure, ventilation may be provided via the side arm of the Stortz bronchoscope, or through a Sanders venturi ventilation system.[55]

Patients undergoing fiberoptic bronchoscopy may receive general endotracheal anesthesia. The procedure is performed by passing the bronchoscope through a special adapter at the end of the endotracheal tube.[56] This allows the patient to be ventilated during the procedure unless the bronchoscope occupies too large a portion of the endotracheal tube lumen.

Complications

Although severe complications such as injury to the subglottic area, asphyxia, and cardiac arrest may occur during bronchoscopy,[57] these complications are uncommon and are often related to the severity of the patient's primary illness. More common complications include laryngospasm, bronchospasm, and tracheal swelling that is manifested as croup postoperatively. These complications may be avoided by minimizing trauma to the trachea during the procedure and ensuring that an adequate depth of anesthesia is maintained during the procedure.

MECHANICAL VENTILATORY SUPPORT

Indications for mechanical ventilation in infants and children include not only support for respiratory failure but also respiratory support for nonpulmonary diseases. These include:

1. resuscitation from circulatory compromise, including circulatory shock and circulatory arrest;
2. maintenance of supranormal blood gases as in hyperventilation and alkalosis for control of intracranial hypertension and for treatment of persistent pulmonary hypertension of the newborn[58];
3. reduced work of breathing where caloric intake is insufficient to support growth as seen in bronchiopulmonary dysplasia; and

4. maintenance of normal lung volumes in conditions that predispose patients to respiratory failure, including marked obesity, massive sepsis, nutritional debilitation, and major thoracic or abdominal trauma or surgery.

Ventilator Therapy

Mechanical respiratory assistance can be accomplished by a variety of positive and negative pressure devices. Positive pressure is applied almost exclusively by way of an endotracheal or tracheostomy tube, whereas negative pressure ventilation does not usually require airway instrumentation.

Positive pressure ventilators can be classified according to their method of controlling ventilator frequency. Volume preset, pressure preset, and time-flow preset ventilators are all commercially available for infants and children. Time-flow or pressure preset ventilators are used most commonly in infants less than 10 kg, and volume preset ventilators are more practical in infants and children greater than 10 kg.[59] Timeflow ventilators offer the advantage of rapid response times at rapid ventilator rates and where high compressible volumes make preset tidal volumes difficult to correlate with delivered tidal volumes in small infants. The major disadvantage of this type of ventilator is that delivered tidal volume will vary with the child's total thoracic and lung compliance.[60] Rapid changes in compliance may result in unrecognized underventilation or overdistension. In children greater than 10 kilograms, the volume preset ventilator becomes more practical. A smaller compressible volume to tidal volume ratio in these older children makes the tidal volume determination more accurate.

Positive end-expiratory pressure capability is available on all modern ventilators regardless of type. In addition, intermittent mandatory ventilation (IMV) is also standard on all infant and pediatric ventilators in use in intensive care units.[61] Pressure present and time-flow preset ventilators often have continuous flow of gas throughout the breathing circuit, allowing spontaneous ventilation at will. Newer volume preset ventilators have synchronized IMV circuits, which necessitates opening and closing "demand" valves to allow spontaneous ventilation. The sensitivity and response time of these valves is crucial in supporting spontaneous ventilation for small children with rapid respiratory rates and small endotracheal tubes.

More recently, additional ventilator modes such as pressure support ventilation have become available and proved efficacious in adults.

Pressure support allows an intermediate degree of respiratory support during spontaneous breaths, which may facilitate weaning from mechanical ventilation in adults and older children with less work of breathing.[62] Again, rapid respiratory rates and small endotracheal tubes make this less likely to be of benefit in smaller patients.

The pattern of positive pressure ventilation can be varied and depends upon the inspiratory and expiratory flow rates, the tidal volume, and the duration of positive pressure. Although philosophies differ among practitioners, it is generally accepted that infants and children with alveolar and pulmonary interstitial disorders are well supported with relatively large tidal volumes (15 to 20 ml/kg) with prolonged inspiratory times (0.8 to 1.5 seconds), a low inspiratory flow rate, and low ventilator frequencies.[3] This pattern is purported to maximize the distribution of gas delivery at the lowest peak airway pressure.

Initiation of Positive Pressure Ventilation

Because practitioners differ in their philosophy of respiratory support, one approach will be offered. In our experience the human hand is an excellent mechanical ventilator. By ventilating the patient's lungs with a non-self-inflating respirator bag (Mapleson circuit) with an airway pressure manometer in line, one can determine the peak airway pressure required to inflate the patient's lungs. This pressure will determine the preset pressure on time-cycled pressure ventilators. In patients with alveolar or interstitial disorders such as hyaline membrane disease, atelectasis, or pneumonia, a prolonged inspiratory time of 0.8 to 1.0 seconds is frequently useful, accompanied by a relatively slow respiratory frequency of ≤ 16 cycles/minute in children.[63]

When initiating mechanical ventilation with a preset volume ventilator, choosing an arbitrary tidal volume of 15 to 20 ml/kg (using the higher number in the smaller child), while observing peak airway pressure, is commonly employed.

Regardless of the type of ventilator used, the most important variables in initiating mechanical ventilation are the adequacy of chest expansion and gas exchange by clinical observation and auscultation, and by the adequacy of alveolar ventilation as determined by the arterial pCO_2. The peak airway pressure should be measured frequently as close to the endotracheal tube as possible.

Positive airway pressure should be initiated at 3.5 cm H_2O as a minimum and be increased in a stepwise fashion by 2 to 3 cm H_2O until arterial oxygenation is maximized. With the initiation of mechanical ventilation, it is not uncommon to see arterial hypotension due to relative hypovolemia. This phenomenon is predictable and usually responsive to an intravenous infusion of 10 to 20 ml/kg of crystalloid. In instances where positive end expiratory pressures are greater than 10 cm H_2O, central venous pressure monitoring is helpful in managing fluid therapy.

NEGATIVE PRESSURE VENTILATION

Body type negative pressure ventilators were popularized by Drinker and associates in 1929 and were used extensively during the polio epidemics of the 1950s.[64,65] These devices have achieved renewed popularity more recently in the management of some forms of respiratory failure in infants and children. Individuals with severe forms of neuromuscular disability, such as Duchenne type muscular dystrophy, and those with chronic obstructive lung disease, such as cystic fibrosis, have been reported to have sustained improvement in their gas exchange and their general clinical condition when subjected to chronic or nighttime home ventilation.[66] Measurements of vital capacity, inspiratory force, and force of diaphragmatic muscle contraction suggest that this therapy will improve gas exchange, reduce the complications of chronic hypoxemia and hypercarbia, and prolong life. In addition, there has been a fundamental change in physicians' attitudes regarding the life expectancy of patients with these types of "fatal" respiratory diseases. This change has been generated in part from the demands of patients and their families as well as the expectation that new forms of therapy, such as lung transplantation, may provide new alternatives for diseases previously considered incurable. In addition, negative pressure ventilation along with other supports at home can provide a tolerable existence for children who previously needed long-term hospitalization.

Negative pressure ventilation is also useful in weaning some patients from positive pressure ventilation in the intensive care unit under certain circumstances. Children requiring prolonged postoperative ventilation due to underlying neuromuscular and pulmonary disease, such as those who have undergone surgical correction of scoliosis or infants with congenital diaphragmatic hernia and severe lung dysplasia, often can be weaned to the negative pressure ventilator and then extubated. Children will nearly always prefer "tank" ventilation to intubation or tracheostomy, and weaning can be done at a more leisurely pace.

Unfortunately, a number of serious conditions limit the efficacy of negative pressure ventilation. For example, a patient's size or deformities can make the patient-machine interface both difficult and uncomfortable, and the ability to provide basic and specialized patient care can be compromised in these devices. Any degree of upper airway obstruction, be it anatomical or due to tracheal secretions, decreases the effectiveness of air flow. Finally, negative pressure ventilation is not effective in patients with very poor lung compliance. Maximal respiratory pressures are -30 cm H_2O, and it is not possible to sustain a reliably constant distending airway pressure. The ideal candidate for negative pressure ventilation is cooperative, has only moderate lung dysfunction, has a normal upper airway, and needs support principally for neuromuscular disability.

REFERENCES

1. Morikawa S, Safar P, DeCarlo J: Influence of the head-jaw position upon upper airway potency. *Anesthesiology* 1961;22:265–270.
2. Backofen J, Rogers M: Emergency management of the airway. In: Rogers MC, ed. *Textbook of Pediatric Intensive Care.* Baltimore Md.: Williams & Wilkins, 1987:57–62.
3. Crone RK: Assisted ventilation in children. In: Gregory GA, ed. *Respiratory Failure in the Child.* New York, NY: Churchill Livingstone, 1981:18.
4. McCormick W, Crone RK: In: *Proceedings of the 8th Annual Conference of the IEEE/Engr Med Biol Society,* 1986;1:140–143.
5. Aberdeen E, Downes JJ: Artificial airways in children. *Surg Clin North Am* 1974;54:1155–1170.
6. Freeland AP, Wright JLW, Ardran GM: Developmental influences of infant tracheostomy. *J Laryngol Otol* 1974;88:927–936.
7. Badgwell JM, McLeod ME, Friedberg J: Airway obstruction in infants and children. *Can J Anaes* 1987; 34(1):90–98.
8. Goldthorn J, Badgwell JM: Upper airway obstruction in infants and children. *Int Anesthes Clin* 1986; 24(1):133–144.
9. Cohen SR, Eavey RD, Desmond MS, May BC: Endoscopy and tracheotomy in the neonatal period. *Ann Otol Rhinol Laryngol* 1977;86:577–583.
10. Schild JA, Holinger LA: Peroral endoscopy in neonates. *Int J Pediatr Otorhinolaryng* 1980;2:133–138.
11. Hans DB, Jensen MH: The hazard of acute epiglottitis. *Inten Care Med* 1978;4:203–206.
12. Maze A, Bloch E: Stridor in pediatric patients. *Anesthesiology* 1979;509:132–145.
13. Carter P, Benjamin B: Ten year review of pediatric tracheotomy. *Ann Otol Rhinol Laryngol* 1983; 92:398–400.
14. Hannallah R, Rosales JK: Acute epiglottitis: Current management and review. *Can Anaes Soc J* 1978; 25:84–91.
15. Adair JC, Ring WH, Jordan WS, Elwyn RA: Ten year

experience with IPPB in the treatment of acute laryngotracheobronchitis. *Anesth Analg* 1971;50:649–655.

16. Herrin TJ, Brzustowicz R, Hendrickson M: Anesthetic management of neck trauma. *South Med J* 1979;72:1102–1106.

17. Seed RF: Traumatic injury to the larynx and trachea. *Anaesthesia* 1971;26(1):55–65.

18. Glover WJ: Nasotracheal intubation and tracheostomy in intensive care in infants. *Acta Anaesthes Scand* 1970;37:62–69.

19. Johnson DG, Stewart DR: Management of acquired tracheal obstructions in infancy. *J Pediatr Surg* 1975;10:709–717.

20. Louhimo I, Grahne B, Pasila M, Suutarinen T: Acquired laryngotracheal stenosis in children. *J Pediatr Surg* 1971;6:730–737.

21. Nau TW, Gates GA, Escobedo MB: Management of neonatal subglottic stenosis. *Otolaryng Clin North Am* 1986;19(1):153–162.

22. Pippin LK, Short DH, Bowes JB: Long-term tracheal intubation practice in the United Kingdom. *Anaesthesia* 1983;38:791–795.

23. Moore P, James O: Guillain-Barré syndrome: Incidence, management and outcome of major complications. *Crit Care Med* 1981;9:549–555.

24. Allen TH, Steven IM: Prolonged endotracheal intubation in infants and children. *Br J Anesth* 1965;37:566.

25. Tepas JJ III, Heroy HH, Shermeta DW, Haller JA Jr: Tracheostomy in neonates and small infants: Problems and pitfalls. *Surgery* 1981;89:635–639.

26. Filston HC, Johnson DG, Crumrine RS: Infant tracheostomy. *AJDC* 1978;132:1172–1176.

27. Stool SE, Beebe JK: Tracheostomy in infants and children. *Curr Prob Pediatr* 1973;3(5):3–33.

28. Chew JY, Cantrell RW: Tracheostomy: Complications and their management. *Arch Otolaryngol* 1972;96:538–545.

29. Webb RW, Johnston JH, Geisler JW: Pneumomediastinum: Physiologic observations. *J Thorac Surg* 1958;35:309–315.

30. Douglas GS, Hoskins D, Stool SE: Tracheotomy in pediatric airway management. *Pediatr Otolaryng* 1976;August:510–516.

31. Freidberg J, Morrison MD: Paediatric tracheotomy. *Can J Otolaryng* 1974;3(2):147–155.

32. Gaudet PT, Peerless A, Sasaki CT, Kirchner JA: Pediatric tracheostomy and associated complications. *Laryngoscope* 1978;88:1633–1641.

33. Padovan IR, Dawson CA, Henschel EO, Lehman RH: Pathogenesis of mediastinal emphysema and pneumothorax following tracheotomy. *Chest* 1974;66:553–556.

34. Diaz JH, Henling CE: Pneumoperitoneum and cardiac arrest during craniofacial reconstruction. *Anesth Analg* 1982;61(2):146–149.

35. Todres ID, Shannon DC: Monitoring occlusion and accidental extubation of tracheostomy tubes in children. *Laryngoscope* 1978;88:130–143.

36. Cameron JL, Reynolds J, Zuidema GD: Aspiration in patients with tracheostomies. *Surg Gynecol Obstet* January 1973;136:68–70.

37. Bonanno PC: Swallowing dysfunction after tracheostomy. *Ann Surg* 1971;174(1):29–33.

38. Rogers LA, Osterhout S: Pneumonia following tracheostomy. *Am Surg* 1970;36(1):39–46.

39. Rosnagle RS, Yanagisawa E: Aerophagia, an unrecognized complication of tracheotomy. *Arch Otolaryngol* 1969;89:537–539.

40. Friman L, Hedenstierna G, Schildt B: Stenosis following tracheostomy: A quantative study of long term results. *Anaesthesia* 1976;31:479–493.

41. Utley JR, Singer MM, Roe BB, et al: Definitive management of innominate artery hemorrhage complicating tracheostomy. *JAMA* 1972;220:577–579.

42. Sasaki CT, Gaudet PT, Peerless A: Tracheostomy decannulation. *AJDC* 1978;132:266–269.

43. Scott JR, Kramer SS: Pediatric tracheostomy: Radiographic features of normal healing. *AJR* 1978;130:887–891.

44. Kirpalani H, Higa T, Perlman M, et al: Diagnosis and therapy of necrotizing tracheobronchitis in ventilated neonates. *Crit Care Med* 1985;13:792–797.

45. Pietsch JB, Nagaraj HS, Groff BD, et al: Necrotizing tracheobronchitis: A new indication for emergency bronchoscopy in the neonate. *J Pediatr Surg* 1985;20:391–393.

46. Rubin SZ, Trevenen CL, Mitchell I: Diffuse necrotizing tracheobronchitis: An acute and chronic disease. *J Pediatr Surg* 1988;23:476–477.

47. Wilson KS, Carley RB, Mammel MC, et al: Necrotizing tracheobronchitis: A newly recognized cause of acute obstruction in mechanically ventilated neonates. *Laryngoscope* 1987;97:1017–1019.

48. Muntz HR: Therapeutic rigid bronchoscopy in the neonatal intensive care unit. *Ann Otol Rhinol Laryngol* 1985;94:462–465.

49. Mantel K, Butenandt I: Tracheobronchial foreign body aspiration in childhood. *Europ J Pediatr* 1986;145:211–216.

50. Schloss MD, Pham-Dang H, Rosales JK: Foreign bodies in the tracheobronchial tree—A retrospective study of 217 cases. *J Otolaryngol* 1983;12:212–216.

51. Barkara A: Bronchoscopic removal of inhaled foreign bodies in children. *Br J Anesth* 1974;46:124–126.

52. Howardy-Hansen P, Berthelsen P: Fiberoptic bronchoscopic nasotracheal intubation of neonate with Pierre Robin syndrome. *Anaesthesia* 1988;43:121–122.

53. Rucker RW, Silva WJ, Worcester CC: Fiberoptic bronchoscopic nasotracheal intubation in children. *Chest* 1979;76(1):56–58.

54. Wood RE, Fink RJ: Applications of flexible fiberoptic bronchoscopes in infants and children. *Chest* 1978;73(suppl):737–740.

55. Carden E, Chir B, Trapp WG, Oulton J: A new and simple method for ventilating patients undergoing bronchoscopy. *Anesthesiology* 1970;33:454–458.

56. Carden E, Phulchand PR: Special new low resistance to flow tube and endotracheal tube adapter for use during fiberoptic bronchoscopy. *Ann Otol Rhinol Laryngol* 1975;84:631–634.

57. Abdulmajid OS, Ebeid AM, Motaweh MM, Kleibo IS: Aspirated foreign bodies in the tracheobronchial tree: Report of 250 cases. *Thorax* 1976;31:635–640.

58. Drummond WH, Gregory GA, Heymann MA, et al: The independent effects of hyperventilation, tolazoline, and dopamine on infants with persistent pulmonary hypertension. *J Pediatr* 1981;98:603–607.

59. Downes JJ, Goldberg AI: Airway management, mechanical ventilation and cardiopulmonary resuscitation. In: Scarpelli EM, Auld P, eds. *Pulmonary Disease of the Fetus, Newborn and Child.* Philadelphia, Pa: Lea and Febiger, 1978:99.

60. Haddad D, Richards CC: Mechanical ventilation of infants: Significance of compression volume and elimination of compression volume. *Anesthesiology* 1968;29:365.

61. Downs JB, Klein EF, Desautels D, et al: Intermittent mandatory ventilation: A new approach to weaning patients from mechanical ventilation. *Chest* 1973; 64:331.

62. Viale JP, Annat GJ, Boufford YM, et al: Oxygen cost of breathing in postoperative patients: Pressure support ventilation vs. continuous positive airway pressure. *Chest* 1988;93:506–509.

63. Crone RK, O'Rourke PP: Pediatric and neonatal intensive care. In: Miller RD, ed. *Anesthesia.* 2nd ed. New York, NY: Churchill Livingstone, 1986:2349.

64. Drinker P, Shaw LA: An apparatus for the prolonged administration of artificial respiration. *J Clin Invest* 1929;7:229–237.

65. Plum F, Lukas DS: An evaluation of the cuirass respirator in acute poliomyelitis respiratory insufficiency. *Am J Med* 1951;221:417–432.

66. Rochester DF, Braun NM: The diaphragm and dyspnea. *Am Rev Respir Dis* 1979;77:199–122.

Intensive Airway and Respiratory Techniques

Didier Moulin, MD

"Intensive Airway and Respiratory Techniques" by David S. Jardine and Robert K. Crone represents the state of the art on the subject and is to be recommended as the standard of care. I take this opportunity to emphasize particular aspects.

ENDOTRACHEAL INTUBATION

Endotracheal intubation is indicated in cardiac arrest, not only to maintain proximal airway patency and adequate lung ventilation during cardiac massage, but also to administer drugs such as epinephrine and xylocaine if a central line is not available. The endotracheal route for drug administration in cardiopulmonary resuscitation is preferred to a peripheral vein catheter and to intracardiac injection.[1]

TRACHEOSTOMY

All attempts are made to avoid a tracheostomy in children younger than 3 years of age because of the related morbidity and mortality. I never perform a tracheostomy for prolonged assisted ventilation in a patient with a curable disease. Some of my patients have been ventilated through a nasotracheal tube for several months without significant laryngeal sequelae. In my experience postintubation stenoses are more often related to the use of tubes that are too large and to their traumatic insertion than to their prolonged use.[2]

I also use prolonged nasotracheal intubation for reversible airway obstruction. Congenital vocal cord paralysis most often resolves spontaneously but may need nasotracheal intubation for several months. Subglottic hemangioma, laryngeal papillomatosis, and inflammatory subglottic stenosis are treated by surgical laser and

temporary intubation.[3] Caustic laryngitis following accidental ingestion is managed by endotracheal intubation very similarly to bacterial epiglottiditis.[4] Any time corrective or palliative surgery can be performed to relieve obstruction, it is performed to avoid the tracheostomy.

Nasopharyngeal intubation is used to maintain the patency of the pharyngeal cavity in situations such as Pierre Robin syndrome and tumors of the buccal or pharyngeal cavity, and for the acute management of the severe form of sleep apnea syndrome until the work-up and surgery are completed.[5-6]

Continuous positive airway pressure or continuous distending pressure through a nasopharyngeal tube is applied in various circumstances: severe tracheomalacia, postextubation croup, recurrent postextubation lobar atelectasis, and diaphragmatic paralysis. The technique is usually well tolerated and successful in the neonate and the very young infant; it is poorly tolerated and unsatisfactory in the child.[7]

The labored breathing secondary to upper airway obstruction may favor gastroesophageal reflux, which may exacerbate the respiratory distress by several mechanisms and necessitate therapy.

BRONCHOSCOPY

Bronchoscopic techniques represent a major diagnostic and therapeutic advance. I still regularly use fluoroscopy with videotape recording to analyze the functional aspects in upper airway obstruction in various conditions: awake, crying, prone, supine. The rigid bronchoscope is used under general anesthesia and is the favored technique for diagnosis of lesions; it is the obligatory method to remove inhaled foreign bodies and the plug associated with the very rare neonatal necrotizing tracheobronchitis. Use of the flexible bronchoscope in the awake patient permits analysis of the motility of the laryngeal and tracheal

Current Topics in General Thoracic Surgery:
An International Series

structures. I use selective bronchial intubation with a protected suctioning catheter after local anesthesia of the larynx and under fluoroscopic control to remove tenacious secretions in small peripheral airways or for diagnostic sampling in pneumonia. This technique is well tolerated and successful.[8]

ARTIFICIAL VENTILATION

In premature newborns with idiopathic respiratory distress syndrome complicated by severe hypoxemia secondary to major interstitial emphysema, predominantly in one lung, I use selective intubation of a main bronchus and positive pressure ventilation of the less affected lung for 36 to 48 hours. This allows the more diseased lung to deflate and to function more effectively. This technique requires deep sedation and muscular relaxation.[9]

Jet ventilation has very limited indication in the pediatric patient. It is useful and lifesaving in the rare patient with tracheopleural fistula secondary to accidental or iatrogenic trauma, but it is limited to patients with almost normal lung parenchyma.[10]

Volume preset respirators are chosen for children who weigh more than 5 kg. In patients with adult type respiratory distress syndrome or with severe interstitial pneumonia, I select the pressure control mode and I/E ratio of 1 in an attempt to avoid high FiO_2 and high peak pressure. With this technique I achieve the same oxygenation and ventilation with a lower FiO_2 and lower peak pressure than is observed with the volume control mode. I have yet to demonstrate an increased survival rate or a reduced morbidity in these severely affected patients.[11]

REFERENCES

1. Standards and guidelines for cardiopulmonary resuscitation (CPR) and emergency cardiac care (ECC): Part V. Pediatric advanced life support. *JAMA* 1986;255:2961–2969.
2. Riggs CD, Lister G: Adverse occurrences in the pediatric intensive care unit. *Ped Clin North Am* 1987; 34:93–117.
3. Richardson MA, Cotton RT: Anatomic abnormalities of the pediatric airway. *Ped Clin North Am* 1984; 31:821–834.
4. Moulin D, Bertrand JM, Buts JP, Nyakabasa M, Otte JB: Upper airway lesions in children after accidental ingestion of caustic substances. *J Pediatr* 1985; 106:408–410.
5. Aubert-Tulkens G, Claus D, Moulin D: Upper airway obstruction during sleep in a child: A polygraphic study. *Acta Pediatr Belg* 1981;34:165–170.
6. Moulin D: Aspects of upper airway obstruction particular to the child. In: Vincent JL, ed. *Update in Intensive Care and Emergency Medicine*, vol. 1. New York, NY: Springer-Verlag, 1986:470–475.
7. Wiseman NE, Duncan PG, Cameron CB: Management of tracheobronchomalacia with continuous positive airway pressure. *J Pediatr Surg* 1985; 20:489–493.
8. Rode H, Millar AJW, Stunden RJ, Cywes S: Selective bronchial intubation for acute postoperative atelectasis in neonates and infants. *Pediatr Radiol* 1988;18:494–496.
9. Brooks JG, Bustamante SA, Koops BL, et al: Selective bronchial intubation for the treatment of severe localized pulmonary interstitial emphysema in newborn infants. *J Pediatr* 1977;91:648–652.
10. Pizov R, Shir Y, Eimerl D, et al: One-lung high frequency ventilation in the management of traumatic tear of bronchus in a child. *Critical Care Medicine* 1987;15:1160–1161.
11. Andersen JB: Inverse I:E ratio ventilation with pressure control in catastrophic lung disease in adults. *Intensive Care World* 1987;4:21–23.

Chapter 4

Extracorporeal Membrane Oxygenation in the Pediatric Thoracic Surgical Patient

Robert J. Attorri, MD and Robert H. Bartlett, MD

INTRODUCTION

Extracorporeal membrane oxygenation (ECMO) is a method of cardiopulmonary bypass using an artificial lung, a mechanical pump, and cannulation of the patient without thoracotomy. The acronym ECMO has gained popular use but implies that oxygenation is its primary function. In fact, cardiac and blood pressure support as well as carbon dioxide removal are equally important functions of the technique, which might be better described as *extracorporeal life support*. ECMO is usually performed on patients with severe cardiac or respiratory failure who are refractory to maximal conventional therapy. Rather than being a treatment, ECMO provides life support during which underlying disease may resolve. The indications for ECMO remain topics of debate, but the experience of the past 15 years has clearly demonstrated that prolonged extracorporeal perfusion of patients is possible and safe.[1–8]

The accomplishments in extracorporeal life support are the result of numerous advances over the past 70 years. Gibbon, the father of extracorporeal circulation, devoted his career to the development of a heart/lung machine, which was first used in the 1950s. This device was intended for cardiopulmonary support of only a few hours' duration.[9,10] More prolonged use of these early machines resulted in lethal changes in the blood. These changes were attributed to the oxygenator, which exposed blood directly to oxygen in order to saturate the hemoglobin. Subsequent investigators developed oxygenators that used a gas-

permeable membrane to effect gas exchange. Kolff noted the gas exchange properties in early dialysis machines, and Clowes developed the first membrane oxygenator in 1956.[11] One year later Kammermeyer described dimethylsiloxane (silicone rubber), a substance with considerably greater gas transfer characteristics than the polyethylene membrane used by Clowes.[12] During the next decade numerous silicone rubber membrane oxygenators were developed, including the Kolobow device, which was the predecessor of the membrane lung used today. Also vital to the development of extracorporeal circulation was McLean's discovery in 1916 of a substance extracted from the liver which was called *heparin*. This reversible anticoagulant allowed the development of artificial organs and prosthetic blood vessels that could be used with whole blood and not result in thrombosis.

INDICATIONS

Acute severe reversible cardiopulmonary failure constitutes the principal indication for ECMO. Within this broad category are numerous disease states encountered in the pediatric thoracic population. Table 4.1 lists some of the conditions that have been successfully treated with ECMO. For neonatal ECMO, specific entry criteria have been developed, the most commonly used being the oxygenation index, which has been shown to correlate with mortality risk.[1,5,13,14]

Neonatal respiratory failure results mainly from diseases that have as their common end point persistent fetal circulation (PFC).[15–18] PFC, also known as persistent pulmonary hyperten-

TABLE 4.1 Etiologies of Cardiopulmonary Failure Treated with ECMO

Congenital heart disease: preoperative and post-
  operative support
  Tetralogy of Fallot
  Transposition of the great arteries
  Idiopathic hypertrophic subaortic stenosis
  Ventricular septal defect
  Atrial septal defect
  Subaortic stenosis
  Ebstein's anomaly
Cardiomyopathy
Cardiac transplant rejection
Pneumonia: bacterial and viral
Bronchiolitis
Hydrocarbon aspiration
Foreign body aspiration
Desquamative interstitial pneumonitis
Near drowning
Goodpasture's syndrome
Posttraumatic ARDS

sion of the newborn (PPHN), may occur as a primary disease or may be secondary to other conditions. Conditions commonly associated with secondary PPHN include meconium aspiration syndrome, respiratory distress syndrome of the newborn (RDS), congenital diaphragmatic hernia (CDH), and neonatal sepsis. The greatest amount of experience and controlled clinical studies has taken place in this patient population. Our experience with clinical ECMO for neonates began in 1972. From 1972 until February 1982 we carried out Phase I trials in moribund infants. These trials to determine efficacy, safety, and morbidity resulted in a 54% survival rate.[19] These encouraging results were the motivation for our Phase II prospective randomized clinical trials, which took place from February 1982 to November 1984. ECMO was compared with conventional therapy in a group of newborns with 80% to 100% mortality risk. Our ECMO survival rate during this period was 90%, and the prospective randomized trial demonstrated statistically significant superiority over conventional therapy.[20] Since 1984 we have treated more than 100 infants, some of whom have been part of our Phase III controlled randomized study to examine efficacy, morbidity, and cost effectiveness in neonates with 50% mortality risk. This study is still under way, but overall survival in neonatal ECMO patients since 1984 exceeds 90%.

There are few clinical trials of ECMO in children and strict entry criteria have not yet evolved with these patients. Successful outcomes in children with other conditions listed in Table 4.1

have been reported.[21-25] Clinical analysis of ECMO in many of these conditions is difficult because of their relative infrequency, but our own experience as well as others' has demonstrated that very high risk children who are failing maximum therapy may be salvaged with ECMO.

Our approach to respiratory failure in the newborn and child has recently been altered by the work of Kolobow, Gattinoni, and others who have stressed that the purpose of mechanical ventilation is carbon dioxide (CO_2) removal rather than oxygenation.[26-30] This work has led us to reconsider venovenous ECMO which is an effective and safe means of CO_2 removal. Gattinoni has been carrying out a clinical trial of venovenous ECMO in adults and children with adult-type respiratory distress syndrome (ARDS), and we have begun clinical trials in adults, children, and neonates. Our early results with neonates is encouraging, and we believe it demonstrates the feasibility of venovenous ECMO.

Venoarterial (VA) bypass is the only mechanical means of cardiac support for children. With the advent of cardiac transplantation, the use of mechanical support for children with cardiac failure becomes even more important. Several groups have reported experience with preoperative and postoperative pediatric cardiac support.[8,21,31-33] Two major problems associated with pediatric cardiac ECMO support have been identified: bleeding and irreversible brain or heart damage. When a child is converted from operating room cardiopulmonary bypass directly to ECMO, bleeding continues at a very rapid rate. It is much more desirable to allow a few hours for restoration of hemostasis before reheparinizing the patient. Irreversible brain or cardiac injury may occur during a long period of cardiogenic shock prior to the use of ECMO. Groups using ECMO for pediatric cardiac support should therefore devise criteria that select high-risk patients but exclude patients who are not salvageable.

In infants long periods of left ventricular distension are well tolerated. However, in older children and adults even a few minutes of left ventricular asystole will result in myocardial injury, subendocardial hemorrhage and elevated left atrial pressure resulting in cardiogenic pulmonary edema. Consequently the left side of the heart must be decompressed when using VA bypass for children whenever the left ventricle does not empty properly. This can be accomplished with balloon atrial septostomy or by direct cannulation of the left atrium or ventricle. Kolobow and colleagues reported decompressing the left side retrograde via the pulmonary artery.[34]

Contraindications to ECMO in pediatric thoracic patients include irreversible end organ damage, mechanical ventilation of greater than 10 days' duration, persistently elevated pulmonary artery pressure, and evidence of irreversible lung disease (ie, extensive fibrosis on lung biopsy). Electroencephalographic evidence of brain death or severe intracranial hemorrhage precludes the potential of normal neurologic function and are also considered contraindications. Because of the prohibitive risk of intracranial hemorrhage, marked prematurity (less than 35 weeks gestational age) is another contraindication.[35] Active bleeding, large burns, and a prognosis of poor quality of life reduce the potential benefit of ECMO and are relative contraindications.

BYPASS TECHNIQUE

Following is a summary of the component techniques used at the University of Michigan.[36] Not all groups perform ECMO exactly the same way, and numerous modifications in the equipment and method of bypass have been made by other groups. The technique at our institution varies depending on the indication for ECMO. Cardiac support is obviously performed with venoarterial bypass, whereas pure respiratory failure is currently treated with venovenous ECMO.

Components

The ECMO circuit consists of several commercially available components that are adapted for ECMO use. Tracing the circuit from intravenous (drainage cannula to perfusion cannula), the first device encountered is a distensible venous reservoir (the bladder) which sits in a servoregulatory device called the *bladder box.* The bladder box sits about 100 cm below the level of the right atrium draining the venous system by siphon effect. The bladder box senses the volume in the bladder, shutting off the roller pump whenever venous return is inadequate to fill the bladder. This is to prevent suction of air into the circuit.

An occlusive roller pump propels blood through the extracorporeal circuit drawing blood from the bladder and perfusing it through the oxygenator and heat exchanger. We use a Kolobow/Sci Med membrane oxygenator with sufficient capacity to fully oxygenate the patient's total cardiac output. The lung size depends upon the total flow that must be obtained in order to achieve satisfactory gas exchange. Table 4.2 describes the common available lung sizes and their rated flows (that amount of venous blood that can be 95% saturated). Oxygen is fed into the gas phase and acts not only to saturate hemoglobin but to

TABLE 4.2 Membrane Lung Sizes and Gas Exchange Capacities

Membrane Lung Surface Area (m^2)	Rated Flow (L/M)	Gas Exchange cc/min
0.4	0.5	30
0.8	1.0	60
1.5	2.0	120
2.5	3.0	180
3.5	4.0	240
4.5	5.0	300

Rated flow = maximal flow of 75% saturated venous blood that can be fully saturated (100%) by lung. Gas exchange = O_2 volume exchange at AVO_2 difference of 6 vol% and RQ of 1.0. Potential CO_2 is higher.

maintain a gradient for CO_2 excretion. Membrane lungs are very efficient CO_2 excretors, and occasionally carbogen (95% O_2, 5% CO_2) is required to prevent hypocarbia. Water vapor is also transferred across the membrane. The final component in the circuit is the countercurrent heat exchanger through which the blood passes on its way to the arterial (perfusion) cannula.

Cannulation and Institution of Bypass

Cannulation is performed at the bedside with an operating room team present. The decision to perform venoarterial bypass or venovenous bypass is determined by the patient's underlying disease. Morphine and pancuronium are administered intravenously and local anesthesia is infiltrated. The patient is heparinized after the vessels for cannulation have been isolated.

Cannulation for venoarterial bypass is accomplished by placing a venous cannula to the right atrium via the right internal jugular vein through a small supraclavicular incision. The arterial cannula can be placed in one of three locations: the right carotid artery via the same supraclavicular incision used for the venous catheter, the right axillary artery, or the femoral artery. Considerable discussion has surrounded the use and subsequent ligation of the carotid artery, but we believe that this can be performed safely in most neonates and children. In older children performing the cannulation under local anesthesia and then testing for movement of the patient's left side allows immediate assessment of the collateral circulation to the brain. The carotid artery allows easy surgical access through a wound that will heal well and delivery of the most highly saturated blood to the carotid and coronary arteries. When using either the axillary or femoral arteries, distal perfusion of the involved limb requires the use of two-way cannulas.

Several methods of venovenous bypass are used.[37,38] Our current preference in newborns is through a single double-lumen catheter placed into the right atrium via the right internal jugular vein. For children with respiratory failure, drainage from the right atrium with perfusion into the femoral vein is most commonly used. Gattinoni and colleagues use bilateral femoral vein cannulas with one cannula passed high into the vena cava near the right atrium and the other returning blood to the lower part of the inferior vena cava.[28] Occasionally during venovenous bypass oxygenation is so poor that conversion to venoarterial bypass is required. When we have performed venovenous bypass, therefore, we also dissect out the corresponding arteries prior to heparinization so that the arteries may be accessed easily and with minimal bleeding if VA conversion is necessary.

Catheter size is determined by the patient's size, but in general the venous catheter must be large enough to deliver the full cardiac output and the arterial (or perfusion) catheter must be large enough to transfer the same flow with pressure in the perfusion line less than a 100 mm Hg above mean arterial pressure. Higher pressures increase the risk of system rupture and may result in hemolysis.

Once the cannulas are in place the ECMO circuit, which has been primed with red blood cells and balanced crystalloid solution, is wheeled to the bedside. Extracorporeal flow is initially increased up to the maximum amount that the venous cannula will deliver. The ventilator is then placed on "rest" settings of 30% FiO_2, inspiratory pressure of 20 to 30 cm H_2O, positive end-expiratory pressure (PEEP) of 0 to 10 cm H_2O, and a rate of 10 breaths per minute. Keszler et al advocated the use of high PEEP in the range of 15 cm H_2O. Their group has presented evidence that this prevents the total alveolar collapse usually seen after institution of bypass and shortens the overall course on ECMO without causing any new complications.[39] We have used these ventilator settings during both venoarterial and venovenous bypass and have achieved total CO_2 and O_2 transfer in neonates and children. In Gattinoni's technique of venovenous bypass, so-called apneic oxygenation is used. The ventilator is set with CPAP around 20 cm H_2O, and 4 breaths a minute with a peak inspiratory pressure of 35 cm H_2O are delivered. The FiO_2 is set to maintain arterial oxygenation at greater than 90%. The patient is usually kept sedated and, in certain cases, paralyzed to minimize oxygen consumption and

CO_2 production. A continuous infusion of heparin into the circuit is used to maintain activated clotting time between 200 and 240 seconds.

Flow

The extracorporeal flow necessary to achieve acceptable gas exchange is determined by either arterial blood gases or by the mixed venous oxygen saturation. In venoarterial bypass we place an Oximetrix catheter in the venous limb of the circuit, which gives a continuous reading of mixed venous oxygen saturation (% SvO_2). Once the patient is stabilized on bypass we adjust flow to maintain an SvO_2 of 70% to 75%. SvO_2 measures the ratio of O_2 delivery to O_2 consumption (normally 4:1, Vsat 71). SvO_2 less than 50% represents DO_2/VO_2 less than 2:1, which is inadequate perfusion in relation to metabolic requirement and results in anerobic metabolism and lactic acidosis.

For patients on venovenous bypass, CO_2 removal is the primary goal.[26–29] Extracorporeal CO_2 removal is limited by the surface area of the membrane lung. Because membrane lungs are efficient CO_2 excretors, all the CO_2 can be removed using relatively low blood flow (usually about $\frac{1}{3}$ of the cardiac output). At low flow some oxygen is provided but some blood oxygenation must take place through the native lung. If adequate oxygenation cannot be achieved through the native lung, then extracorporeal flow must be increased or the patient must be converted to venoarterial bypass. Venous saturation is artificially high during venovenous bypass, but is still a useful trend and safety monitor.

Extracorporeal oxygenation and carbon dioxide clearance are accomplished by the flow of oxygen ("sweep gas") through the membrane lung, usually 100% oxygen at 1–2 l/min. When a lung of proper size is used the perfusate blood is 100% saturated.

PATIENT MANAGEMENT DURING ECMO

The typical ECMO patient is initially fluid overloaded from aggressive resuscitation. Return to dry weight (or to birth weight in the case of neonates) while still providing necessary calories becomes the paramount goal of fluid management while on ECMO. Renal function usually improves soon after bypass beings and diuresis is stimulated in an attempt to return to dry weight within 24 to 48 hours. Fluid loss through the membrane lung aids in this process. If urine output is insufficient to affect this diuresis, a hemofiltration device can be easily added to the ECMO circuit.[40]

Total parenteral nutrition is begun as soon as the patient is stabilized on bypass.

Blood products are usually required during each ECMO run. Red blood cells are administered to maintain a hematocrit of 45 to 50 cc and the platelet count is maintained at a level of 80 000 or greater. Bleeding problems increase significantly after the seventh day of bypass and in longer ECMO runs. Bleeding from the chest tubes, cannula sites, and surgical wounds can become very copious.[41]

Surgery in the patient who is on bypass presents special problems. Situations in which this may arise include the newborn who requires ligation of a patent ductus arteriosus (PDA) in order to be weaned from bypass, the patient who requires ECMO prior to repair of congenital diaphragmatic hernia, the patient who is placed on ECMO and is later found to have a surgical cause of cardiopulmonary failure, and the patient who had an emergent condition requiring surgical correction. In each of these cases liberal use of electrocautery and meticulous hemostasis is mandatory. We have successfully ligated 20 PDAs on ECMO patients with minimal postoperative bleeding and no deaths. There are now reports of patients who have undergone successful repair of congenital diaphragmatic hernia while being supported on ECMO. The Neonatal ECMO Registry documents two patients placed on ECMO originally for presumed respiratory failure who were later found to have pulmonary arterial venous malformations. Both of these patients underwent successful lobectomy. The most common surgical problem of the patient on ECMO is abnormal bleeding.[42] Our initial approach in these patients is to increase the platelet count to at least 100 000 and to decrease the activated clotting time to 180 to 200 seconds. We believe it is important to explore immediately any patient who bleeds persistently from cannula sites, incisions, and chest tube sites. We have experience with one patient who underwent placement of a chest tube into the parenchyma of the lung who required thoracotomy for control of his bleeding.

Weaning and Decannulation

An ECMO run can last from two days to several weeks. A typical neonatal respiratory failure support lasts for an average of four days, and a patient with adult-type respiratory distress syndrome may require nearly a month of extracorporeal support. Extracorporeal flow is weaned throughout the course as indicated by blood gases. Once extracorporeal flow is reduced to a level of 10% to 20% of cardiac output the patient is ready for a trial off bypass. The cannulas are clamped and ventilator settings are increased to supportive but not harmful levels. The patient's vital signs are closely observed and arterial blood gases are checked every 5 to 10 minutes during the trial. The ventilator settings are then weaned as tolerated. Good blood gases (PO_2 greater than 100, PCO_2 less than 45 with an FiO_2 less than 60%) and a mean airway pressure less than 12 cm H_2O (or peak airway pressure less than 40 cm H_2O) indicate that decannulation can proceed.

Decannulation is performed at the bedside. In newborn patients the proximal carotid and internal jugular stumps are ligated. Repair of the artery is technically possible but we believe that the risk of thrombosis at the site of repair with subsequent embolization into this route of circulation exceeds the risk of ligation. The internal jugular vein is repaired only in cases of heart transplantation candidates who will later require central venous access for endocardial biopsy. Axillary and femoral vessels that are used for cannulation require repair. Following decannulation the patient is weaned from the ventilator and extubated in a conventional fashion. Occasionally there appears to be no hope of recovery and ECMO must be discontinued before flow has been satisfactorily weaned, as in the case of irreversible end organ failure.

RESULTS, COMPLICATIONS, AND FOLLOW-UP

Due largely to the neonatal ECMO registry, excellent data regarding neonatal population are now available. The registry recorded 2830 cases from over 57 centers as of August 1989, with a survival rate of 82%. Meconium aspiration was the most common diagnosis and also had the greatest survival rate, whereas congenital diaphragmatic hernia had the poorest outcome. Factors associated with significantly lower survival include PDA ligation during ECMO (46%), other surgery while on ECMO (59%), and cardiac arrest as the indication for ECMO (27%). Complications associated with the worst outcomes include intracranial hemorrhage (50%), gastrointestinal bleeding (61%), renal failure (60%) and thrombocytopenia requiring more than 5 units of platelets in 24 hours (51%).

Because neonatal ECMO patients are selected from a population with a very high mortality risk there is no readily available control group with which to compare follow-up data. There are reports on neonates with severe respiratory failure treated with mechanical ventilation and tolazaline.[43] In one of these reports,

77% of three-year survivors were normal, the remaining sustaining some developmental or neurologic impairment. Several of the more experienced ECMO centers have published their initial follow-up studies, and all of these have reported that the majority of their ECMO patients are normal at one year of age.[1,44–48] Bartlett et al[1] reported on their first 72 survivors. In a follow-up period ranging from 3 months to 11 years 63% were considered normal. Seventeen percent had significant developmental delay and 8% had significant pulmonary problems. Krummel and colleagues[46] identified one patient among their first six survivors with significant neurologic deficit one year following treatment with ECMO. Glass et al[45] reported a series of 42 ECMO patients evaluated at one year of age showing that 10% had significant developmental or neurologic abnormality. Andrews et al[44] reported one- to three-year follow-up of 14 patients in which 50% were considered completely or near normal and 71% were mentally normal. Towne et al[48] evaluated 16 children between the ages of 4 and 11 years who were treated as newborns with ECMO. Of these children, 13 (79%) were normal or near normal with expected mental and physical capacity. These results are all comparable to those reported for conventionally treated patients who did not require ECMO, suggesting that pre-ECMO events are at least partly responsible for suboptimal outcomes. Current experience indicates that newborns with high mortality risk can be effectively and safely treated with ECMO and that the majority of children who survive have normal or near-normal growth and development.

The treatment of patients with congenital diaphragmatic hernia has yielded very encouraging results.[49–53] Between January 1981 and January 1988 the Pediatric Surgery Service at the University of Michigan treated 39 patients with congenital diaphragmatic hernia, 31 of whom are now long-term survivors (79%). Twenty-four of these patients were treated with surgery and mechanical ventilation; 18 (75%) survived and 6 died. All 6 who died had specific contraindications to ECMO: two were less than 35 weeks gestational age, two had no honeymoon period, and two had severe congenital anomalies incompatible with prolonged survival. Fifteen patients were unresponsive to conventional therapy and were placed on ECMO postoperatively. Thirteen of these survived (87%). One patient died 1½ years postoperatively from sepsis and respiratory failure, and the other died shortly after repair of tetralogy of Fallot while still on ECMO.

The most common complications during ECMO are physiologic, including seizures, hemorrhage, hypertension, pneumothorax, and renal insufficiency. Approximately two-thirds of the patients in the ECMO registry have experienced at least one physiologic complication, with the majority of these patients (75%) surviving. Technical complications are less common, occurring in 23% of the patients in the registry.[41] Less common complications occur as a consequence of anticoagulation. The most ominous of these is intracranial hemorrhage, which occurs predominantly in children who are less than 35 weeks gestational age. Other bleeding complications include cardiac tamponade and gastrointestinal, retroperitoneal, and intrathoracic bleeding secondary to surgery and thoracostomy. In our experience, about 12% of patients have bleeding complications.

Data concerning older children on ECMO for cardiac support are more scattered, though efforts to establish a pediatric ECMO registry are currently under way. We have treated 33 children with cardiac and respiratory failure, all of whom were judged by their physicians to have virtually no possibility of survival with conventional treatment.[21] We have had a total of 14 survivors in this group. Outcome by diagnostic group is depicted in Table 4.3. In this experience, complications occurred in nearly every case. Bleeding was a ubiquitous problem and, if measured in terms of blood and platelet transfusion, worsens after the sixth day of bypass. Renal failure was common, occurring in nearly one-third of these patients, and no patient who developed ATN while on bypass survived. We had nearly 20 membrane lung changes and 3 raceway ruptures. Neurologic complications in this group included two

TABLE 4.3 Diagnosis and Outcome of Children Treated with ECMO

	Patients	Survivors
Congential heart disease	10	2
Postoperative support	9	2
Preoperative support	1	0
Infectious pneumonia	6	1
Heart transplant rejection	3	2
Cardiomyopathy	3	0
Bronchiolitis	2	2
Posttraumatic ARDS	2	0
Near drowning	2	1
Desquamative interstitial pneumonitis	1	1
Goodpasture's syndrome	1	1
Foreign body aspiration	1	1
Turpentine aspiration	1	1
Malignant histiocytosis	1	0
	33	14

episodes of intracranial hemorrhage, two cases of left-sided weakness and paresthesia, and four patients who experienced seizures.

Several other groups have reported their experiences with similar conclusions: ECMO can be safely and effectively used to treat reversible cardiopulmonary failure in children.[21,25,32,33] Survival and reversibility are improved by starting ECMO early in the course of the disease before barotrauma, acidosis, shock, cardiac arrest, and multiple organ failure occur.

CLINICAL UPDATE AND FUTURE AREAS OF INVESTIGATION

Development of a heparin-coated system, which would avoid systemic anticoagulation, will mark the next milestone in extracorporeal circulation. The use of heparin-coated systems should significantly lessen bleeding complications and will allow expansion of research in clinical practice (eg, pulmonary support in premature infants).

Studies in our laboratory and intensive care unit have demonstrated the feasibility and efficacy of venovenous bypass, and this can be performed with existing ECMO equipment without special modifications. Because of recirculation, higher flows are required with venovenous bypass to achieve full oxygenation support, but with the emphasis on CO_2 removal, venovenous access through a single catheter will probably be the direction of the future for most infants, children, and adults with respiratory failure.

The development of safe autoservoregulating pumping systems is the first important step in making the ECMO simple enough that it does not require continuous technician attendance. When such pumping systems are routinely available, and when it is no longer necessary to give heparin or measure activated clotting time, it is reasonable to expect that a single bedside nurse with appropriate training will be able to care for the patient and the ECMO machine, similar to the method in which nurses now care for patients on mechanical ventilators or hemofiltration.

REFERENCES

1. Bartlett RH, Gazzaniga AB, Toomasian JM, et al: Extracorporeal membrane oxygenation (ECMO) in neonatal respiratory failure: 100 cases. *Ann Surg* 1986;204:236–245.
2. Kirkpatrick BV, Krummel TM, Mueller DG, et al: Use of extracorporeal membrane oxygenation for respiratory failure in term infants. *Pediatrics* 1983; 72:872–876.
3. Krummel TM, Greenfield LJ, Kirkpatrick BV, et al: Extracorporeal membrane oxygenation in neonatal pulmonary failure. *Pediatr Annals* 1982;11:905–908.
4. Krummel TM, Greenfield LJ, Kirkpatrick BV, et al: Clinical use of an extracorporeal membrane oxygenator in neonatal pulmonary failure. *J Pediatr Surg* 1982;17:528–531.
5. Krummel TM, Greenfield LJ, Kirkpatrick BV, et al: Alveolar-arterial oxygen gradients versus the neonatal pulmonary insufficiency index for prediction of mortality in ECMO candidates. *J Pediatr Surg* 1984;19:380–384.
6. Loe WA, Graves ED, Ochsner JL, et al: Extracorporeal membrane oxygenation for newborn respiratory failure. *J Pediatr Surg* 1985;20:684–688.
7. Short BL, Pearson GD: Neonatal extracorporeal membrane oxygenation: A review. *J Int Care Med* 1986;1:47–54.
8. Trento A, Griffith BP, Hardesty RL: Extracorporeal membrane oxygenation experience at the University of Pittsburgh. *Ann Thorac Surg* 1986;42:56–59.
9. Gibbon JH Jr: Artificial maintenance circulation during experimental occlusion of pulmonary artery. *Arch Surg* 1937;34:1105.
10. Lee WH, Krumhaar D, Fonkalsrud EW, et al: Denaturation of plasma proteins as a cause of morbidity and death after intracardiac operations. *Surgery* 1961;50:29.
11. Bartlett RH, Gazzaniga AB: Extracorporeal circulation for cardiopulmonary failure. In: *Current Problems in Surgery*. Chicago, Ill.: Year Book Medical Publishers, 1978.
12. Kammermeyer K: Silicone rubber as a selective barrier. *Ind Eng Chem* 1957;49:1685.
13. Bartlett RH, Drinker PA, Hill JD, et al: Indications for extracorporeal membrane oxygenation support: Quantitating pulmonary insufficiency (Presented at the First International Conference on Membrane Lung Technology, Copenhagen). In: Zapol and Quist, eds. *Artificial Lungs for Acute Respiratory Failure*. San Diego, Calif: Academic Press, 1976.
14. Beck R, Anderson KD, Pearson GD, et al: Criteria for extracorporeal membrane oxygenation in a population of infants with persistent pulmonary hypertension of the newborn. *J Pediatr Surg* 1986;21:297–301.
15. Cornish JD, Gerstmann DR, Clark RH, et al: Extracorporeal membrane oxygenation and high-frequency oscillatory ventilation: Potential therapeutic relationships. *Crit Care Med* 1987;15:831–840.
16. Fox WW, Duara S: Clinical management of persistent pulmonary hypertension of the newborn. *J Pediatr* 1983;103:505–511.
17. Lyrene RK, Phillips JB: Control of pulmonary vascular resistance in the fetus and newborn. *Clin Perinat* 1984;11:581–584.
18. Wung JT, James LS, Kilchevsky E, et al: Management of infants with severe respiratory failure and persistence of the fetal circulation without hyperventilation. *Pediatrics* 1985;76:488–494.
19. Bartlett RH, Andrews AF, Toomasian JM, et al: Extracorporeal membrane oxygenation for newborn respiratory failure: Forty-five cases. *Surgery* 1982; 92:425–433.
20. Bartlett RH, Roloff DW, Cornell RG, et al: Extracorporeal circulation in neonatal respiratory failure: A prospective randomized study. *Pediatrics* 1985; 76:479–487.
21. Anderson HL, Attorri RJ, Custer JR, et al: Extracorporeal membrane oxygenation for pediatric cardio-

pulmonary failure. *J Thorac Cardiovasc Surg* (in press).

22. Hanson EL, Drinker PA, Don HF, et al: Venoarterial bypass with a membrane oxygenator: Successful respiratory support in a woman following pulmonary hemorrhage secondary to renal failure. *Surgery* 1974;75:557–565.

23. Hicks RE, Kenney TR, Raphaely RC, et al: Successful treatment of varicella pneumonia with prolonged extracorporeal membrane oxygenation in a child with leukemia. *J Thorac Cardiovasc Surg* 1977; 73:297–301.

24. Kanter KR, Pennington DG, McBride LR, et al: Mechanical circulatory assistance after heart transplantation. *J Heart Transplant* 1987;6:150–154.

25. Klein MD, Arensman RM, Weber TR, et al: Pediatric ECMO: Directions for new developments. *Trans ASAIO* 1988;34:978–985.

26. Gattinoni L, Kolobow T, Agostoni A, et al: Clinical application of low frequency positive pressure ventilation with extracorporeal CO_2 removal (LFPPV-$ECCO_2R$) in treatment of adult respiratory distress syndrome (ARDS). *Int J Artif Organs* 1979;2:282–283.

27. Gattinoni L, Kolobow T, Damia G, et al: Extracorporeal carbon dioxide removal ($ECCO_2R$): A new form of respiratory assistance. *Int J Artif Organs* 1979;2:183–185.

28. Gattinoni L, Pesenti A, Mascheroni D, et al: Low-frequency positive-pressure ventilation with extracorporeal CO_2 removal in severe acute respiratory failure. *JAMA* 1986;256:881–886.

29. Gattinoni L, Pesenti A, Pelizzola A, et al: Reversal of terminal acute respiratory failure by low frequency positive pressure ventilation with extracorporeal removal of CO_2 (LFPPV-$ECCO_2R$). *Trans ASAIO* 1981;27:289–293.

30. Snider MT, Campbell DB, Kolke WA, et al: Venovenous perfusion of adults and children with severe acute respiratory distress syndrome. *Trans ASAIO* 1988;34:1014–1020.

31. Pennington DG, Codd JE, Merjavy JP, et al: The expanded use of ventricular bypass system for severe cardiac failure and as a bridge to cardiac transplantation. *Heart Transplant* 1984;3:170–175.

32. Pennington GD, Merjavy JP, Codd JE, et al: Extracorporeal membrane oxygenation for patients with cardiogenic shock. *Circulation* (suppl) 1984;I:130–137.

33. Redmond CR, Graves ED, Falterman KW, et al: Extracorporeal membrane oxygenation for respiratory and cardiac failure in infants and children. *J Thorac Cardiovasc Surg* 1987;93:199–204.

34. Kolobow T, Rossi F, Borelli M, et al: Long-term closed chest partial and total cardiopulmonary bypass by peripheral cannulation for severe right and/or left ventricular failure, including ventricular fibrillation. *Trans ASAIO* 1988;34:485–489.

35. Cilley RE, Zwischenberger JB, Andrews AF, et al: Intracranial hemorrhage during extracorporeal membrane oxygenation in neonates. *Pediatrics* 1986;78:699–704.

36. Bartlett RH: Extracorporeal membrane oxygenation. In: *Technical Specialist Manual.* Ann Arbor, Mi.: University of Michigan Department of Surgery, 1987.

37. Andrews AF, Klein MD, Toomasian JM, et al: Venovenous extracorporeal membrane oxygenation in neonates with respiratory failure. *J Pediatr Surg* 1983;18:339–346.

38. Klein MD, Andrews AF, Wesley JR, et al: Venovenous perfusion in ECMO for newborn respiratory insufficiency: A clinical comparison with venoarterial perfusion. *Ann Surg* 1985;201:520–526.

39. Keszler M, Subramanian KNC, Smith WA, et al: Pulmonary management during ECMO. *Crit Care Med* 1989;17:495–500.

40. Heiss KF, Pettit B, Hirschl RB: Renal insufficiency and volume overload in neonatal ECMO managed by continuous ultrafiltration. *Trans ASAIO* 1987; 33:557–560.

41. Toomasian JM, Snedecor SM, Cornell RG, et al: National experience with extracorporeal membrane oxygenation for newborn respiratory failure: Data from 715 cases. *Trans ASAIO* 1988;34:140–147.

42. Anderson HL, Cilley RE, Zwischenberger JB, et al: Thrombocytopenia in neonates after extracorporeal membrane oxygenation. *Trans ASAIO* 1986; 32:534–537.

43. Cohen RS, Stevenson DK, Malachowski N, et al: Late morbidity among survivors of respiratory failure treated with tolazoline. *J Pediatr* 1980;97:644.

44. Andrews AF, Nixon CA, Roloff DW, et al: One-to-three year outcome of fourteen neonatal ECMO survivors. *Pediatrics* 1986;78:692–698.

45. Glass P, Miller M, Short B: Morbidity for survivors of ECMO: Neurodevelopmental outcome at one year of age. *Pediatrics* 1989;83:72–78.

46. Krummel TM, Greenfield LJ, Kirkpatrick BV, et al: The early evaluation of survivors after extracorporeal membrane oxygenation for neonatal pulmonary failure. *J Pediatr Surg* 1984;19:585–590.

47. Schumacher RE, Barks JDE, Johnston MV, et al: Right-sided brain lesions in infants following unilateral carotid ligation for extracorporeal membrane oxygenation. *Pediatrics* 1988;82:155–161.

48. Towne BH, Lott IT, Hicks DA, et al: Long-term follow-up of infants and children treated with extracorporeal membrane oxygenation (ECMO): A preliminary report. *J Pediatr Surg* 1985;20:410–414.

49. Hardesty RL, Griffith BP, Debski RF, et al: Extracorporeal membrane oxygenation: Successful treatment of persistent fetal circulation following repair of congenital diaphragmatic hernia. *J Thorac Cardiovasc Surg* 1981;81:556–563.

50. Heiss K, Manning PB, Oldham KP, et al: Reversal of mortality rate for CDH with ECMO. *Ann Surg* 1989; 209:225–230.

51. Langham MR, Krummel TM, Greenfield LJ, et al: Extracorporeal membrane oxygenation following repair of congenital diaphragmatic hernias. *Ann Thorac Surg* 1987;44:247–252.

52. Stolar CJ, Dillon PW, Stalcup SA: Extracorporeal membrane oxygenation and congenital diaphragmatic hernia: Modification of the pulmonary vasoactive profile. *J Pediatr Surg* 1985;20:681–683.

53. Weber TR, Connors RH, Pennington DG: Neonatal diaphragmatic hernia: An improving outlook with extracorporeal membrane oxygenation. *Arch Surg* 1987;122:615–618.

DISCUSSION

Extracorporeal Membrane Oxygenation in the Pediatric Thoracic Surgical Patient

Yves Durandy, MD and Jean-Yves Chevalier, MD

In the 1970s prolonged extracorporeal lung support was probably a dream for some medical doctors, but it was surely a nightmare for those who dared do it. At that time, however, Bartlett, the pioneer of pediatric membrane lung support, developed a new technique—ECMO. When applied to moribund patients, the ECMO rate of success was progressively raised to 50%. In the early 1980s the acronym ECMO became popular, but its wide clinical application began later, in the late 1980s. The use of this sophisticated treatment then increased exponentially (more than 3000 patients have been treated) and the overall success rate exceeded 80%. ECMO is now a conventional therapy. The main facts that have been demonstrated during this 20-year period follow:

It is possible to treat hypoxia unresponsive to ventilation with a membrane lung—that is, maximal mechanical conventional ventilation is ineffective in preventing lethal hypoxia when intrapulmonary and/or intracardiac shunts are large enough. In these cases the answer is ECMO.

It is possible to bypass the natural lungs for days or weeks; cardiopulmonary bypass does not invariably induce lethal complications such as metabolic disturbances, infection, or hemorrhage.

An ECMO circuit runs safely with the activated clotting times (ACTs) lower than those used for cardiac surgery. Hence risk from hemorrhage can be reduced.

A venous cannula inserted via the jugular vein into the right atrium can divert about 80% of the total cardiac output.

In neonates the ligation of the carotid results in an acceptable neurological risk.

ECMO therapy is routinely manageable in a pediatric intensive care unit.

When predicted mortality is 80% with maximal conventional therapy, ECMO outcome is more than 80% survival.

Nonetheless, and despite these amazing results, therapeutic improvements must always be considered. Attorri and Bartlett list in their review three main areas of investigation: (1) A heparin-coated system is proposed which will decrease the need for systemic heparinization. This step reduces bleeding and allows clinical trials of membrane lung support in premature infants. (2) Neonatal venovenous bypass should prevent systemic embolization, the need for carotid artery ligation, and their potential neurological side effects. Furthermore, in older children it may be a logical alternative to arterial cannulation. (3) Simpler bypass circuits should be managable by a single trained nurse and should cut the cost of ECMO therapy.

We agree with all these remarks, and while waiting for a "magic drug" that will treat pulmonary hypertension and parenchymal lung disease, we have developed an original device directed to answering most of the abovementioned concerns: *assistance respiratoire extracorporelle* (AREC).[1] To a great extent the development of AREC was inspired by the work of Gattinoni and colleagues.[2]

The AREC technique dissociates oxygenation from CO_2 removal. Oxygenation mainly depends on apneic oxygenation through the motionless natural lungs. Oxygen is infused (1 l/min/ m^2) through a catheter introduced in the tracheal tube. The lungs are inflated with continuous positive pressure (8 to 14 cm H_2O) to prevent alveolar collapse and are ventilated 4 to 6 times

Current Topics in General Thoracic Surgery:
An International Series

per minute with a limited peak pressure (35 cm H_2O) to increase alveolar recruitment. Because there is no CO_2 elimination during apnea, an extracorporeal lung circuit is added to extract CO_2. For this purpose we have described a single-lumen cannula and tidal flow venovenous circuit (Fig. D4.1). This circuit consists of a 7 to 12 French single-lumen catheter (Jostra Inc., Hechigen, Germany), a pressure-time controlled alternative clamp (Gamgro Inc., Colombes, France), a nonocclusive roller pump (Collin Cardio Inc., Arceuil, France), a membrane lung (Sci-Med Life Systems Inc., Minneapolis, Minnesota), a heat exchanger (Jostra Inc., Hechingen, Germany), a circulating liquid heater (Granulab Inc., Illfurth, France), and a Doppler (Medicorp Inc., Nancy, France). This circuit is very simple because the tidal flow is generated by alternative clamping without interposition of a venous bladder and with a pump running at a constant rotor speed. The silicon tubing of the rotor is collapsible and acts as a venous bladder. The blood is pooled in this tubing during the drainage phase and reinjected during the infusion phase (Fig. D4.2). To minimize recirculation, the total cycle time is 6 seconds and the ratio of drainage to infusion time is 2:1. The perfusion circuit is primed with fresh citrated blood with added heparin (1 unit/ml) and $CaCl_2$ (1 g/l). When the patient's spontaneous activated clotting time (ACT) is above 150 seconds prior to cannulation, heparin injection is delayed; otherwise a 25 unit/kg bolus of heparin is given as the priming dose. During perfusion we maintain a continuous infusion of heparin to obtain an ACT between 150 and 180 seconds.

The aims of AREC are:

1. To obtain lung rest through apneic oxygenation and low-frequency positive-pressure ventilation.

2. To avoid the neurological risk of systemic embolization and carotid ligation.[3,4]

3. To achieve CO_2 removal through a simple extracorporeal membrane lung circuit with a low extracorporeal blood flow (total CO_2 removal is possible with a flow of 30% of the total cardiac output).

4. To decrease systemic heparinization. We believe this simple circuit with no stasis area is a factor in lowering the coagulation risk and the need for heparin.

5. To maintain a normal pulmonary blood flow (pulmonary devascularization has been considered as a negative factor for the recovery of the natural lung).

6. To inject oxygenated blood directly into the pulmonary artery, oxygen being probably the best selective pulmonary vasodilator.

7. To obtain a simple bypass circuit manageable in any medical pediatric intensive care unit with only one trained nurse for each patient.

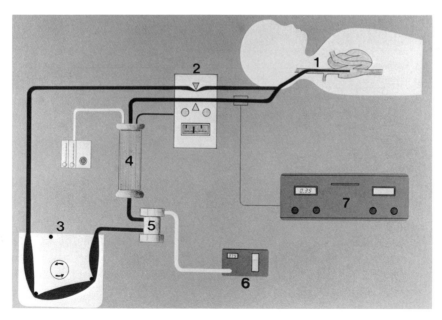

FIGURE D4.1 Perfusion circuit. **1.** Single-lumen cannula. **2.** Alternative clamp. **3.** Nonocclusive roller pump. **4.** Membrane lung. **5.** Heat exchanger. **6.** Liquid heater. **7.** Doppler.

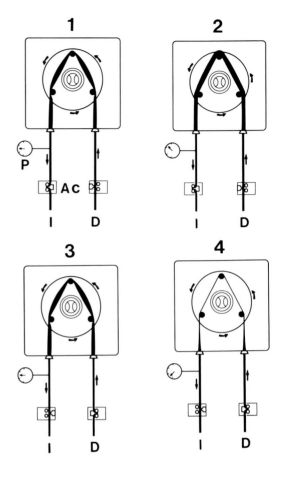

FIGURE D4.2 One cycle of the alternative clamp. D = drainage line; I = infusion line; AC = alternative clamp; P = pressure transducer of the alternative clamp. **1.** Drainage line = open, infusion line = closed. Blood is pooled in the tubing of the pump. Pressure increases downstream from the pump. **2.** Drainage line = open, infusion line = closed. Outflow of the pump is zero. Alternative clamp is activated. **3.** Drainage line = closed, infusion line = open. Blood is infused. Pressure decreases downstream from the pump. **4.** Drainage line = closed, infusion line = open. Outflow of the pump is zero, alternative clamp is activated.

TABLE D4.1 Patients Treated with AREC

Group	Gestational Age	Age	Weight (kg)	PaO_2 (mm Hg)	$AaDO_2$ (mm Hg)	Diagnosis
Neonates (n = 33)	38 ± 1.9 wk (35–41)	37.4 ± 27 hr	3.11 ± 0.68 (2.00–5.65)	42.3 ± 14.5 (20–63)	637 ± 16 (599–667)	MAS (9) PFC (7) Sepsis (8) RDS (7) CDH (1)
Infants and children (n = 18)		1 mo to 14 yr	16.7 ± 8.3 (1.8[a]–30)	64 ± 19 (44–80)		AIDS (4) Severe hypoxia post lung transplant (2) SCID (1) Postop. RDS (3) RDS sepsis (8)
Immunocompromised children (n = 8)		12 mo to 10 yr	16.7 ± 8.3	64 ± 19		Interstitial pneumonias patients with malignant hemopathies and bone marrow graft (8)

[a] The patient weighing 1.8 kg was a premature infant whose birth weight was 0.9 kg.

AIDS = acquired immunodeficiency syndrome; CDH = congential diaphragmatic hernia; MAS = meconium aspiration syndrome; PFC = persistent pulmonary hypertension of the newborn; RDS = respiratory distress syndrome; SCID = severe combined immunodeficiency.

We have already treated 59 patients divided into three groups (Table D4.1): 33 neonates, 18 infants and children, and 8 immunocompromised children with bone marrow grafts and interstitial pneumonias, most often of unprecise etiology. Although initially we treated moribund patients, our AREC inclusion criteria have become similar to those followed in centers with an ECMO program. Currently 50% of the patients are referred from other pediatric ICUs specifically for AREC.

Two patients, or even three in some instances, have been treated at the same time in our unit with a single bedside nurse for each; 28 neonates (85%) and 12 infants and children (67%) were successfully treated, but there was no success in the group of immunocompromised patients. Mean total duration of AREC was 101.5 ± 64 hours for neonates, 194 ± 143 hours for infants and children, and 256 ± 220 hours for immunocompromised patients. The mean duration of mechanical ventilation after discontinuation of AREC was 7.8 ± 6 days for neonates and 7.2 ± 5.8 days for older children. In neonates, the 12-month follow-up of 10 survivors suggests normal growth and development, and neurological examination failed to reveal any deficit.

We have noticed that the PaO_2 increases immediately and sustainably after initiation of AREC. We maintain an arterial PaO_2 between 70 and 100 mm Hg by lowering FiO_2, first on the ventilator, then on the tracheal catheter, and at last on the membrane. In most patients better oxygenation is associated with improvement of the chest roentgenogram: "white lungs" are well aerated 12 to 24 hours after initiation of AREC. CO_2 elimination is always adequate. The $PaCO_2$ is maintained around 30 to 35 mm Hg, and we have never had to add CO_2 to the membrane gas.

The most common complications during AREC are weight gain and renal insufficiency. When necessary, we have treated these complications very successfully with continuous hemodialysis. Because we have progressively decreased systemic heparinization, local bleeding at the cannulation site is rare and we have never experienced any other consequence of anticoagulation.

CONCLUSION

AREC has been successful in the treatment of pediatric respiratory insufficiency resistant to conventional management (except for immunocompromised patients with bone marrow graft and interstitial pneumonias, most often of unknown etiology).

The survival rates of this series—85% for neonates and 67% for older infants and children—are equivalent to the survival rate obtained with ECMO therapy.[5] These encouraging results prompt us to carry on with this technique. Our final hope is to prove that it will compare favorably, at least for most patients, with venoarterial ECMO.

REFERENCES

1. Durandy Y, Chevalier JY, Lecompte Y: Single cannula venovenous bypass circuit for respiratory membrane lung support. *J Thorac Cardiovasc Surg* 1990;99:404–409.
2. Gattinoni L, Pesenti A, Rossi JP, et al: Treatment of acute respiratory failure with low-frequency positive-pressure ventilation and extracorporeal removal of CO_2. *Lancet* 1980;II:292–294.
3. Hammerman C, Yousefzadeh D, Choi JH, Bui KC: Persistent pulmonary hypertension of the newborn. *Clin Perinat* 1989;16:137–155.
4. Babcock D, Han BK, Weiss RG, Ryckman FC: Brain abnormalities in infants on extracorporeal membrane oxygenation: Sonographic and CT findings. *AJR* 1989;153:571–576.
5. Moront H, Katz N, Keszler M: Extracorporeal membrane oxygenation for neonatal respiratory failure: A report of 50 cases. *J Thorac Cardiovasc Surg* 1989;97:706–714.

PART II

Bronchopulmonary and Foregut Malformations

Chapter 5

Intrathoracic Malformations of Foregut Derivatives

Stephen W. Gray, PhD and
John E. Skandalakis, MD, PhD, FACS

INTRODUCTION

The development of an embryo from a single fertilized ovum into a complex organism capable of leading an independent existence is one of the great mysteries of life. We are able to describe, but not always explain, the changes taking place before our eyes.

Certain conventions in terminology should be noticed. Reference to organs such as the thyroid gland or the lungs is to a group of cells which will become the thyroid gland or the lungs. To be strictly correct, we should use the expression "presumptive thyroid gland," for it is not yet a functioning organ. Even this has its caveats; most of those "organs" are represented by their epithelium, in the case of the foregut by endoderm. We know that in many cases it is the mesenchyme underlying the epithelium that controls local development. Nevertheless, the changes we can see are largely epithelial in expression.

Broadly, embryonic development starts with cell movements, foldings, rotations, separations, migrations, and splitting. Once the organ is roughly in place, differentiation of specific cells and tissues begins. The final step is the appearance of function, achieved in many organs only at or soon after birth.

In some of the following tables we have used nonscientific terms for the frequency of particular malformations: *common, uncommon, rare,* and *very rare.* These terms are relative to the total number of malformations that occur, not to the total number of live births.

© 1991 Elsevier Science Publishing Co., Inc.
655 Avenue of the Americas, New York, NY 10010
Current Topics in General Thoracic Surgery:
An International Series

BOUNDARIES OF THE FOREGUT

The embryonic foregut is the result of overgrowth of the cranial end of the embryo, the head fold. The cranial limit is the buccopharyngeal membrane (oral membrane), the posterior edge of Rathke's pouch, and the cranial end of the notochord (Fig. 5.1). The membrane ruptures early in embryonic life, leaving no visible boundary between oral ectoderm and pharyngeal endoderm.

The caudal end of the foregut is the point at which the liver diverticulum arises. In practice, the end is taken to be at a line through the axis of the loop of the future duodenum.

From the foregut thus defined arise a number of organs: pharynx and derivatives, esophagus, trachea, lungs, and stomach. In this presentation only thoracic anomalies will be discussed.

DEVELOPMENT OF THE ESOPHAGUS, TRACHEA, AND LUNGS

The cranial end of the esophagus and trachea is demarcated with the appearance of a median, ventral diverticulum of the foregut about 22 or 23 days after fertilization. Shortly after this, the spindle-shaped enlargement of the stomach appears immediately caudal to it. The esophagus will develop from the small area between the tracheal diverticulum and the stomach dilatation (Fig. 5.2).

The tracheal diverticulum rapidly becomes a groove in the floor of the esophagus, and elongation of both structures begins. Ridges of cells appear on the lateral walls, and beginning at the posterior end of the tracheal groove, the union of these ridges divides the foregut into tracheal

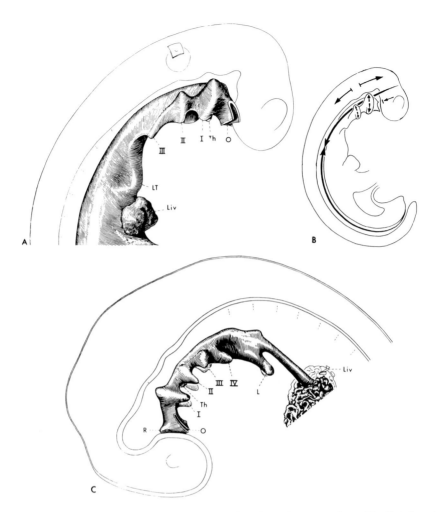

FIGURE 5.1 Development of the pharynx. **A.** The foregut of a 2.5 mm human embryo. The first three branchial pouches are present (I, II, III). The thyroid diverticulum (th), oral membrane (o), laryngotracheal groove (LT), and liver (Liv) are indicated. **B.** Chief directions of growth. **C.** The foregut of a 4.2 mm human embryo. Four pouches are present (I, II, III, IV). Rathke's pouch (R), thyroid gland (Th), and lung buds (L) have appeared. *Reproduced from Blechschmidt E: The stages of human development before birth. Philadelphia, PA: WB Saunders, 1961, with permission.*

(ventral) and esophageal (dorsal) channels (Fig. 5.3). At the distal end of the tracheal primordium, the lung buds are visible. Although separation proceeds toward the head, simultaneous elongation of both trachea and esophagus prevents the completion of the process before 34 to 36 days of age. The elongation involves the first lower portion of the esophagus, and later the upper portion. At the level of the tracheal bifurcation the esophageal diameter is reduced so that it actually is smaller than it was at an earlier stage. It is here that most esophageal atresias will occur.

Elongation of the esophagus appears to carry the stomach primordium down 16 segments to a position below the diaphragm. Descent is actually accomplished by growth of the body craniad, away from the transverse septum and pericardium. Elongation results from "ascent" of the pharynx, rather than "descent" of the stomach (Fig. 5.4).

ANOMALIES OF THE ESOPHAGUS, TRACHEA, AND LUNGS

Tracheoesophageal Fistulae, Esophageal Stenoses, and Atresias

The separation of the trachea from the esophagus in the fourth week is a major developmental ma-

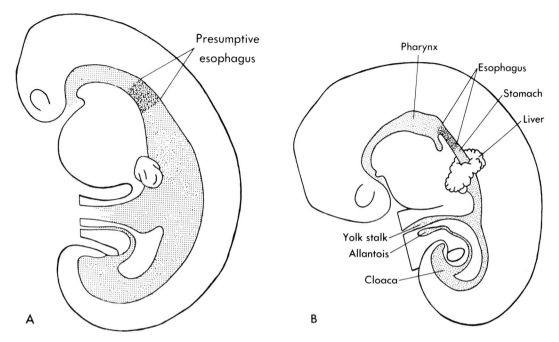

FIGURE 5.2 Elongation of the esophagus by cranial growth of the embryo at **A.** 2.5 mm and **B.** 4.2 mm. The pharynx occupies the greater part of the foregut. *Reproduced from Gray,[6] with permission.*

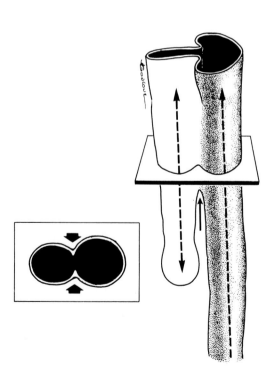

FIGURE 5.3 Morphogenetic movements involved in the division of the foregut into trachea and esophagus. *Reproduced from Gray,[6] with permission.*

neuver that provides a number of opportunities for malformations to occur[1] (Tables 5.1 and 5.2).

There are three simultaneous but independent processes occurring: (1) appearance of separate organ-forming fields, probably from mesoderm on opposite sides of the foregut, which will control differentiation of the endoderm into anterior tracheal mucosa and posterior esophageal mucosa; (2) appearance of the lateral ridges, which project into the foregut lumen to physically separate the tracheal and esophageal tubes; and (3) elongation of both primordia (Fig. 5.5).

Should the balance between the organ-forming fields be upset, the division of endoderm will become inequitable. In such cases, it is usually the tracheal field that dominates the esophageal field.[2] Esophageal atresia, complete (Fig. 5.6A) or segmental (Fig. 5.6 B, C), results when a disproportionate amount of endoderm becomes organized into the trachea, leaving too little from which to form an esophagus. Apparently, it is more difficult to preserve an esophagus than to form a trachea.

The minimal defects are of two varieties:

(1) *Arrest of cranial growth of the septum.* The septum between the trachea and esophagus grows craniad and may stop before it reaches its normal termination. Fusion has failed to keep up with elongation.

(2) *Local failure of fusion of the lateral ridges.* If fusion fails to occur, with no other

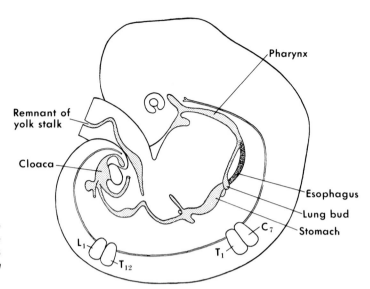

FIGURE 5.4 Elongation of the esophagus by cranial growth of the embryo during the sixth week (6.3 mm). *Reproduced from Gray,[6] with permission.*

changes taking place, a simple tracheoesophageal fistula without esophageal atresia results (Fig. 5.7). More often, the unclosed portion falls under the influence of the tracheal mesoderm, and a short section of the foregut becomes entirely trachea, with a corresponding segment of esophagus absent. A fistula to either the upper or lower portion, or both, is present as well. It is these more common lesions with which the surgeon is chiefly concerned (Fig. 5.8 A, B, C).

Not all of these defects are equally common. Among lesions of the middle esophagus, atresia is more common than is stenosis, tracheal fistula accompanies most atresias, and the fistula is usually from the lower esophageal segment.[3] In spite of these statements, the surgeon must keep in mind that variations, even among the most common types of malformations, may require that changes in procedure be adapted to the particular patient. Fig. 5.9 is a clinical classification of these defects.

About 50% of infants with esophageal atresia or tracheoesophageal fistula will have other anomalies.[1,2] The most common single defect as-

TABLE 5.1 Anomalies of the Esophagus

Anomaly	Origin of Defect	First Appearance	Sex Chiefly Affected	Relative Frequency	Remarks
Esophageal atresia, stenosis, and tracheoesophageal fistula	Between 21 and 34 days	At birth	Equal	Common	
True duplication	7th week	Any age	?	Very rare	May never produce symptoms
Enterogenous cysts	End of 3rd	Birth to any age	Female ?	Rare	
Diverticula (excluding traction diverticula)	5th month to birth?	Any age	Male	Uncommon	Muscular weakness may exist indefinitely without herniation occurring
Heterotopic gastric mucosa	5th month to birth	Any age (if at all)	Equal ?	Common	May never produce symptoms
Short esophagus	7th week	At birth	Male	Rare	
Infantile hiatal hernia	?	At birth	Equal ?	Rare in infants	

Reprinted from Gray,[6] with permission.

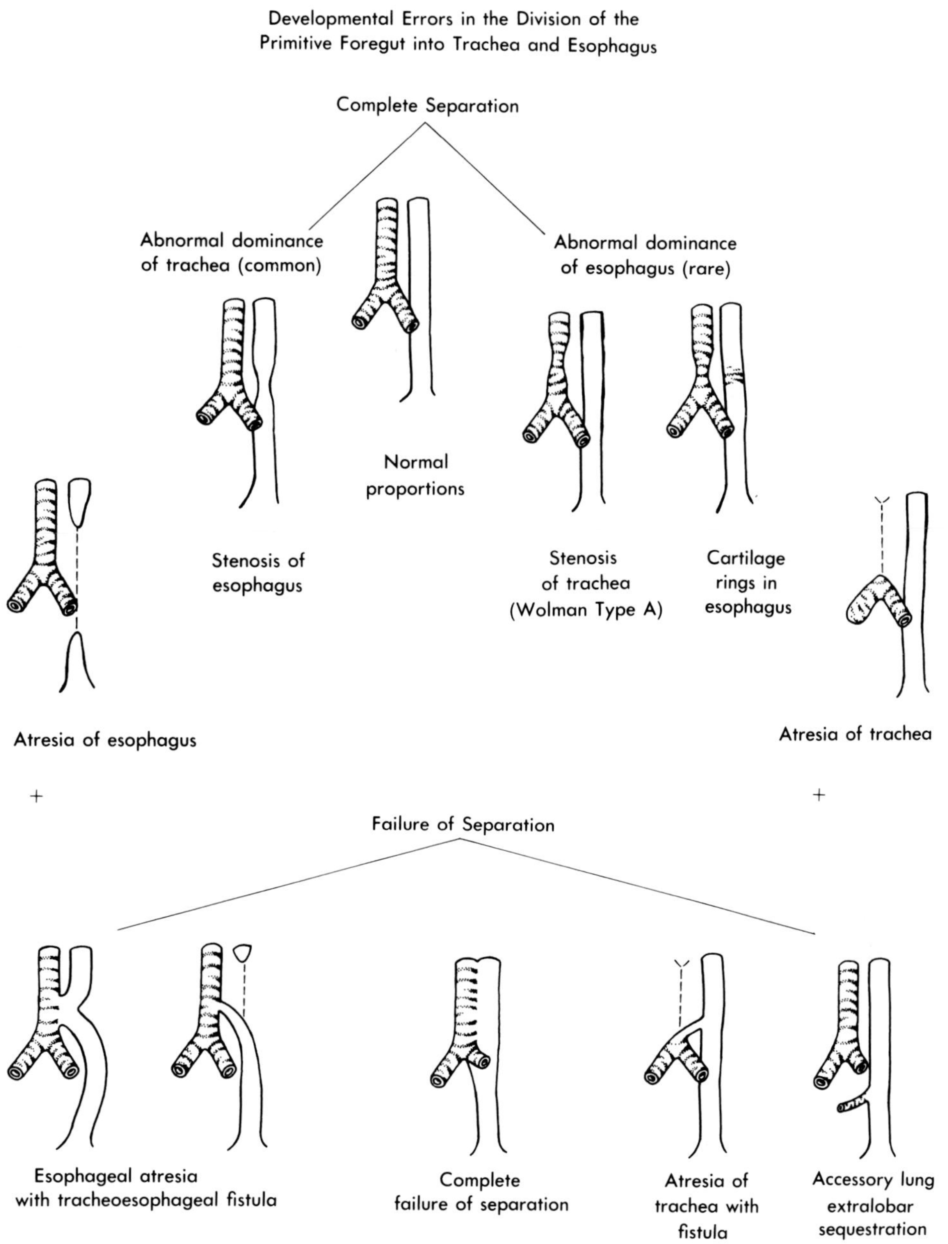

FIGURE 5.5 Patterns of developmental errors in the division of the embryonic foregut. *Reproduced from Gray,*[6] *with permission.*

sociated with esophageal lesions is imperforate anus, with or without fistula.[4] Down's syndrome is not unusual. Hydramnios is frequently encountered in infants with esophageal atresia; inability to swallow and excrete the fluid permits its accumulation.

Short Esophagus

If esophageal elongation is permanently arrested short of its normal relation with the diaphragm,

the stomach never fully descends and a portion of it may lie in the thorax. This condition exists at birth, and the thoracic stomach cannot be reduced. This is the congenital "short esophagus," which in some ways resembles the acquired hiatal hernia of later life.[5]

Thoracic Cysts

Cysts, usually lined with ciliated (respiratory) epithelium, may lie in the posterior mediastinum

TABLE 5.2 Anomalies of the Trachea and Lungs

Anomaly	Origin of Defect	First Appearance (or other diagnostic clues)	Sex Chiefly Affected	Relative Frequency	Remarks
Tracheal atresia	3rd to 4th week	At birth	?	Very rare	Fatal at birth
Bilateral agenesis of the lungs	4th week	At birth	?	Very rare	Fatal at birth
Congenital tracheal stenosis	3rd to 4th week	At birth	?	Rare	Usually fatal soon after birth
Tracheobronchomegaly	5th month?	Late childhood or later	?	Rare	
Unilateral agenesis and hypoplasia of the lungs	Late 4th week	Infancy and child-hood	Female	Uncommon	50% die in first five years
Anomalies of lobulation	10th week	None	Male ?	Common	Asymptomatic
Pulmonary isomerism	Unknown	None	?	Uncommon	Associated with hetero-taxy, asplenia, and anomalous pulmo-nary veins
Congenital cysts of the respiratory tract: bronchogenic cysts	6th to 7th	Infancy (if at all)	?	Uncommon	Compression of trachea may be fatal
Pulmonary cysts	24th week	Infancy and child-hood	Male	Uncommon	Eventually fatal if un-treated

Reprinted from Gray,[6] with permission.

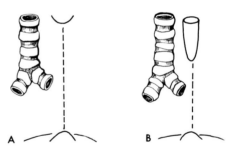

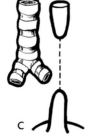
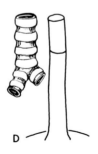
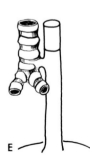

FIGURE 5.6 Atresia of the esophagus. **A.** Complete absence. **B, C.** Segmental absence. **D.** Membranous atresia without fistula. **E.** Membranous atresia with fistula. *Reproduced from Gray,[6] with permission.*

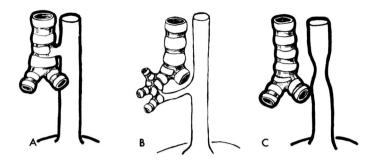

FIGURE 5.7 A, B. Tracheoesophageal fistula without esophageal atresia. **C.** Esophageal stenosis without fistula. In this and following illustrations the more frequently encountered lesions are drawn with bolder lines. *Reproduced from Gray,[6] with permission.*

with or without an esophageal fistula (Fig. 5.10, Table 5.3). They are attached cranially to the ventral surface of the vertebrae. Caudally, they open into the esophagus, occasionally passing through the diaphragm to enter the duodenum. These structures are known as *dorsal enteric remnants.*

Small cysts with ciliated epithelium lying on the trachea, bronchi, or bronchioles are of tracheal origin. They may open into the respiratory tract.

Accessory Lung and Sequestration

A pulmonary lobe that is separately supplied by a large anomalous artery arising from the aorta or one of its branches and drained by anomalous veins is said to be sequestered. Such a lobe is usually composed of one or more cysts. The artery is of the elastic type resembling a normal pulmonary artery rather than a systemic branch of the aorta. The conditions may be divided into intralobar sequestration in which the sequestered portion is anatomically part of the normal lung and extralobar sequestration (accessory lung) in which the anomalous tissue is anatomically separated from the normal lung. The lesions may be classified as follows:

(1) *Intralobar sequestration* (Fig. 5.11). Type I: The anomalous artery supplies normal lung tissue. Type II: The anomalous artery supplies nor-

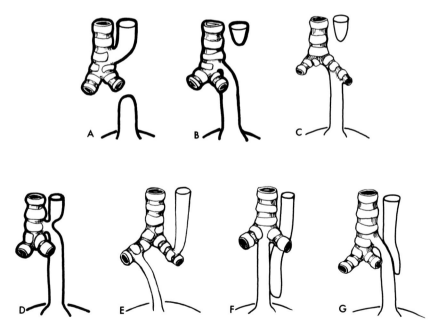

FIGURE 5.8 Atresia of the esophagus with fistula. **A.** Fistula from proximal esophageal segment. **B.** Fistula from distal esophageal segment. **C.** Fistula from distal segment to bronchus. **D, E.** Fistula from both segments of esophagus. **F, G.** Fistula from distal segment with elongated proximal segment. *Reproduced from Gray,[6] with permission.*

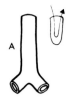

Clinical Group I
Excessive salivation

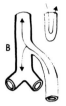

Clinical Group II
Excessive salivation,
with coughing,
choking and cyanosis

Clinical Group III
Coughing, choking
and cyanosis at
feeding

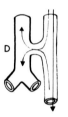

Clinical Group IV
Episodic coughing
and choking, may
persist into adulthood

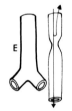

Clinical Group V
Partial regurgitation
and dysphagia

FIGURE 5.9 Differential diagnosis among five clinical groups of esophageal defects. *Reproduced from Gray,[6] with permission.*

TABLE 5.3 Key to Thoracic Cysts Lined with Respiratory Epithelium

Cysts	Origin	Location	Communication	Blood Supply
Dorsal enteric cysts of the embryonic foregut ("duplications of the esophagus")	2nd week	Posterior mediastinum	None, or with esophagus	Esophageal arteries
Bronchogenic paratracheal cysts (duplication of the trachea)	6th week	Right lateral tracheal wall	None, or with trachea or bronchus	Bronchial arteries or aorta
Intralobar sequestration of the lung	8th week or later	Usually part of posterior basal segment of left lung	None, or with trachea or bronchus	Anomalous elastic artery from aorta; drainage through pulmonary veins
Extralobar sequestrations of the lung (accessory lungs)	6th week or later	Separated from lung; posterior; usually on left; rarely subdiaphragmatic	None, or with trachea or bronchus, esophagus, or stomach	Anomalous artery from aorta; drainage into azygos veins

Reproduced from Gray,[6] with permission.

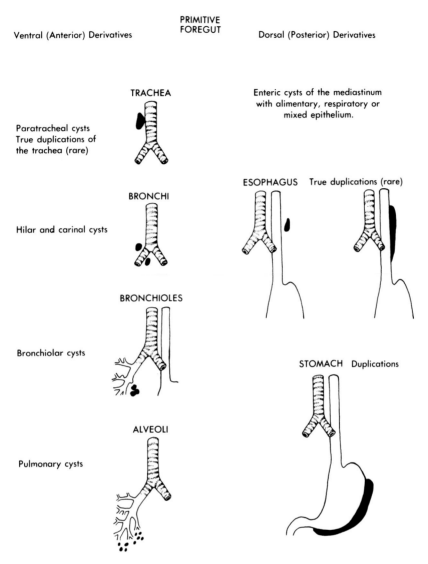

FIGURE 5.10 Duplication and cysts associated with tracheopulmonary (ventral) and esophageal (dorsal) portion of the foregut. *Reproduced from Gray,[6] with permission.*

mal lung tissue and the sequestered lobe. Type III: The anomalous artery supplies the sequestered lung tissue only.

(2) *Extralobar sequestrations* (Fig. 5.12). Most extralobar lesions are found in the posterior, basal segment of the lower lobe of the left lung.

The affected lobe is anatomically as well as physiologically sequestered. Extralobar anomalies may be found in the thorax or abdomen. There may be a bronchial connection between the sequestered lobe and the esophagus, or even with the stomach below the diaphragm. These rare cases have been called *bronchopulmonary*

foregut malformations (Fig. 5.6, lower right). Fowler et al in 1988 reviewed the embryological development of sequestration.[2]

Unilateral Aplasia and Hypoplasia of the Lung

Radiologically, two groups of lesions may be diagnosed in life: (1) aplasia—no lung tissue visible; and (2) hypoplasia (primary)—lung greatly reduced in size and may or may not be contained within the mediastinum. In complete unilateral agenesis there is no pleural cavity on the affected side, but the heart and remaining lung fill the

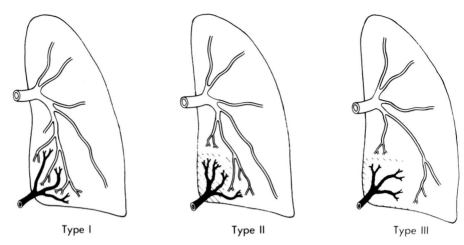

FIGURE 5.11 Three types of intralobar sequestration. Unshaded vessel is normal pulmonary artery; shaded vessel is anomalous artery. *Reproduced from Gray,[6] with permission.*

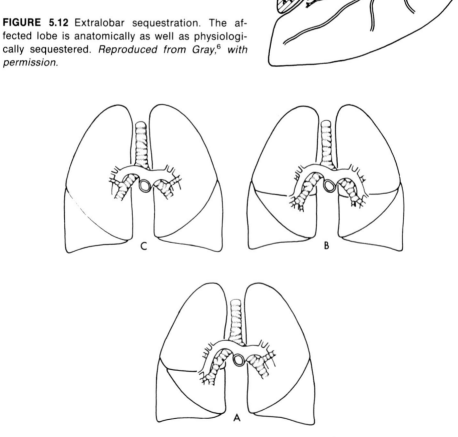

FIGURE 5.12 Extralobar sequestration. The affected lobe is anatomically as well as physiologically sequestered. *Reproduced from Gray,[6] with permission.*

FIGURE 5.13 Pulmonary lobulation. **A.** Normal asymmetry: right lung with three lobes, left lung with two. **B.** Two "right" lungs with three lobes each. **C.** Two "left" lungs with two lobes each. *Reproduced from Gray,[6] with permission.*

thorax. Most of the increase results from hyper-plasia.[6]

In primary hypoplasia, the rudimentary lung is usually without air. This hypoplasia is very different from the hypoplasia found secondary to diaphragmatic hernia, in which the growth retardation of the affected lung results from lack of normal room to develop in the thorax. In such secondary hypoplasia, the lung is usually aerated and often achieves its normal size following reduction of the herniated viscera and repair of the diaphragmatic defect.

The rarity of bilateral agenesis of the lung, compared with unilateral agenesis, indicates that the latter is not a simple arrest of normal development but rather a failure to maintain the developmental balance between the two lung buds. Normal development requires that the bronchial anlage be divided reasonably equally between the two buds. If this balance is not established, one side will develop normally whereas the other will fail completely (aplasia) or undergo only limited development (dysplasia or hypoplasia). We must not think that the normal balance depends on an exact equal division of the bronchial primordium. The division need leave only an adequate cell population, not necessarily of the same size, on each side. The minimum population needed for normal development is not known, but it is probably much less than one-half of the developing lung bud. Both lungs are affected in equal proportion, although patients with aplasia of the left lung have a considerably better prognosis.[7]

Pulmonary Patterns and Splenic Anomalies

In the absence of the spleen (asplenia syndrome) both lungs have three lobes and eparterial bronchi. There are thus two "right" lungs. Similarly, in the presence of multiple spleens (polysplenia syndrome), both lungs have two lobes and hy-parterial bronchi. There are thus two "left" lungs (Fig. 5.13).

These configurations of the lungs function normally and are of no importance by themselves. They are, however, associated with severe cardiac malformations.[1,3,4]

SUMMARY

Congenital defects of the embryonic foregut are numerous. Many are asymptomatic and are found incidentally at surgery or at autopsy. Others are readily correctable by simple surgery. Most of the severe malformations, however, are associated with other equally severe anomalies. What can be done for the infant with both tracheoesophageal fistula and imperforate anus? Either defect can often be cured, but some combinations present a nearly impossible challenge. Unfortunately, there will always be some who cannot be saved.

REFERENCES

1. Bergsma D: *Birth Defects Compendium.* 2nd ed. New York: Alan R. Liss, Inc, 1979.
2. Fowler CL, Pokorny WJ, Wagner ML, Kessler MS: Review of bronchopulmonary foregut malformations. *J Pediatr Surg* 1988;23:793–797.
3. Martin LW, Alexander F: Esophageal atresia. *Surg Clin North Am* 1985;65:1099–1113.
4. Manning PB, Morgan RA, Coran AG: Fifty years' experience with esophageal atresia and tracheoesophageal fistula. *Ann Surg* 1986;204:446–451.
5. Treacy J, Jamieson GG: Para-oesophageal hernias. In Jamieson GG, (ed.): Surgery of the oesophagus. Edinburgh: Churchill Livingstone, 1988, pp. 149–157.
6. Gray SW, Skandalakis JE: Embryology for surgeons. Philadelphia, WB Saunders, 1972.
7. Schechter DC: Congenital absence of deficiency of lung tissue: The congenital subtractive bronchopneumonic malformations. *Ann Thorac Surg* 1968; 6:286–313.

Intrathoracic Malformations of Foregut Derivatives

Francis Jaubert, MD and Claire Danel, MD

We agree with the clinical data reported in Chapter 5, and rather than repeat them, we will develop a few points of interest or of controversy.

The regulation of embryonal development is beginning to surface. Growth factors are involved in a multistep process.[1] The blastocyst of the mouse elaborates three growth factors: two transforming growth factors (TGF α and TGF β) and the platelet derived growth factor A (PDGF-A).[2] On one hand, these factors act on the blastula itself as mitotic and differentiating agents, and on the other hand they induce early angiogenesis and deciduation of the uterus for nesting. At the blastulation stage, in Xenopus, fibroblast growth factor (FGF) and TGF β induce mesoderm differentiation.[3] Later on, after implantation in the endometrium, there is an intermingling of embryonal and maternal derived growth factors acting on the embryo. For example, stimulation by PDGF-A induces the expression of c-*myc* oncogene in the receptive cells.[4] An enhanced c-*myc* expression is found in the intestine (30 per 100 cells) and lung (20 per 100 cells) of the human embryo.[5] Other growth factors may stimulate various oncogenes. The action of growth factors and of the surrounding connective tissue on cell differentiation is called *paracrine action,* in contrast to the endocrine action of hormones.[1] For insects, it is demonstrated that specialized organizers (Homeo box) with a segmental (metameric) specificity are switched on for a while during differentiation.

The DiGeorge syndrome is the consequence of a developmental abnormality involving the third and fourth pharyngeal pouches. The abnormalities include midline cardiac defects, absent parathyroid glands leading to neonatal tetany, an atypical facies including hypertelorism and high arched palate, auricular maldevelopment, and absence of the thymus gland.

Such a syndrome may be experimentally produced in the chick by the elimination of limited areas of the cephalic neural crest in stage 9 or 10 of chick embryos.[6] Such an experiment demonstrates the role of neural crest elements in the development of thymus, parathyroid, aortic arches, and the face. However, the neural crest elements differentiate appropriately only in response to extracellular matrix elements,[7] which suggests that the DiGeorge syndrome pathogeny is more complicated than a focal defect of neural crest derivative. Genetic data demonstrate that the DiGeorge syndrome may be sporadic or familial with an inheritance linked to a chromosomal deletion 22q11.[8] Such data suggest that the DiGeorge syndrome is a disease of segmental organizers (or homeobox) of differentiation in humans. Complete DiGeorge syndrome is rare, and there is a spectrum of third and fourth pharyngeal pouch maldevelopment. Our experience with DiGeorge syndrome is that the thymus is not found in the thorax, but if you do serial sections of the whole cervical area you always find two to four remnants of maldeveloped thymus having the size and the macroscopy of a lymph node.

For esophageal atresia the association of congenital abnormalities ranges between 40% and 57% of patients and is not linked to the existence of a fistula.[9] The VATER association is the occurrence of three or more anomalies—vertebral defect, anorectal malformation, tracheoesophageal fistula, renal anomalies and radial dysplasia—and occurs in 10% of cases. The level of the rectoanal malformation is not associated with the type of esophageal atresia but is related to tissue derived from the endoderm and mesoderm, which differentiate actively and synchronously during the fourth and fifth embryonic week. Most cases of esophageal atresia are sporadic, but familial cases exist, suggesting a genetic basis. A careful study produced the conclusion that apart from cases occurring as part of a known chromosomal abnormality (various trisomies and monogenic abnormalities), these cases are multifactorial despite being familial.[10] However, a strain of mouse possesses an autosomal recessive gene for the development of a laryngoesophageal cleft without any other morphological congenital abnormalities.[11] The pathogenesis of esophageal atresia itself is discussed. It is generally hypothesized that there is a tracheoesophageal septum and that atresia is a disturbance of the process of closure of the septum.

But there is no anatomic proof of the existence of such a septum either in the chick[12] or in humans.[13] Another hypothesis is that there is a gap in the esophageal vascularization at the level of the aortic arch and that vascular insufficiency causes esophageal atresia with a fistula as a complication.[14] If this were true, esophageal atresia would have the same mechanism as the other intestinal atresias, and the poor vascularization of the lower portion of the esophagus would explain problems in surgical repair. Squamous cell metaplasia of the trachea would be acquired[15] and linked to an abnormal blood supply.

Lung development may be split into two main parts: the bronchial tree and lesser circulation.

Bronchial tree development follows the glandular, canalicular, and alveolar stages of development. The main pathological lesions are cystic development and atresia. Cysts are the end result of an imbalance between epithelial growth or the budding process and the extracellular matrix.[16] Abnormal budding from the primitive esophagus produces enteric cysts (or duplications) that are always associated with vertebral abnormalities and considered the consequence of a split notochord.[17] At the glandular stage an abnormal bud is the cause of a bronchogenic cyst. These cysts are usually located in the anterosuperior part of the thorax with a preponderance in the mediastinum. At the canalicular stage cystic adenomatoid malformation arises with its three subtypes.[18] Type III, with numerous membranous bronchioles, is lethal. Type II, which is characterized by multiple small cysts is associated with a high frequency of other anomalies. Type I, with simple or multiple cysts, has a good prognosis. Later, bronchial arterial obstruction may cause bronchial atresia with malformative emphysema. These lesions predominate in the left upper lobe, which has the more variable pattern of development for the bronchial tree and arteries.[19]

The lesser circulation development involves on the one hand the involution of the systemic supply of the primitive lung and on the other hand the individualization of the pulmonary arteries and veins.

The pulmonary arteries derive from the sixth aortic arches under the influence of neural crest derivatives.[20] In the chick, ablation of specific segments of the neural crest results in persistent truncus arteriosus and/or in anomalies of the aortic arches.[21] Other pulmonary artery abnormalities of less well known pathogenesis may arise in similar fashion to hypoplasia or a retrotracheal path of the left branch. In the latter case there is an associated tracheal maldevelopment with stenosis linked to a circular cartilagenous ring. The remnants of the systemic circulation are the bronchial arteries and arteries of the lung ligament.[22] A persistant systemic supply of a lung segment is called *sequestration.* Intralobar sequestrations are the most frequent type and occur predominantly in the left lower lobe.[23] Clinically they are considered to be malformations linked to failure of involution of a systemic artery. In favor of such a hypothesis are cases of ectopic pancreas,[24,25] aberrant lung segmentation, and accompanying esophageal or gastric diverticulum.[26,27] However, in other cases it may be an acquired disease with lung ligament artery development in response to a bronchial or pulmonary artery obstruction in a lung segment.[22] Extralobar sequestrations are always malformative and are frequently linked to diaphragmatic maldevelopment, such as diaphragmatic hernia.[23] However, a few cases of purely subdiaphragmatic sequestration are reported.

Pulmonary vein development involves the loss of the splanchnic connection and their capture by a bud from the left atrium. Such a process is surmised from pathological data such as cor triatriatum and anomalous pulmonary drainage. The scimitar syndrome combines a complete but hypoplastic right lung with anomalous pulmonary drainage into the inferior vena cava and a systemic artery supplying the lower lobe.[28] The left lung is usually enlarged.

Experimentally it can be demonstrated that the surgical inversion of 80% of the lung bud, in chick embryo stage 28, results either in an isolated anomalous venous drainage of the lung or in the combination of an anomalous venous drainage and a systemic arterial supply.[29] Such data suggest that separation of arterial and venous supply is artificial because they may share the same cause or may be associated. For example, some sequestrations have an abnormal venous drainage, whereas in the scimitar syndrome is a systemic artery.[16] That is the reason some authors consider these malformations as a spectrum.[30]

It can be deduced from the previous data

that if normal embryonal development is a subtle balance among epithelial cells, mesenchyme, and neural derivatives, its pathologic variants rarely have a single cause. This favors a multifactorial or multistep pathogenesis and explains the difficulties encountered in postulating preventive measures.

ACKNOWLEDGMENTS

The authors thank H. Martelli, A. L. Delezoide, and M. Grimal for their help.

REFERENCES

1. Milner RDG, Hill DJ: Fetal growth signals. *Arch Dis Child* 1989;65:53–57.
2. Rappolee DA, Brenner CA, Schultz R, et al: Developmental expression of PDGF, TGF-α, and TGF-β genes in preimplantation mouse embryos. *Science* 1988;241:1823–1825.
3. Mercola M, Melton DA, Stiles CD: Platelet-derived growth factor A chain is maternally encoded in xenopus embryos. *Science* 1988;241:1223–1225.
4. Schmid P, Schulz WA, Hameister H: Dynamic expression pattern of the myc protooncogene in midgestation mouse embryos. *Science* 1989;243:226–229.
5. Pfeifer-Ohlsson S, Rydnert J, Goustin AS, et al: Cell-type-specific pattern of myc protooncogene expression in developing human embryos. *Proc Natl Acad Sci USA* 1985;82:5050–5054.
6. Bockman DE, Kirby ML: Dependence of thymus development on derivatives of the neural crest. *Science* 1984;223:498–500.
7. Perris R, Von Boxberg Y, Lofberg J: Local embryonic matrices determine region-specific phenotypes in neural crest cells. *Science* 1988;241:86–89.
8. de la Chapelle A, Herva R, Koivisto M, Aula P: A deletion in chromosome 22 can cause DiGeorge syndrome. *Hum Genet* 1981;57:253–256.
9. Chittmittrapap S, Spitz L, Kiely EM, Brereton RJ: Oesophageal atresia and associated anomalies. *Arch Dis Child* 1989;64:364–368.
10. Van Staey M, Debie S, Matton MT, De Roose J: Familial congenital oesophageal atresia: Personal case report and review of the literature. *Hum Genet* 1984;66:260–266.
11. Essien FB, Maderious A: A genetic factor controlling morphogenesis of the laryngo-esophageal complex in the mouse. *Teratology* 1981;24:235–239.
12. Kluth D, Steding G, Seidl W: The embryology of foregut malformations. *J Pediatr Surg* 1987;22:389–393.
13. Zam-Tun HA: The tracheo-esophageal septum—Fact or fantasy? Origin and development of the respiratory primordium and esophagus. *Acta Anat* 1982;114:1–21.
14. Lister J: The blood supply of the oesophagus in relation to oesophageal atresia. *Arch Dis Child* 1964;39:131–137.
15. Emery JL, Haddadin AJ: Squamous epithelium in respiratory tract of children with tracheo-oesophageal fistula. *Arch Dis Child* 1971;46:236–242.
16. Stovin PGI: Early lung development. *Thorax* 1985;40:401–404.
17. Kirwan WO, Walfaum PR, McCormack RJM: Cystic intrathoracic derivatives of the foregut and their complications. *Thorax* 1973;28:424–428.
18. Stocker JT, Madewell JE, Drake RM: Congenital cystic adenomatoid malformation of the lung: Classification and morphologic spectrum. *Hum Pathol* 1977;8:155–171.
19. Landing BH, Dixon LG: Congenital malformations and genetic disorders of the respiratory tract. *Am Rev Respir Dis* 1979;120:151–185.
20. Le Lievre C, Le Douarin N: Embryologie expérimentale: Contribution du mésectoderme à la genèse des arcs aortiques chez l'embryon d'oiseau. *CR Acad Sci Paris* 1973;276:383–386.
21. Nishibatake M, Kirby ML, Van Mierop LHS: Pathogenesis of persistent truncus arteriosus and dextroposed aorta in the chick embryo after neural crest ablation. *Circulation* 1987;75:255–264.
22. Stocker JT, Malczak HT: A study of pulmonary ligament arteries: Relationship to intralobar pulmonary sequestration. *Chest* 1984;86:611–615.
23. Savic B, Birtel FJ, Tholen W, et al: Lung sequestration: Report of seven cases and review of 540 published cases. *Thorax* 1979;34:96–101.
24. Beskin CA: Intralobar enteric sequestration of the lung containing aberrant pancreas. *J Thorac Cardiovasc Surg* 1961;41:314–317.
25. Corrin B, Danel C, Allaway A, et al: Intralobar pulmonary sequestration of ectopic pancreatic tissue with gastropancreatic duplications. *Thorax* 1985;40:637–638.
26. Gerle RD, Jeretzki A, Ashley CA, Berne AS: Congenital bronchopulmonary-foregut malformation: Pulmonary sequestration communicating with the gastrointestinal tract. *N Engl J Med* 1968;278:1413–1419.
27. Heithoff KB, Sane SM, Williams HJ, et al: Bronchopulmonary foregut malformations: A unifying etiological concept. *AJR* 1976;126:46–55.
28. Farnsworth AE, Ankeney JL: The spectrum of the scimitar syndrome. *J Thorac Cardiovasc Surg* 1974;68:37–42.
29. Clark EB, Martini R, Rosenquist GC: Spectrum of pulmonary venous connections following lung bud inversion in the chick embryo. In: Pexieder T, ed. *Perspectives in Cardiovascular Research.* New York: Raven Press, 1981;5:419–428.
30. Clements BS, Warner JO: Pulmonary sequestration and related congenital broncho-pulmonary vascular malformations: Nomenclature and classification based on anatomical and embryological considerations. *Thorax* 1987;42:401–408.

Chapter 6

Intrapulmonary Lesions

Yves P M. Chavrier, MD

Congenital bronchopulmonary lesions were first described by Delarue et al in 1959.[1] However, the pathologic anatomy of these conditions is still difficult to understand.

A review of tracheobronchopulmonary development sheds some light on the nature of these malformations. Some are due to ectopic or supernumerary bronchial buds and others appear to be secondary to the defective transformation of the bronchial outline during the transition from the alveolar to the canalicular stage of lung development. The ectopic or supernumerary lung buds end up as bronchogenic cysts and pulmonary sequestrations. These latter defects produce distal bronchial dysgenesis and inflation cysts, as well as pulmonary adenomatoid malformations.[2] On occasion both these processes are associated.

PULMONARY SEQUESTRATIONS

The term *sequestration,* suggested in 1946 by Pryce, defines a zone of pulmonary lobar or segmental tissue separated from its normal bronchial and vascular connections and supplied by one or more systemic arteries (Fig. 6.1).

Most authors use the term sequestration for a segment of pulmonary tissue in which the connections with the normal bronchial tree and pulmonary artery are absent and the tissue is supplied with an aberrant systemic artery. Other criteria are also recognized by some.[3]

In 1974, Sade introduced the term *spectrum sequestration,* which comprises all the different combinations that can result from abnormalities in bronchial connection, arterial supply, or venous drainage. Gerle et al[4] applied the term sequestration or bronchopneumointestinal malformation whenever pulmonary parenchyma had

lost its normal bronchial, arterial, or venous connections and had retained other foregut or systemic vascular connections. Although several theories have been put forward to explain the development of sequestrations, the most appealing is still the theory of the supernumerary bronchial bud that retains its own systemic blood supply.[3]

If the supernumerary bud develops early in gestation it will be enveloped within the normal tracheobronchial bud during its caudal migration and will result in intralobar sequestration (ILS). If, on the other hand, it appears late, it will remain separated from the normal lung (extralobar sequestration, or ELS). In some cases a sequestration is connected to the normal lung by a fibrous string or by a true bronchus.[4–7]

Anatomical Survey

The systemic abnormal artery most often originates from the lower thoracic aorta or from the upper abdominal aorta or one of its branches (diaphragmatic, intercostal, celiac trunk). It often has a short course, and it penetrates into the sequestration through the inner part of the triangular ligament. Abnormal anastomoses with other vessels can occur.[8] Venous return from the sequestered lung is generally by way of the pulmonary veins in the case of ILS or by the azygos, hemiazygos, and inferior vena cava in the case of ELS. As noted by Merlier et al,[9] it is logical to distinguish between ILS and ELS. One form of ILS appears as an ovoid or quadrangular mass and is readily distinguished macroscopically from the normal lung parenchyma by its pinkish white, reddish, or yellowish coloration, without anthracotic pigmentation. Frequently the sequestration is cystic and is easy to appreciate. Less obvious are the rarer pseudo-tumoral forms. The histological appearance of the parenchyma varies from normal[10] to dysembryoplasic as described by Le Brigand.[9]

One form of ELS is isolated from the normal lung by its own pleural sac. It appears as a dark

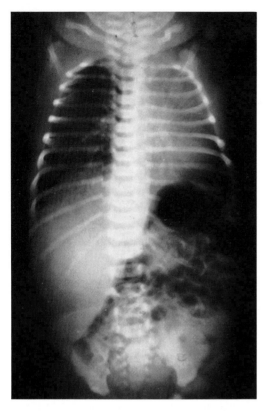

FIGURE 6.1 Sequestration in right lower lobe.

red liver-like pyramid or oval and is easily detected at thoracotomy (Figs. 6.2 and 6.3).

Localization

Savic et al[11] have shown that 97% of intralobar sequestrations are in the left lower lobe (Fig. 6.4) whereas the ELS sequestrations are nearly always situated between the left lower lobe and the diaphragm. However, sequestrations in the upper[12] and middle lobes and, sometimes, in an entire lung or in both lungs[13] can be found. Rarely the sequestration is in the retroperitoneum.[14]

Other congenital malformations are often seen in ELS. These include cardiopericardial, digestive, genitourinary, osseous, and other pulmonary malformations (cystic adenomatoid disease, pulmonary hypoplasia).[15]

Clinical Features

This rare anomaly affects boys and girls equally. It most frequently is detected in the young child and 10% of cases are found in neonates. They account for about 1.5% of all thoracotomies needed in childhood.

The diagnosis is reached by several meth-

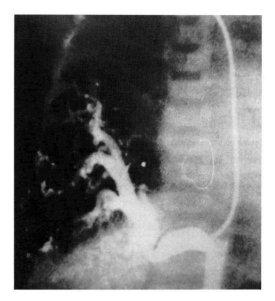

FIGURE 6.2 Arteriography of this same sequestration.

ods. Antenatal diagnosis by ultrasound is theoretically possible, though I have no experience in this. Usually the child has a history of repeated bronchopulmonary infection with bronchorrhea, coupled with radiological abnormalities in the lower posterior chest region.[16] Rarely a sequestration is detected because of an isolated cough or an acute pneumonia.

Thirty percent of diagnosed sequestrations are asymptomatic and are discovered during the

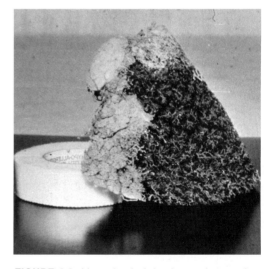

FIGURE 6.3 After plastic injection and corrosion, the part without a bronchus is clearly evident (dark portion).

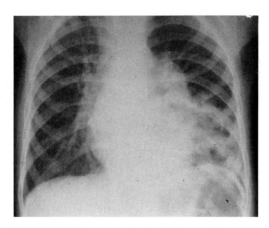

FIGURE 6.4 Sequestration in left lower lobe.

investigation of another abnormality (Chapter 15). Occasionally the lesion is discovered during surgery for diaphragmatic hernia. Rarely a sequestration presents with neonatal respiratory distress and heart failure.[9] Clinical examination is generally normal. A simple chest roentgenogram may show single or multiple densities near the diaphragmatic cupola (Fig. 6.5). Sometimes an air-fluid level or an air-fluid cyst is seen, which may suggest a large esophageal bronchus.[17] Rarely, the plain roentgenogram is entirely normal. I wish to emphasize the importance of the use of filtered mediastinal x-ray. Almost 50% of sequestrations demonstrate the scimitar sign radiographically.

Ultrasound can confirm the diagnosis when it reveals a large systemic artery,[18] but the absence of this finding does not rule out sequestration.

Bronchography may show the absence of Lipiodol in the sequestration and it may lead to the diagnosis of Pryce's intralobar type if the bronchi are counted. Bronchoscopy is of little use.

Barium swallow can reveal a latent communication[19] and can help to eliminate esophageal diseases that may be included in the differential diagnosis.

Angiography by venous injection will show if the lesion is not vascularized by the pulmonary artery but by a systemic artery,[20] and demonstrate its site of origin. I think that in infants, angiocardiopneumography is far less dangerous than aortography (see Fig. 6.2). In some institutions computed tomography (CT) has replaced angiography. Experience with magnetic resonance imaging (MRI) for diagnosis is lacking.

Treatment

Treatment is exclusively surgical. Because of superinfection and inadequate drainage of the sequestration, surgical resection is the only suitable treatment. It is also needed to eliminate the systemic artery to pulmonary vein shunt, which may not be well tolerated. Surgery should be performed as soon as the diagnosis is made to limit the incidence of infection[16] and lead to better functional recovery.[21]

Although the ideal treatment for ILS is segmentectomy, it is rarely possible, and in most cases of ILS a lobectomy is performed.

For ELS excision of only the sequestrated segment with ligation of the abnormal vessels is required. After freeing the many adhesions identification of the lesion is usually easy. A communication with the esophagus among the many adhesions must be recognized. Surgery is generally uncomplicated as soon as the systemic artery has been controlled. Venous return should be identified before excising the sequestration to avoid venous infarction. The abnormal artery

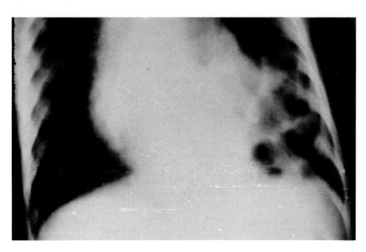

FIGURE 6.5 Tomography of this same sequestration.

should be systematically oversewn. One must avoid trauma to the artery by hemostatic clamps.

Results

There were no deaths in our series. However, one expects the mortality to be a little higher in ELS because other malformations are more frequent with ELS. In a joint series of 31 cases published with Jaubert de Beaujeu,[21] we carried out 11 right lower lobectomies, 6 left lower lobectomies, 2 right upper lobectomies, 1 left upper lobectomy, 2 pneumonectomies, 4 segmentectomies, and 5 extralobar sequestrectomies. Seven cases were associated with the treatment of a diaphragmatic hernia. Two children required reoperations, one for a hemothorax due to bleeding near the diaphragmatic suture and the other for an abscess due to an esophageal fistula leak at the site of an esophageal suture.

BRONCHOGENIC CYSTS

Bronchogenic cysts develop from abnormal buds from the primitive esophagus or tracheobronchial tree, which do not extend to the site where alveolar differentiation occurs. If the aberrant bud separates early from the tracheobronchial outline, it will result in a mediastinal cyst; if it separates later it will lead to an intraparenchymal cyst.[2]

The epithelial wall of the cyst is that of the bronchus, which explains the mucoid content of the lesion. Usually these cysts occur along the aerodigestive axis (Fig. 6.6). In exceptional cases they are found subcutaneously. The later the separation of the bud, the closer the cyst's structure will simulate normal bronchoalveolar structures. The volume of the cyst varies from 1 or 2 ml to 10 to 15 ml. Large cysts are often polylobed and of a whitish or pinkish color.

The cyst may communicate with the airways either at its inception or, more often, because of

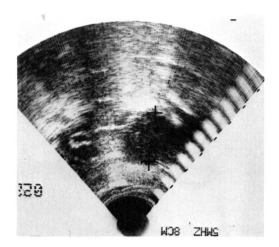

FIGURE 6.7 Ultrasonography showing a paratracheal cyst.

superinfection (Figs. 6.7, 6.8, 6.9). The radiological appearance varies from a cyst with an air-fluid level, to an air-filled cyst under tension.[20] In some cases, a bronchogenic cyst can present as a pneumothorax or as a typical lobar emphysema with respiratory distress with compression of the contralateral lung. In exceptional cases, the cyst wall becomes calcified because of an inflammatory reaction. In contrast to esophageal or neuroenteric cysts, which have a digestive epithelium, bronchogenic cysts are never associated with vertebral malformations.

Investigations

Ultrasonography may confirm the liquid nature of the cyst contents (see Fig. 6.8). CT scan may indicate the variations in density and echogenicity if the contents are heterogeneous or if there is infection (Fig. 6.10). This information should assist in differentiating cyst from solid tumors.[22]

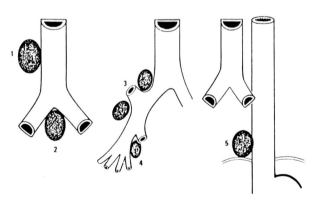

FIGURE 6.6 Bronchogenic cyst topography. 1. paratracheal. 2. Subcarinal. 3. Hilar. 4. Parenchymatous. 5. Inferomediastinal.

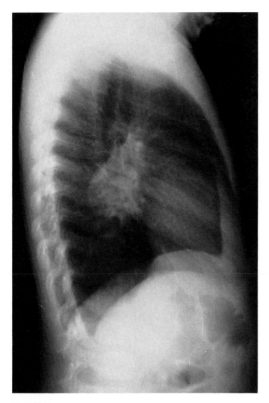

FIGURE 6.8 Perihilar lateral roentgenogram.

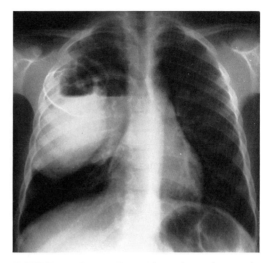

FIGURE 6.9 Superinfected bronchogenic cyst in right upper lobe.

Barium esophagography will often show extrinsic esophageal compression by the cyst. Bronchoscopy often demonstrates extrinsic compression of the aerodigestive axis by the cyst. When the diagnosis remains obscure bronchography may help in the differential diagnosis. MRI can be extremely useful in these cases.[23]

In cysts that are asymptomatic (30%), radiographic features vary according to whether or not it communicates with the airway.[24] Commonly, infection in the cyst leads to its detection. Bronchogenic cysts represent 6.5% of mediastinal tumors in children (see Fig. 6.7). Many may ultimately be diagnosed by antenatal ultrasonography.

Paratracheal Cysts

Paratracheal cysts are situated more commonly on the right than on the left (Fig. 6.7). Although they are often asymptomatic and may be discovered during a routine examination, they can also cause neonatal respiratory distress.[22] Radiographically, they appear as an oval image in the middle mediastinum, often deviating or compressing the trachea[25] or even extending posteriorly toward the vertebral column.

Barium esophagogram often shows lateral compression of the esophagus or the presence of an intertracheoesophageal mass. The differential diagnosis includes an abnormal aortic arch with a posterior esophageal indentation, a foregut cyst with associated vertebral lesions, and lymphadenopathy.

Subcarina Trachea Cysts

These cysts are situated in a space where they can remain latent for a long time, becoming evident only when their size results in bronchial compression. They are mainly situated in the posterior mediastinum.[26]

Radiological diagnosis is not easy if the cyst is small and is not accompanied by blunting or widening of the subcarinal angle. Diagnosis is more obvious when it causes bronchial compression with obstructive emphysema. Barium esophagogram can confirm the existence of such a mass and a CT scan will differentiate the cyst from a large right atrium. Sonogram may confirm the diagnosis by revealing the image of a retrocardiac, liquid-filled cyst.

Perihilar Cysts

Perihilar cysts are often subbronchial and retrobronchial, thus explaining the frequency of extrinsic compressions.[26] They are situated more commonly on the left, where the bronchus is longer and the aortic arch prevents the cyst from expanding. Radiographically one usually notes a hilar shadow (see Fig. 6.7), often accompanied by obstructive emphysema. Barium esophagogram will confirm the presence of the mass, its

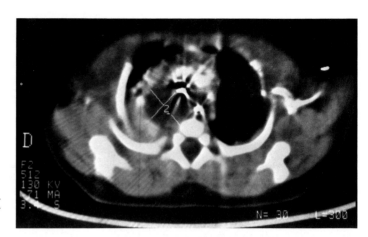

FIGURE 6.10 The same bronchogenic cyst as in Figure 6.9 in a CT scan.

topography, and its effect on mediastinal structures. Mediastinal lymphadenopathy, dilatation of the pulmonary artery, and bronchial atresia with a bronchocele are all in the differential diagnosis.

Inner Mediastinal Cysts

Inner mediastinal cysts are situated behind the heart and are often not detected because they are usually asymptomatic. Occasionally they can cause esophageal compression. Diagnosis depends on a filtered x-ray of the mediastinum and a barium esophagogram. Paraesophageal intramural cysts can be attached to it.

Intraparenchymal Cysts

These balloon-cysts represent 30% of all lung cysts. They can be found in any lobe and appear as a solitary pulmonary mass. Without complications, they remain asymptomatic. The existence of a communication with the bronchial tree can lead to infections, and the radiological picture will then become one of a cavity showing an air-fluid level. Precise diagnosis of this lesion can be difficult. A one-way valve mechanism can cause rapid expansion of a cyst under tension. Urgent thoracotomy and lobectomy or drainage of the cyst may be needed.

Treatment

Risks from gradual expansion with compression of adjacent lung infection and hemorrhage, or sudden death from rapid enlargement under tension, justify excision.[26] Generally these lesions are approached through a posterolateral thoracotomy. The surgeon should preserve the maximum amount of pulmonary tissue. When excising the cyst there is risk of entering a small bronchus if the surgeon attempts to remove the cyst

wall in its entirety. Should this occur, the leak must be repaired. It is safer to open into the cyst and leave a portion of the wall adherent to lung.[25] Care must be taken to preserve the phrenic nerve. Certain laterotracheal cysts have been approached by sternotomy, whereas others require lateral thoracotomy.[27] It is true that in pulmonary cystic disease of the child, sequestrations, and cystic adenomatoid malformations coexist.[24]

In the newborn child and the young infant, the decision to operate is easy. All "liquid boyles" hanging from the tracheobronchial tree should be removed. In older children, in the case of a large cyst or in the presence of a superinfection, the indication to operate is equally clear, though excision is more difficult. Preservation of the maximum amount of parenchyma remains the rule and segmentectomy will be preferred to lobectomy.

The results of surgery are excellent. DiLorenzo et al[28] report 26 patients in 10 years. All had excellent results without sequellae in spite of preexisting pneumonia. There was one transitory phrenic paralysis.

CONGENITAL CYSTIC ADENOMATOID MALFORMATION

Described by Ch'In and Teang in 1949, and confirmed by Craig in 1956, congenital cystic adenomatoid malformation (CCAM) is defined according to the histological criteria (Kwitten and Reiner).[29] These include adenomatoid proliferation of terminal respiratory structures, appearing as cysts of varying size (Figs. 6.11, 6.12), communicating among themselves and lined with a cylindrical or cuboidal epithelium; polypoid configuration of the mucous membrane and increased elastic fibers in the cystic walls lined with a typical bronchial epithelium; absence of car-

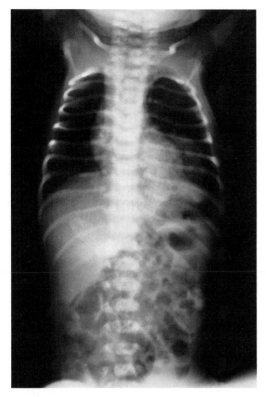

FIGURE 6.11 X-ray of congenital cystic adenomatoid malformation in left lower lobe.

tilaginous structure in the cystic parenchyma; absence of inflammation.

The anomaly responsible for the CCAM seems to appear toward the end of the fifth week or at the beginning of the sixth week of embryonic development. Its nature has not yet been per-fectly established though the lesion is considered to be a focal dysplasia rather than a hamartoma.

This is a relatively rare anomaly. Nevertheless, reports have been increasing with Esposito et al[30] recording 279 cases in 1985. Initial cases were in stillborn infants with anasarca, or in premature babies with respiratory distress, whose mothers displayed polyhydramnios. CCAM is recognized most often clinically in the perinatal period.[31] There is no racial or ethnic predominance, but boys seem affected more than girls.

CCAM is one of the four major congenital pulmonary malformations that appear as cystic spaces. Others include lobar emphysema, sequestration, and bronchogenic cysts.[32] With the exception of a report by Stocker et al,[33] associated malformations are not usually considered to be significant.

The CCAM generally affects a single lobe—more commonly, a lower one (Fig. 6.13) in most cases, it is unilateral. The malformed lobe is clearly increased in volume and weighs two to five times normal. Stocker et al,[33] among others, distinguish three types of lesions. Type 1 contains single or multiple cysts of more than 2 cm diameter. These cases have a good prognosis. In type 2 there are multiple cysts of less than 1 cm diameter. Type 3 lesions are large; either a few or no cysts are evident and the lesion appears solid. These carry a very bad prognosis.

Diagnosis

Clinical Presentation

Respiratory distress is common usually beginning in the neonatal period after a few hours or days of birth. Symptoms are due to cyst inflation and mediastinal displacement. In the more

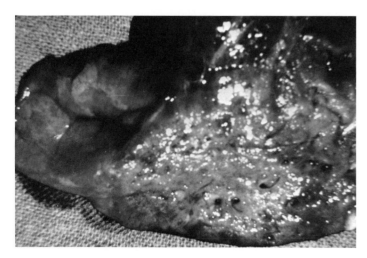

FIGURE 6.12 Cystic adenomatosis with the appearance of a rubber ball.

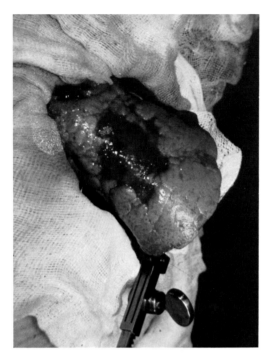

FIGURE 6.13 Solid adenomatosis.

chronic form one notes recurrent pneumonia with persistent radiological signs. At times symptoms worsen in spite of medical treatment. In some cases the small lesions produce no symptoms.

Radiological Diagnosis

In the neonatal period the appearance is that of a unilateral multicystic lesion (see Fig. 6.11), which can be either completely or partially opaque or translucent and which displaces the mediastinum. Torsion of pulmonary vessels and atelectasis around the cystic lesions modify the contours of the lesion.[34] In the solid form's presentation, a homogenous opacity at birth may aerate progressively. In several days microcysts give a spongy appearance.

When discovered in older children there are air-filled cysts surrounded by chronic infiltration, sometimes with a beehive appearance, or an air-fluid level simulating an abscess. Rarely a cyst is completely filled with liquid, giving it a solid appearance.

The antenatal ultrasound shows an intrathoracic mass of liquid nature, which is multicystic and independent of the heart. After birth, ultrasound can demonstrate liquid that cannot be verified on roentgenogram and, possibly, an abnormal vessel, as in sequestration. CT scan, which confirms the cystic nature, demonstrates the thickness of the walls and distinguishes it from a giant lobar emphysema. Barium eosphagogram, angiogram, and bronchoscopy may be needed to aid in the differential diagnosis. It is necessary to rule out a diaphragmatic hernia, a classic pitfall in diagnosis.

Treatment

Treatment is surgical and usually consists of lobectomy. When the whole lung is affected a pneumonectomy may be needed. Segmentectomy is rejected by some because of more frequent complications[32–36]; however, one should attempt segmentectomy whenever it appears possible in order to conserve pulmonary tissue.

It is important to remember that there can be an anomaly of pulmonary vascularization and/or an abnormal communication with the digestive tract[36] and that the surgical exposure must always be generous.

Prognosis is determined by the promptness of diagnosis and by the existence of contralateral pulmonary hypoplasia, especially in the neonatal period. It is recommended that treatment be carried out before acute respiratory distress develops, at which time emergency operation must be carried out.[34]

Because antenatal ultrasound is now routine, prenatal diagnosis is common[36] and has led to intrauterine drainage procedures in selected cases.

Postoperative Course

The postoperative course can be straightforward with recovery of a normal roentgenogram as soon as the operation is over. In such cases the drain is removed on the third or fourth day, when it stops functioning and contains merely a little yellowish serofibrinous liquid. Occasionally the course is more difficult, especially after a partial excision with a temporary air leak, which requires longer drainage time. After pneumonectomy, mediastinal equilibration can be of great concern, though this may be greatly improved by the installation of a prosthesis at surgery.

In difficult cases, particularly in the very small neonates and in the fatigued child, respiratory support should be used without hesitation during the first two days. It is important to insist on immediate postoperative physiotherapy and to continue it for several weeks in children who cannot cough satisfactorily. Complications are essentially due to superinfection, but with prenatal diagnosis and early treatment this is less common. In the majority of cases, there are no other sequellae except for a scar on the thorax.

REFERENCES

1. DeLarue J, Paillas J, Abelanet R, Chomette G: Les broncho-pneumopathies congénitales *Bronches* 1959;9:114–211.
2. Baudain P, Martin G: Les malformations congénitales des voies aériennes intrathoraciques de l'enfant. *Encycl Med Chir (Paris France) radio diagnostic III*, 1984;32496.
3. Gerbeaux J, Couvreur J, Tournier G: *Pathologie respiratoire de l'enfant.* Paris: Flammarion Médecine Sciences Édit., 1979.
4. Gerle RD, Jaretzki A, Ashley CA, Berne AS: Congenital bronchopulmonary foregut malformation: Pulmonary sequestration communicating with the gastrointestinal tract. *N Engl J Med* 1968;278:1413–1419.
5. Clements BS, Warner JO, Shinebourne EA: Congenital bronchopulmonary vascular malformations: Clinical application of a simple anatomical approach in 25 cases. *Thorax* 1987;42:409–416.
6. Clements BS, Warner JO: Pulmonary sequestration and related congenital broncho-pulmonary-vascular malformations: Nomenclature and classification based on anatomical and embryological considerations. *Thorax* 1987;42:401–408.
7. Ferre P, Courpotin C, Fourne JP: Kyste enterique et séquestration pulmonaire: Une association non fortuite à propos d'un cas. *Arch Fr Pediatr* 1985;42:455–458.
8. Pernot C, Simon P, Hoeffel JC, et al: Fistule artère systémique—veine pulmonaire—A propos d'une observation. *J Radiol* 1988;69:437–441.
9. Merlier M, Verley JM, Rochainzamir A, et al: Formes anatomocliniques des séquestrations pulmonaires. *Rev Prat* 1970;20:405.
10. Schilling B: Séquestration pulmonaire intralobaire à révèlation néonatale par une défaillance cardiorespiratoire. Université Jean Tonnet-Saint-Etienne; 1980. Thesis.
11. Savic B, Birtel FJ, Tholen W, et al: Lung sequestration: Report of seven cases and review of 540 published cases. *Thorax* 1979;34:96–101.
12. Bernard C, Hoeffel JC, Bretagne MC, et al: Séquestrations pulmonaires du sommet chez l'enfant à propos de 3 cas. *Ann Pediatr (Paris)* 1985;32:512–519.
13. Wimbish KJ, Aghaf P, Brady TM: Bilateral pulmonary sequestration: Computed tomographic appearance. *AJR* 1983;140:589–690.
14. Baker EL, Gore RM, Moss AA: Retroperitoneal pulmonary sequestration: Computed tomographic findings. *AJR* 1982;138:956–957.
15. Choplin RH, Siegel MJ: Pulmonary sequestration: Six unusual presentations. *AJR* 1980;134:695–700.
16. Colhin PP, DesJardins JG, Khan AH: Pulmonary sequestration. *J Pediatr Surg* 1987;22:750–753.
17. Cazaban A, Sarban S, Bacques O, Bonnard V: L'échotomographie dans les séquestrations pulmonaires postérobasales chez l'enfant—A propos de 8 enfants dont 4 séquestrations. *J Radio* 1987;68:39–44.
18. Kaude JV, Laurin S: Ultrasonographic demonstration of systemic artery feeding extrapulmonary sequestration. *Pediatr Radiol* 1984;14:226–227.
19. Stanley P, Vachon L, Gilsanz V: Pulmonary sequestration with congenital gastro-oesophageal communication—Report of two cases. *Pediatr Radiol* 1985;15:343–345.
20. Chirio R, Besancon MC, Lepercq G, Fortier-Beaulieu M: A propos d'une opacité thoracique postérobasale. *Arm Pediatr,* 1986;33:543–545.
21. Jaubert de Beaujeu M, Chavrier Y, Riou RJ, et al: Séquestrations pulmonaires chez l'enfant—A propos de 31 cas. *Lyon Chirurgical* 1982;78:11–16.
22. Jaubert de Beaujeu M, Chavrier Y: Duplications digestives—A propos de 2 kystes oesophagiens intra muraux. *Ann Chir Infant* 1974;5:15–22.
23. Konig R, Herold U: Nuclear magnetic resonance detection of a mediastinal bronchogenic cyst. *Radiology* 1986;26:464–466.
24. Dibden LJ, Fischer JD, Zuberbuhler PD: Pulmonary sequestration and congenital cystic adenomatoid malformation in an infant. *J Pediatr Surg* 1986;21:731–733.
25. Richard O, Teyssier G, Rayet I et al: Kystes Bronchogéniques comprimant la trachée, une cause inhabituelle de détresse respiratoire néonatale. *Pédiatrie* 1988;43:521–523.
26. Blaquet P: Kystes bronchogéniques comprimant la trachée et les bronches souches. *Chir Pédiatr* 1984;25:270–275.
27. Synder ME, Luck SR, Hernandez R, et al: Diagnostic dilemmas of mediastinal cysts. *J Pediatr Surg* 1985;20:810–815.
28. DiLorenzo M, Collin PP, Vaillancourt R, Duranceau A: Bronchogenic cysts. *J Pediatr Surg* 1989;24:988–991.
29. Maisonneuve D: Malformation adénomatoide pulmonaire—A propos de 22 observations. Université Claude Bernard-Lyon 1; 1985. Thesis.
30. Esposito G, DeLuca U, Cigliano B, et al: La malformation adénomateuse kystique congénitale du poumon. *Chir Pédiatr* 1985;26:321–342.
31. Adzick NS, Harrisson MR, Glick P et al: Fetal cystic adenomatoid malformation: Prenatal diagnosis and natural history. *J Pediatr Surg* 1985;20:483–488.
32. Buntain WL, Isaacs H, Paynev C, et al: Lobar emphysema, cystic adenomatoid malformation, pulmonary sequestration, and bronchogenic cyst in infancy and children: A clinical group. *J Pediatr Surg* 1974;9:85–93.
33. Stocker JT, Drake RH, Madwell JE: Cystic congenital lung disease in the newborn. In Rosenberg HS and Bolaride RP, eds. *Perspectives in Pediatric Pathology.* Vol 4. Chicago, Ill.: Year Book Medical Publishers, 1978:93–148.
34. Nishibayashi SW, Andrassy RJ, Wooley MM: Congénital cystic adenomatoid malformation: A 30-year experience. *J Pediatr Surg* 1981;16:704.
35. Chavrier Y, Gounot J, Gounot R, et al: Malformation adénomateuse kystique congénitale du poumon—A propos de 4 cas chez le nouveau-né. *Pediatrie* 1980;35:537–540.
36. Deffrenne P, Coicaud C, Pracros JP, et al: Malformation adénomatoide pulmonaire—Diagnostic prénatal. *Chir Pédiatr* 1985;26:287–294.

Intrapulmonary Lesions

Leon K. Lacquet, MD, FRCS(C)

The preceding chapter on intrapulmonary lesions, pulmonary sequestrations, bronchogenic cysts, and congenital cystic adenomatoid malformation (or, in general, lung bud anomalies) gives an excellent overview of the literature—though mainly the French literature—on embryology, clinical presentation, and surgical treatment of those interesting congenital lung anomalies.

I agree completely with the distinction between intralobar sequestration (ILS) and extralobar (ELS) sequestration, though I have also encountered atypical forms in my pediatric cardiac surgery practice. In the childhood series of Jaubert de Beaujeu et al[1] in 1982, there were only five cases of ELS (16%), apparently without pulmonary symptoms. In our much smaller series[2] of 5 children and eight adults in 1982 there were also 5 cases of ELS (38%), of which three were in children—two with pulmonary symptoms and one without—discovered fortuitously. Of the two adults with ELS, one presented pulmonary symptoms and in the other the anomaly was discovered by screening. Finally, all our patients with ILS presented pulmonary symptomatology. One adult of 38 years with pleurisy, and one adult of 60 years with empyema were treated in a sanatorium for pulmonary tuberculosis, though their sputum remained negative. This difference in incidence and symptomatology reflects the difference between a series with only children and a series with children and adults. Although there is an anatomical separation of the lung tissue and no bronchial communication in ELS, pulmonary infection is also possible via lymphatic or hematogenous pathways, and three of our five patients with ELS were symptomatic, in contrast with the literature.

© 1991 Elsevier Science Publishing Co., Inc.
655 Avenue of the Americas, New York, NY 10010
Current Topics in General Thoracic Surgery:
An International Series

Chavrier stresses the association of lung sequestration with other congenital malformations, especially with diaphragmatic hernia. In the series of Jaubert de Beaujeu et al[1] there were seven cases of diaphragmatic hernia, more with ELS than with ILS, as is reported in the literature. Of our five cases of ELS,[2] one child also had a pericardial defect and one child, a funnel chest. Lung sequestration and funnel chest are both congenital anomalies, and both are frequently associated with other anomalies, but their mutual association seems rare. In my series[3] of 210 operations for congenital deformities of the anterior chest wall, I encountered multiple other congenital anomalies. However, as far as lung bud anomalies are concerned, only one child with ELS and two cases with bronchial atresia and associated emphysema (one child and one adult) were encountered.

In that series a case of combined lung sequestration and funnel chest was in a boy 6 years of age with a long history of recurrent bronchopulmonary infections. A persistent shadow on the x-ray film, just above the right diaphragm, led to the suspicion of lung sequestration (Fig. D6.1). A Seldinger arteriography showed the abnormal artery from the thoracic aorta to the abnormal pulmonary tissue, and during the venous run-off there was opacification of the systemic azygos vein (Fig. D6.2). Thus, the diagnosis of ELS was established. Because of concern about adhesions and infection I elected for operative treatment in two stages. Via a right lateral thoracotomy I carried out the surgical resection of the abnormal sequestrated lung tissue (Fig. D6.3) by dividing and oversewing the abnormal vessels. The postoperative course was uneventful and some months later I corrected the funnel chest via a bilateral submammary incision, using my usual Daniel[4] technique, with excellent result (Fig. D6.4). At the first operation there were no adhesions and no signs of infection and the sequestration was completely free and easily re-

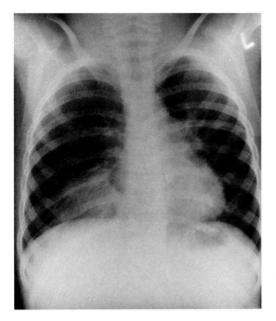

FIGURE D6.1 Frontal chest roentgenogram shows a persistent shadow above the right diaphragm.

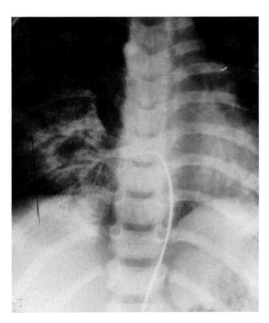

FIGURE D6.2 Seldinger arteriography shows an abnormal systemic artery from the thoracic descending aorta and venous run-off through the systemic azygos vein.

sectable. I regretted the decision to operate in two stages, as the sequestration could have been removed without complications via the funnel chest incision.

Interesting is Iwa and Watanabe's[5] paper, which reports 10 cases of pulmonary sequestration (9 children, 1 adult) with other anomalies. The low incidence of ELS (one case: 10%) in this Japanese series of anomalies with pulmonary sequestration is surprising. The case of ELS is associated with an esophageal duplication cyst. Another surprising observation is the absence of diaphragmatic hernia. Four children showed the unusual combination of ILS and funnel chest. Two were operated on by segmentectomy and sternoturnover,[6] one in two stages a month apart, and one had both procedures in the same operation. The two others underwent only lung resection as the thoracic deformity was mild and even improved afterward. Iwa and Watanabe suggest that there may be a connection between pulmonary sequestration and the formation of funnel chest, given that physiologic and anatomic factors combine in the formation of a funnel. They support their speculation by noting the improvement in the thoracic deformity following lung resection in two cases of mild deformity. I think that congenital anomalies are frequently associated without related cause and effect.

In the section on bronchogenic cysts, the intramural esophageal cyst merits more attention, as in the author's original publication with Jaubert de Beaujeu.[7,8] This cyst is rare and frequently asymptomatic. However, when in the also rare cervico mediastinal location between the trachea and the esophagus, an urgent operation can be necessary, as my colleagues and I[8] experienced in an adult patient.

A 57-year-old woman presented with acute dyspnea and stridor and was urgently intubated. A firm, smooth mass was palpated in the neck. On chest roentgenogram an opacity was seen at the thoracic inlet with dorsal compression of the trachea and right-sided displacement of the nasogastric and tracheal tube. Subsequently the patient was operated on through cervical and median sternal approaches. A smooth mass was found between the trachea and the proximal third of the esophagus. The cyst was opened and the wall almost entirely removed from its intramural esophageal location, without opening into the esophageal lumen. Histology revealed a cyst with esophageal lining and active inflammation.

This case was unusual in that the patient was asymptomatic for many years but needed an emergency operation when the cyst became acutely inflamed. Our experience confirms the in-

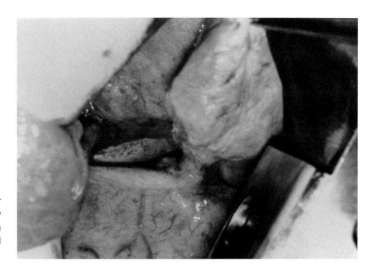

FIGURE D6.3 Operative view after right posterolateral thoracotomy shows sequestrated lung tissue in forceps pediculated on abnormal artery and vein.

creased risk of complications with age. Therefore, when a mediastinal mass is found, diagnosis and treatment should always be performed as recommended by Chavrier. Also, as shown in our case, esophageal mucosal injury must be avoided and I agree completely with Chavrier that some cystic wall without cystic mucosa should be left in situ. After removal of the intramural esophageal cyst there is a muscular defect and long term follow-up is indicated because esophagitis, without relation to the primary localization of the cyst, may develop. Salo and Ala-Kulju[9] speculate that the removal of the cyst may damage neurogenic and myogenic mechanisms.

Finally, in instances of aberrant right subclavian artery and dysphagia lusoria in children, my colleagues and I[10] favor the translocation of this vessel to the ascending aorta without graft interposition, thus reestablishing the normal flow in the subclavian artery.

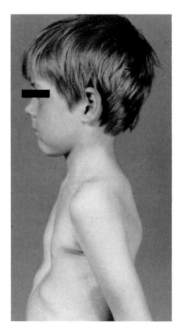
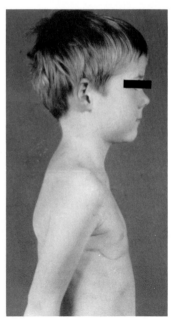

FIGURE D6.4 Left: 6-year-old boy with funnel chest and lung sequestration before operation. **Right:** Result 10 months after sequestrectomy and 5 weeks after corrective operation for funnel chest.

REFERENCES

1. Jaubert de Beaujeu M, Chavrier Y, Riou RJ, et al: Séquestrations pulmonaires chez l'enfant: A propos de 31 cas. *Lyon Chirurgical* 1982;78:11.
2. Koolen MGJ, Moulijn AC, Jongerius CM, Lacquet LK: Longsekwestratie. *Ned T Geneesk* 1982;126:1398.
3. Lacquet LK: Congenital deformities of the anterior chest wall. In: Delarue N, and Eschapasse H, eds. *International Trends in General Thoracic Surgery.* Vol. 2. Philadelphia, Penn: WB Saunders Co, 1987:328–337.
4. Daniel RA: The surgical treatment of pectus excavatum. *J Thorac Surg* 1958;35:719.
5. Iwa T, Watanabe Y: Unusual combination of pulmonary sequestration and funnel chest. *Chest* 1979;76:314.
6. Wada J, Ikeda T, Iwa T, et al: Sternoturnover: An advanced new surgical method to correct funnel chest deformity. *J Int Coll Surg* 1965;44:69.
7. Jaubert de Beaujeu M, Chavrier Y: Duplications digestives: à propos de deux kystes oesophagiens intra-muraux. *Ann Chir Inf* 1974;15:15.
8. Morshuis WJ, van Son JAM, Lacquet LK et al: Intramural esophageal cyst as a cause of acute respiratory distress. *Europ J Cardio-Thorac Surg* 1990; 4:454.
9. Salo JA, Ala-Kulju KV: Congenital esophageal cysts in adults. *Ann Thorac Surg* 1987;44:135.
10. Van Son JAM, Vincent JG, Van Oort A, Lacquet LK: Translocation of aberrant right subclavian artery in dysphagia lusoria in children through a right thoracotomy. *Thorac Cardiovasc Surg* 1989;37:52.

Chapter 7

Malformations of the Lung Mass

Jean-François Dyon, MD, Philippe Baudain, MD, and Jean-Pierre Alibeu, MD

Lung tissue malformations include various lung abnormalities (except for bronchial and vascular malformations, bronchogenic cysts, and extralobar pulmonary sequestrations). These lung tissue malformations may result in an increase in size of the whole, or part, of a lung—for instance, localized infantile pulmonary emphysema, which will be considered first. However, such abnormalities can also affect lung morphology, resulting in malformations such as complete lack of lung tissue (bilateral agenesis) or variations in lung segmentation and incisures.

CONGENITAL OR INFANTILE LOBAR EMPHYSEMA

Definition

Lobar emphysema is an anatomicopathological entity. It is a localized emphysematous distension of a pulmonary lobe and may be responsible for respiratory distress in the newborn or infant. Although this macroscopic definition is commonly accepted, there is no consensus concerning the classification of the different causative factors.[1] According to some authors[2] the primary anomaly is an alveolar parenchymal lesion. However, most authors believe that emphysema can also be due to more or less complete bronchial obstruction occurring early on. Moreover, the lobar characterization of this disease is thought to be inappropriate by some authors, who prefer the term *localized pulmonary emphysema;* indeed, its topography varies, affecting anything from a single segment to a whole lung.[3]

Historical Aspects

The first cases apparently were reported by Bartholinus (1687) and Kaufman (1904), but Nelson (1932) was really the first to have described this disease precisely. The earliest case reports insisted on the association between emphysema and cystic lesions. Cases of emphysema alone have been reported only since 1939, when it was noticed that the natural evolution of emphysema was not toward pulmonary cystic formation.[41] In 1943, Gross and Lewis[5] carried out the first curative lobectomy on a 4-year-old girl. Murray[4] analyzed 166 case reports published in English-language journals. In France, Binet et al[6] reported in 1974 the largest series of patients treated surgically (84 cases).

Topography

The upper lobe, especially on the left, is most frequently involved. The middle lobe is occasionally involved, but the lower lobe is involved only very rarely. Hendren and McKee[7] reviewed 113 cases and found the following distribution: left upper lobe 46: right upper lobe 24; right middle lobe 38; lower lobe 2; bilateral lesions 3. Murray[4] recorded 11 cases of lower lobe involvement in his analysis of 166 cases. Most reports confirm this distribution of lesions.

Pathological Anatomy and Pathogenesis

Macroscopically, the lobe is uniformly distended, smooth, pale, pink, and hypercrepitant and pillowy on palpation; it looks like a ball of moss. Even when the bronchus is widely open, the lobe does not usually deflate, confirming pulmonary air trapping.

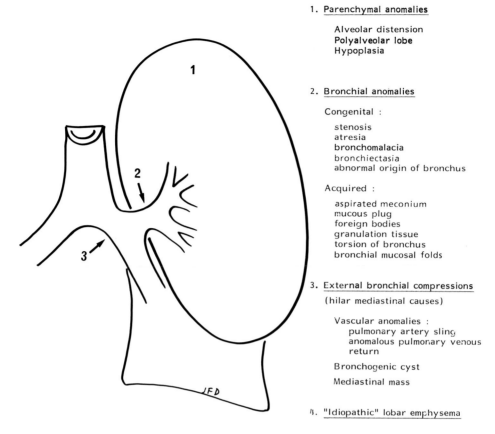

1. <u>Parenchymal anomalies</u>

   Alveolar distension
   Polyalveolar lobe
   Hypoplasia

2. <u>Bronchial anomalies</u>

   Congenital :

   stenosis
   atresia
   bronchomalacia
   bronchiectasia
   abnormal origin of bronchus

   Acquired :

   aspirated meconium
   mucous plug
   foreign bodies
   granulation tissue
   torsion of bronchus
   bronchial mucosal folds

3. <u>External bronchial compressions</u>
   (hilar mediastinal causes)

   Vascular anomalies :
   pulmonary artery sling
   anomalous pulmonary venous
   return

   Bronchogenic cyst

   Mediastinal mass

4. "Idiopathic" lobar emphysema

FIGURE 7.1 Causes of infantile lobal emphysema.

Histologically, there is alveolar distension without any structural anomalies. Nevertheless anatomical lesions are frequent. Some authors describe two different anatomical aspects of lobar emphysema: (1) typical giant lobar emphysema, with an increase in lobar volume, as described earlier (17/23 cases for Jaubert de Beaujeu and Chavrier[8]); and (2) giant bullous emphysema, with regular thin-walled bullae without any epithelium, within which are small fibers with small pulmonary vessels running along them, making it look like a "puffed doughnut" (6/23 cases).[8]

Classification of lobar emphysema has always been controversial because the original definition is imprecise.[9-10] Nowadays, most authors[2-12] include several mechanisms: a congenital origin is more than likely in the newborn and infant but quite uncertain in older patients. The following classification, subdividing the disease into two groups of pulmonary parenchymal and structural anomalies and primary bronchial anomalies, seems to be the one used most (Fig. 7.1):

1. Parenchymal lesions correspond to the classical definition. Reid[2] includes in this group so-called congenital lesions because these exist before birth and are linked to embryonic development. A polyalveolar lobe is an overdeveloped lobar mass, with normal alveolar and vascular histology and an excessive number of alveoli. This voluminous lobe will compress adjacent lung.[12-14] It may seem paradoxical to include localized lobar hypoplasia here; however, the affected lobe may be increased in size because of an increased air space, though the number of alveoli is reduced.[13] Other authors also include fibrous alveolitis with abnormal collagen accumulation on the alveolar wall (eg, Bolande's fibrous dysplasia).[15] Still other authors have recently considered some cases of congenital localized pulmonary lymphangiectasis as part of the group of lobar emphysema.

2. Lobar emphysema may also be secondary to obstructive bronchial lesions. These may be:
   a. Endoluminal, such as mucous plug, bron-

chial foreign body, or viscous secretions in the newborn.

b. Parietal, resulting in a unidirectional valve effect: mucosal folds, bronchial stenosis or kinking, or inflammation. The frequent lobar or segmental bronchial cartilage anomalies are responsible for obstructive emphysema by bronchomalacia. Cases of congenital bronchiectasis causing emphysema have even been described in the newborn.[16]

c. Extrinsic compression of the bronchus, either mediastinal or hilar. A mediastinal tumor, especially a bronchogenic cyst, can compress the main, or the upper lobe, bronchus. Other causes have been described: aortic arch malformations, aberrant blood vessels (aberrant left pulmonary artery), venous ectasia, and cardiomegaly due to cardiopathy. Some cases of compression of an ectopic tracheal bronchus by a normal blood vessel have also been reported.[17] Emphysema can also be due to an ectopic segmental bronchus implanted on the left main bronchus.[18]

3. Fifty percent of cases of emphysema are of unknown origin. Several different mechanisms may be involved. According to Demos and Teresi,[19] anomalies of bronchial cartilage are the most frequent etiology; they emphasized that precise histopathological examination of surgical specimens is needed to obtain better data concerning the etiological factors.

Although lobar emphysema is often the result of a lesion too vague to define precisely, it is the degree of localized hyperinflation that leads to the clinical symptoms that need to be treated. To conclude, there is ambiguity in the literature concerning the classification and etiology of the disease. Moreover, the limits between congenital emphysema, pulmonary adenomatoid malformation, pulmonary and bronchogenic cysts, and even some intralobar sequestrations can be difficult to define. In fact, some authors simply regroup these lesions into one common "clinical group."[19-22]

Incidence

The incidence of this disease is not well known. The sex ratio appears to be about 2 boys for 1 girl. Some familial cases have been described. Associated anomalies are rare but include cardiovascular malformations (14% of cases from Pierce et al),[23] ductus arteriosus, interventricular septal defect, pectus excavatum, and other bronchial, pulmonary and mediastinal malformations.

Clinical Features

Symptoms occur during the first days of life in 50% of cases and nearly always before the fourth month. The severity and time of onset of these symptoms depend on the degree of parenchymal distension. The lobe overinflates quickly by trapping inspired air, thus inducing homolateral lung compression and mediastinal displacement. There usually is no history of any birth trauma or antenatal maternal illness. There are intermittent and repetitive episodes of acute respiratory failure set off by feeding or crying. Clinical signs are not always uniform, and dyspnea, tachypnea, wheezing, coughing, and cyanosis are seen in the worst cases. Infections have not been reported. Physical findings often include recession of the intercostal spaces, hyperresonant percussion, and diminished breath sounds on the affected side. Unilateral distension of the chest may be seen in neonates and infants.

The plain chest roentgenogram is mandatory for diagnosis.[3] It shows overdistension of the affected lobe and reveals an asymmetry in parenchymal transparency with a hyperlucent zone. The distended lobe contains small blood vessel markings that are best seen in the peripheral zone; it compresses adjacent lung tissue, which is pushed flat against the mediastinum and in the lower part of the thorax. The diaphragmatic dome is lowered, and intercostal spaces are enlarged. These characteristics increase on expiration, confirming air trapping. Sometimes, the degree of distension can be such that the x-ray film shows what looks like a clear hemithorax, with contralateral hernia and mediastinal displacement. The presence of blood vessels within this distended lobe is an important radiological sign, distinguishing lobar emphysema from pulmonary cystic lesions and pneumothorax, in which peripheral bronchovascular markings are absent (Fig. 7.2).

It must be noted that the plain chest roentgenogram taken soon after birth can be particularly misleading: because of bronchoalveolar retention of amniotic fluid, it can show a distended lobe, full of fluid, which becomes radiolucent when the fluid is absorbed (Fig. 7.3).

In a few cases, the emphysema is due to bronchial atresia, especially in the left upper lobe.[24-26] Bronchial obstruction can cause emphysema by ventilation through collateral channels and interalveolar pores (Kohn's pores). Accumulation of postatretic secretions constitutes a bronchocele, which is radiologically recognizable.

Other investigations may need to be carried out, depending on the clinical picture:

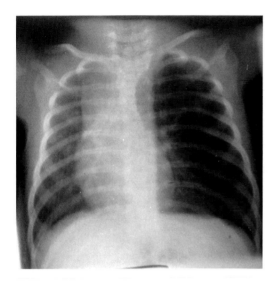

FIGURE 7.2 Giant lobar emphysema in a 2-month-old infant. Hyperlucent left hemithorax deviating the mediastinum to the right. Lung parenchyma pushed against the inferior part of the mediastinum. The signs are increased on the expiratory roentgenogram.

Esophagography can help to diagnose extrinsic compression, a mediastinal lesion, or an anomaly in a main bronchus.

Bronchography may also be of help if both inspiratory and expiratory films are taken, as long as there is no opacification of the distal bronchi. Bronchial lesions such as stenosis, bronchomalacia, atresia, extrinsic compression (most often by a bronchogenic cyst) can thus be diagnosed (Fig. 7.4).

Bronchoscopy, which can be carried out just before starting surgery, is often used to rule out other etiologies, especially intrabronchial foreign bodies.

Other investigation is not very useful unless other associated malformations—mostly cardiovascular—are suspected. When angiography is carried out, it can reveal stretched, displaced and compressed pulmonary vessels.

Computed tomography or magnetic resonance imaging can be of use in a few cases to help find hilar or mediastinal lesions, which are difficult to see.

The different age-dependent clinical forms must be considered separately because of their therapeutic implications.

Hyperacute neonatal respiratory distress is rare but life threatening. It appears and deteriorates very quickly. Clinical examination and a plain chest roentgenogram are enough to make the diagnosis. Conservative treatment is absolutely ineffective, and a fatal outcome can occur within a few hours. Surgery must therefore be performed immediately.

The usual course is one of progressive respiratory distress, which develops more slowly. It may appear during the first days of life, the clinical picture becoming worse relatively quickly, usually before the fourth month. Dyspnea is the main symptom, and a plain chest film should be ordered. Assessment of the patient should be

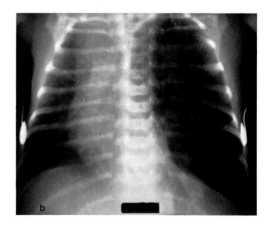

FIGURE 7.3 Giant lobar emphysema in a neonate. **A.** Left-sided lobar emphysema hidden by delayed resorption of amniotic fluid. The left hemithorax is blurred; there is deviation of the mediastinum and inferior lung parenchyma. The inferior and outer angle between the ribs and the diaphragm remains clear. **B.** A few hours later, the x-ray film shows signs of typical lobar emphysema involving the left upper lobe.

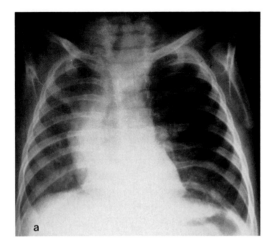

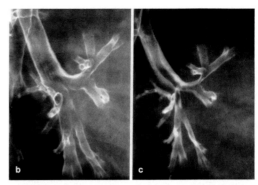

FIGURE 7.4 Left-sided pulmonary emphysema in a 6-month-old infant. **A.** Standard AP chest film. The entire left hemithorax is hyperlucent, with expiratory air trapping. **B.** Bronchography. Normal inspiratory film. **C.** Bronchography. Expiratory film: collapse of the distal end of the left main bronchus and of the proximal ends of the lobar bronchi. Diagnosis: primary bronchomalacia.

complete before deciding on the need for surgical treatment, which is almost always necessary.

Rarely, a chest roentgenogram can reveal asymptomatic forms in children (4% of cases) or adults. In these patients, the emphysema may regress spontaneously; treatment will depend on the clinical course, which requires careful monitoring. Lung function tests may be useful here.

Differential Diagnosis

This difficult clinical problem has to be solved for every case of respiratory distress; etiologies differ according to the patient's age.

In the first few days of life, a tension pneumothorax is the most serious pitfall, as this needs to be drained quickly. However, puncture or drainage of pulmonary emphysema will lead to an air leak or a serious pneumothorax. Diaphragmatic hernia must also be excluded; it produces bullous intestinal images within the thorax.

In the newborn, radiological features due to amniotic fluid inhalation can be confusing. Indeed, the compensatory emphysematous expansion adjacent to a zone of atelectasis can be misleading. Similarly, pulmonary agenesis or hypoplasia can lead to erroneous lesional and topographic diagnoses.

In infants and young children, the following lesions must be ruled out: intrabronchial foreign body, poststaphylococcal and postinfectious emphysema, pseudo-emphysematous unilateral hyperlucent lung,[27] pneumomediastinum, and congenital lung cyst. However, the main cause of error is attributable to localized emphysema resulting from distal inflammatory bronchial sten-

oses occurring after an infectious or a viral illness; this type of emphysema regresses slowly. When the diagnosis is not certain, it is the lack of clinical and radiological improvement that points to a malformative anomaly, and so to surgical treatment.

Treatment

A few cases of spontaneous regression have been reported, but morbidity and mortality would seem to be too high to accept this as current practice. However, it may be appropriate for asymptomatic patients. Eigen et al[28] reported 14 cases treated conservatively, resulting in a return to normal respiratory function in 12 cases within a period of five days to one year. Murray,[4] however, found a 50% mortality for conservative treatment, and 75% of the survivors had residual emphysema.

In most cases, emergency surgery is required, consisting of the removal of the emphysematous parenchyma. In young children, the respiratory distress can rapidly become life threatening, and one must be ready to carry out emergency thoracotomy. Most authors agree that chest puncture or drainage is contraindicated, except perhaps just before operation. Anesthesia is difficult to carry out, because it can worsen the respiratory distress syndrome by increasing pressure within the emphysematous lung. The surgeon must be gowned and have his or her instruments ready before induction of anesthesia. As soon as the lung has herniated out of the chest cavity, there usually is a spectacular respiratory improvement.

Lobectomy is to be preferred with respect to other possible techniques, such as segmentectomy or excision of the bullae. The bronchial pedicle can be easily dissected, as it is not inflammed, and the surgery will be quite simple. The remaining lung parenchyma will then be able to expand to its normal volume. The thoracotomy wound can then be closed over one or two pleural drains with an underwater seal on low suction. The postoperative course is usually smooth if the lesion was single and there was no sepsis.

In the rare cases of bilateral lobar emphysema, both sides should be operated on together for definitive cure, so as to avoid possible contralateral worsening when one side is operated on before the other.[6-29]

Even more rarely, a conservative surgical procedure may be possible: removal of a mucous plug by bronchotomy or partial bronchial resection in case of stenosis. However, treatment of the bronchial lesion may not cure the emphysema, in which case removal of the emphysematous lung tissue will be necessary.

Treatment Results

Results of treatment are generally satisfactory. Long-term follow-up results are good in most cases. There was 7% mortality in Murray's review of 166 patients.[4] Nevertheless, some children presented with minor chronic bronchial problems, which were made worse by respiratory tract infections.

In the last few years, cases of "acquired" lobar emphysema have been reported. These were premature infants with a respiratory distress syndrome treated by long-term mechanical ventilation. There is interstitial and often diffuse emphysema. Occasionally, an affected segment or lobe may require removal. In 20 cases reported by Martinez-Frontanilla et al,[30] results were good for 14 patients with localized lesions (11 recoveries, 1 failure, 2 deaths); diffuse forms had a much worse prognosis: 5 of 6 patients died. This condition is a result of progress in neonatal intensive care.

Lobar emphysema almost always requires surgical excision, but treatment must be guided by the volume of the emphysematous lung and the degree of pulmonary compression. Its acquired or congenital origin is not always very clear.

DEFICIENT LUNG PARENCHYMA DEVELOPMENT

The malformations in this group are due to a congenital deficiency in lung tissue development. No classification is completely satisfactory, as it depends on organogenesis, pathogenesis, and clinical and radiological features (Table 7.1). Schneider and Schwalbe's[31] classification is the most useful; it distinguishes among *agenesis:* a complete absence of bronchus, pulmonary tissue and blood vessels; *aplasia:* a bronchial stump without any parenchyma or pulmonary vessels (the difference between agenesis and aplasia is only radiological and endoscopic); and *hypoplasia:* poor lung development (this term is imprecise).

Agenesis and Aplasia

Here, the lung is completely absent, on one or on both sides. Due to a defect in subdivision of the growing lung bud, agenesis and aplasia are always associated with a lack of arterial and venous vessels (Fig. 7.5).[2,3,32]

The causative agent is not known; most likely, it is due to a problem during organogenesis. Nevertheless, this anomaly has been described in monozygotic twins and in cases of chromosomal defects, such as trisomy 18. Experimentally, pulmonary agenesis has been produced in the offspring of rats fed a vitamin A-deficient diet.[33]

Bilateral lung agenesis is extremely rare, 10 cases only having been reported in the world literature.[34] It is a lethal malformation which corresponds to agenesis of the distal trachea.

Unilateral lung agenesis is more frequent: about 250 cases have been reported so far.[35] True agenesis and aplasia can be combined in this group, because the result is the same. In 80 cases reported by Delarue et al, there were 43 cases of agenesis and 37 of aplasia.[36]

Anatomically, the pulmonary blood vessels are always absent, because their development depends on bronchial organogenesis. The hemithorax is filled by heart and mediastinal structures. The pleura is often absent. The opposite lung often has abnormal segmentation and is hypertrophied, though the number of bronchial subdivisions may be reduced. According to some authors, however, even though the number of al-

TABLE 7.1 Factors Influencing Pulmonary Developmental Arrest

1. Bronchial developmental fault
   → agenesis
   → aplasia
2. Pulmonary vessels developmental fault
   → harmonious lung hypoplasia
3. Extrinsic factors of lung compression
   → localized hypoplasia
4. Unknown

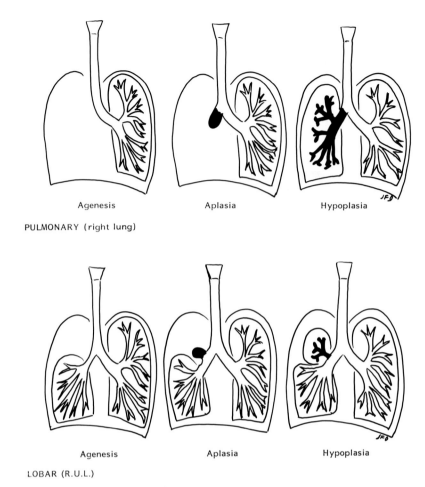

Agenesis   Aplasia   Hypoplasia

PULMONARY (right lung)

Agenesis   Aplasia   Hypoplasia

LOBAR (R.U.L.)

FIGURE 7.5 Developmental arrests in the lung.

veoli is twice the usual number, the total number of alveoli is in fact what it should have been with two normal lungs.[37]

The sex ratio varies from author to author as does the incidence of the commonly involved side, though it would seem to be predominantly left-sided. Associated malformations are common, being present in 50% to 70% of cases. They occur mostly in cases of right-sided pulmonary agenesis. In decreasing order of incidence, these include malformations of the heart and great vessels; malformations of bones (hemivertebrae, fused ribs); malformations of the alimentary canal (tracheoesophageal fistula, esophageal atresia, imperforate anus); and malformations of the urogenital tract. Some cases of lung agenesis also have agenesis of the diaphragm.[38]

Clinical Features

Most cases are diagnosed postmortem in neonates who died soon after birth. Only half the patients with lung agenesis survive, mostly when there is no other associated malformation. In those that survive, the condition is generally discovered radiologically. A plain chest x-ray film is taken for diagnosis of a lung infection, exertional dyspnea, a suspected malformation, or as a routine investigation. In fact, agenesis may be asymptomatic. In the neonate, the thorax often appears normal, because the single lung has expanded to fill almost both sides of the chest. However, in the older child, there often is asymmetry, with scoliosis, displaced heart sounds, absent breath sounds on one side, and an apparently distended normal side.

The chest roentgenogram shows a dark, retracted hemithorax.[3] The cardiac shadow is included within this opacity, and a transmediastinal hernia of the lung to the opposite side is often seen. This picture can make one think this is a small, air-filled lung (Fig. 7.6). The diaphragm is raised, and the intercostal spaces are variably

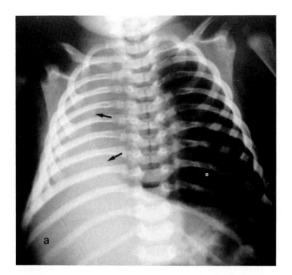
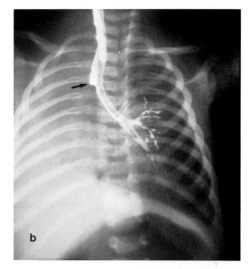

FIGURE 7.6 Right-sided lung aplasia. **A.** Standard film. Dark retracted hemithorax, which includes the cardiac and mediastinal shadows. Transmediastinal hernia due to a compensatory hypertrophy of the left lung. (→) **B.** Bronchography. Opacification of a right-sided bronchial dead-end. (→)

narrowed. It is important to make a radiological diagnosis, especially when there is an associated malformation requiring urgent surgical treatment, such as an esophageal atresia. The congenital origin of this picture must also be determined; associated vertebral and rib malformations tend to indicate this. The differential diagnosis includes atelectasis, bronchial obstruction by foreign body or tumor, and sometimes lobar or pulmonary emphysema on the opposite side in a neonate or infant; rarely, this picture can suggest complete lung sequestration, with agenesis of the main bronchus, systemic blood vessels being present, or sequestration in the presence of an esophageal bronchus.[38]

Other investigations are mandatory: esophagography, to rule out a lung sequestrated esophageal bronchus; bronchography to make the diagnosis and label the anomaly agenesis or, when there is a bronchial diverticulum, aplasia; bronchoscopy; and lung function tests to assess the functional status of the lung.

One must look for other associated malformations. The lung vasculature on the other side must be studied; a cardiopathy with a pathological shunt must be sought using cardiac ultrasonography, electrocardiography, computerized tomography, nuclear magnetic resonance imaging, or angiography. In unilateral pulmonary agenesis there are never pulmonary blood vessels on the affected side.

Treatment consists of the prevention and cure of possible lung infections. Surgery is of little use but can be indicated to treat tracheobron-chial compressions by abnormal or deviated blood vessels, or for resecting a chronically infected bronchial diverticulum in aplasia.[39] The presence of a single lung must be known before surgery is carried out for an associated malformation, such as a tracheoesophageal fistula or esophageal atresia, because there is an important risk of respiratory distress during the operation.[40] In some cases, cardiac and mediastinal displacement is poorly tolerated, and an intrathoracic prosthesis may be required to restore equilibrium.

Prognosis is poor in most cases, as patients die from respiratory infections; these are always very serious in a patient with a single lung.

Segmental or Lobar Agenesis and Aplasia

Segmental or lobar agenesis and aplasia are rather rare, and probably remain undetected or classified as hypoplasia. Indeed, they are asymptomatic when no other malformations are associated.[3]

The radiological picture is one of a small lung of reduced volume on one side, with a raised diaphragm and narrowed intercostal spaces (Fig. 7.7). There are differences according to the side involved: a right-sided agenesis is partially filled in by fibrous tissue, which obscures the right side of the heart shadow; this fibrous band is best seen on the lateral film. A left-sided agenesis makes the left side of the heart shadow more visible, and the fibrous tissue itself is less visible. This

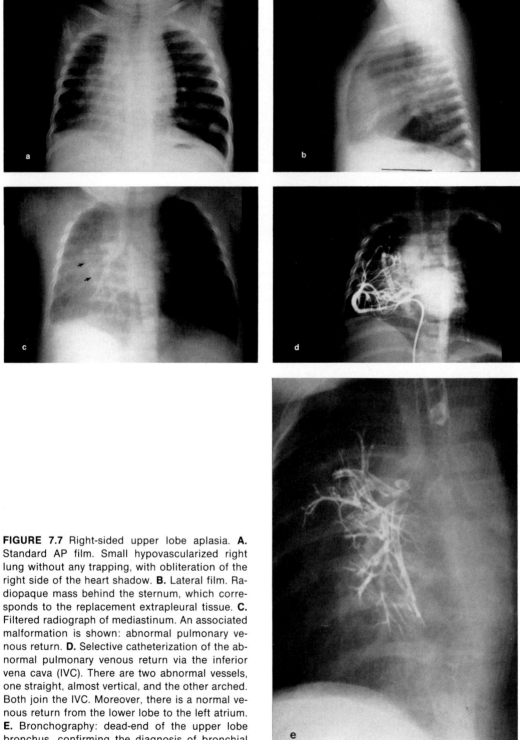

FIGURE 7.7 Right-sided upper lobe aplasia. **A.** Standard AP film. Small hypovascularized right lung without any trapping, with obliteration of the right side of the heart shadow. **B.** Lateral film. Radiopaque mass behind the sternum, which corresponds to the replacement extrapleural tissue. **C.** Filtered radiograph of mediastinum. An associated malformation is shown: abnormal pulmonary venous return. **D.** Selective catheterization of the abnormal pulmonary venous return via the inferior vena cava (IVC). There are two abnormal vessels, one straight, almost vertical, and the other arched. Both join the IVC. Moreover, there is a normal venous return from the lower lobe to the left atrium. **E.** Bronchography: dead-end of the upper lobe bronchus, confirming the diagnosis of bronchial aplasia.

This differs from the radiological picture given by bronchial atresia, as there is no bronchocele.

Important and useful investigations include a bronchography, to look for a missing lobar bronchus, or an aplastic cul-de-sac.[5] Other associated malformations, especially cardiovascular ones, must be sought. A missing lobar or segmental pulmonary artery is demonstrated by angiography. An anomalous pulmonary venous return (scimitar syndrome) is quite frequent. Nowadays, nuclear magnetic resonance imaging sometimes replaces angiography. Treatment is linked to pulmonary infection, bronchial pathology, and cardiovascular abnormalities.

Pulmonary Hypoplasia

The definition of pulmonary hypoplasia remains imprecise in the literature. The lesion is usually said to be a reduced number of alveoli and bronchial subdivisions. Some authors[36] also include in this group of abnormalities poor differentiation of lung parenchyma. This remains controversial, because these lesions are mostly made up of cystic dysplasias or adenomatoid malformations, dealt with elsewhere. At present, most authors agree in defining pulmonary hypoplasia as a defect in lung parenchyma development with a reduced number of bronchiolalveolar units.

The anatomical characterization of this malformation is often difficult and variable. The principal diagnostic techniques described in the literature are[34]: the ratio of lung weight to total body weight; the radial alveolar count; and the most sophisticated method for determining lung growth, the study of lung DNA with gestational age. There is hypoplasia when there is less than 100 mg lung DNA per kilogram weight. All these require advanced histopathological methods.

Classification

Isolated pulmonary hypoplasia: According to Luck,[33] this rather rare lesion is primary if there are no other lesions. Death of the neonate can be expected. Histopathological studies show an important reduction in lung volume, as well as a hypertrophy of the pulmonary arterial smooth muscle which has not undergone normal postnatal involution. The number of alveoli, alveolar ducts and bronchioles are reduced. Death occurs rapidly because of persisting fetal circulation, with pulmonary arterial hypertension.

Pulmonary hypoplasia associated with another lesion: This is the more common type. Luck considers it secondary.[33] Anything that reduces the size of the fetal chest cavity can cause pulmonary hypoplasia. Oligohydramnios is the chief cause and this is confirmed by experimental procedures.[41-43] Pulmonary hypoplasia is seen after

TABLE 7.2 Etiologic Factors in Pulmonary Hypoplasia

Intrathoracic mass with compression effect
Extrathoracic compression of thorax
Abnormal or absent fetal breathing movements
Decreased blood flow to the lung
Primary mesodermal defect
Unknown

(Reprinted from Stocker, 1988,[34] with permission.)

a leak of amniotic fluid has occurred or after its production has been reduced by a fetal urethral obstruction. Clinically, this is a well-known fact: major bilateral pulmonary hypoplasia is seen in patients with renal agenesis or dysplasia due to fetal compression (Potter's syndrome). Any thoracic compression, rigidity, or reduction in the size of the chest can give rise to more or less severe pulmonary hypoplasia. The list of possible causes is long. However, it probably is of multifactorial origin.

Anatomical studies have shown that there is delayed alveolar and bronchiolar growth, anomalous vascular growth, and a delay in maturation such that neonates may develop hyaline membrane disease. (Tables 7.2 and 7.3).

TABLE 7.3 Anomalies Associated with Pulmonary Hypoplasia

Frequent
    Diaphragmatic hernia
    Renal agenesis, bilateral
    Renal dysgenesis, bilateral
    Obstructive uropathy
    Renal polycystic disease
Unusual
    Diaphragmatic hypoplasia or eventration
    Extralobar pulmonary sequestration
    Hemolytic disease
    Musculoskeletal abnormalities such as thoracic dystrophies
    Oligohydramnios caused by prolonged amniotic fluid leakage
    Chromosomal including trisomy 13, 18, 21
    Anencephaly
    Scimitar syndrome
Rare
    Pleural effusion
    Ascites secondary to congenital infection
    Thoracic neuroblastoma
    Phrenic nerve agenesis
    Right-sided cardiovascular malformation as with hypoplastic right heart
    Gastroschisis
    Upper-cervical spinal cord injury
    Laryngotracheoesophageal cleft

(Reprinted from Stocker, 1988,[34] with permission.)

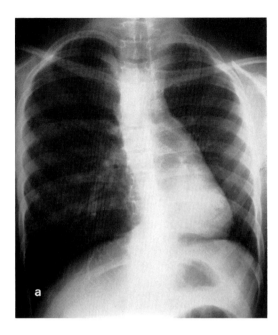

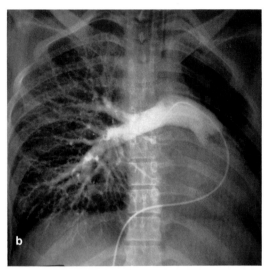

FIGURE 7.8 Harmonious left-sided lung hypoplasia associated with a deficient vasculature. **A.** Standard AP film. There is a small clear left lung, with right-sided compensatory hypervascularity. A right-sided aorta and the lack of a left-sided pulmonary arterial bulge leads to the diagnosis of absent left pulmonary artery. **B.** Pulmonary angiography, AP film. Lack of opacification of the left pulmonary artery.

Clinical features

The diagnosis may be suspected during pregnancy from changes in the ultrasonic image of lung parenchyma.[44] The diagnosis may also be suspected when there is evidence of lung compression, such as a cystic mass within the chest, a liquid effusion,[45] a diaphragmatic hernia, oligohydramnios, or a small chest. The best criterion for diagnosis and prognosis is a reduced fetal circumference, in the absence of an intrathoracic effusion.[46] The amplitude of respiratory movements does not seem to be a useful sign.[47,48]

After birth, the clinical picture is variable. In the most serious forms, death is immediate or very quick. The diagnosis of bilateral neonatal hypoplasia has been suggested by Schwishuk et al[49] for the combination of early respiratory distress, early and repeated pneumothoraces, with an x-ray picture of a small hyperlucent lung, associated with signs of refractory hypoxemia and persisting fetal circulation. On the other hand some forms of pulmonary hypoplasia are asymptomatic.

The diagnosis here is mainly radiological. The plain chest roentgenogram shows a reduced unilateral or bilateral lung volume, often associated with a reduced pulmonary vasculature, giving a hyperlucent lung. There often are as-

sociated abnormalities.[50–53] Other investigations must be carried out in accordance with the clinical picture (Fig. 7.8).

Treatment

This is most difficult, especially when there is neonatal respiratory distress. Knowing the diagnosis before birth allows for better immediate neonatal care. Resuscitative measures are usually required; all the modern techniques of mechanical respiration may be used to improve oxygen transport and eliminate the persisting fetal circulation (high frequency ventilation, pulmonary dilators, extracorporeal membrane oxygenation). Treating associated malformations, such as diaphragmatic hernia, may be a great help.

Prognosis

Outcome cannot be predicted. Patients with severe pulmonary hypoplasia die quickly, despite treatment. However, some patients do well; the decrease in pulmonary volumes seems to lessen with growth, at least until the age of 2 to 3 years. The pediatrician is still somewhat at a loss when faced with severe pulmonary hypoplasia. Attempts at fetal surgery—for example, to remove an obstruction in utero—cannot yet be carried out, and the deficient parenchyma appears too early on to hope for recovery.

ABNORMAL LUNG SEGMENTATION

These are usually asymptomatic, except when they are associated with other lesions[34]: pulmonary isomerism with asplenia or polysplenia; an azygos lobe associated with an anomalous bronchial insertion, which may lead to lung pathology[54]; horseshoe lung; ectopic lung.

Horseshoe lung is rare[55] and is similar to the horseshoe kidney. The two lungs are fused in the middle behind the heart. Distribution of the bronchi and blood vessels is sometimes abnormal; venous drainage can look like the scimitar syndrome. Surgical separation of the two lungs is recommended, though it may sometimes lead to vascular dysfunction because of the abnormal vascular supply.

Ectopic lung is also very rare. Acquired herniation of the lung outside the thoracic cavity is seen mostly in adults (emphysema, chronic cough, asthma). In the newborn, however, it is extremely rare: cervical ectopia has been described in some multiple anomaly syndromes (iniencephaly, Klippel-Feil syndrome, cat's cry syndrome), as has protrusion through the diaphragm. Although an accessory pulmonary lobe can also exist, this is more of an extralobar pulmonary sequestration.

ACKNOWLEDGMENT

The authors wish to thank Dr. N. Drouet, MA (Cantab.) for his very valuable assistance in reading and correcting the manuscript.

REFERENCES

1. Gerbeaux J, Couvreur J, Tournier G: Emphysème lobaire congénital. In: *Pathologie respiratoire de l'enfant.* Paris; Flammarion Ed., 1979;146–148.
2. Reid L: The lung: Its growth and remodeling in health and disease. *AJR* 1977;129:777–788.
3. Baudain P, Martin G: Les malformations congénitales des voies aériennes intrathoraciques de l'enfant. *Encycl Méd-Chir (Paris). Radiodiagnostic III,* 1984;32496A10.
4. Murray GF: Congenital lobar emphysema. *Surg Gynecol Obstet* 1967;124:611–625.
5. Gross RE, Lewis JE: Defects of the anterior mediastinum. *Surg Gynecol Obstet* 1945;80:549–554.
6. Binet JP, Langlois J, Miranda A, et al.: Le traitement chirurgical des emphysèmes pulmonaires malformatifs: A propos de 84 cas opérés. *Ann Chir Thorac Cardiovasc* 1974;13:109–112.
7. Hendren HW, McKee DM: Lobar emphysema of infancy. *J Pediatr Surg* 1966;1:24–39.
8. Jaubert de Beaujeu M, Chavrier Y: Emphysème pul-
monaire de l'enfant. *Ann Chir Thorac Cardiovasc* 1974;13:119–122.
9. Luck SR: Congenital bronchopulmonary malformation. *Curr Probl Surg* 1986;23:256–275.
10. Gray SW, Skandalakis JE: Congenital pulmonary lobar emphysema: Congenital cysts of the lung. In: *Embryology for Surgeons.* Philadelphia, Penn: WB Saunders, 1972.
11. Binet JP: Grandes cavités aériennes, d'origine dystrophique de l'enfant et du nourrisson. *Ann Chir Thorac Cardiovasc* 1962;1:1107–1139.
12. Hislop A, Reid L: New pathological finding emphysema in childhood: 1. Polyalveolar lobe with emphysema. *Thorax* 1970;25:682–690.
13. Hislop A, Reid L: New pathological finding in emphysema in childhood: 2. Overinflation of a normal lobe. *Thorax* 1971;26:190–194.
14. Munnell ER, Lambird PA, Austin RL: Polyalveolar lobe causing lobar emphysema of infancy. *Ann Thorac Surg* 1973;16:624.
15. Bolande RB, Schneider AF, Bogg SJB: Infantile lobar emphysema. *Arch Pathol* 1956;61:289.
16. Shafir R, Jaffe R, Kalter Y: Bronchiectasis: A cause of infantile lobar emphysema. *J Pediatr Surg* 1976;11:107–108.
17. Canty TG: Congenital lobar emphysema resulting from bronchial sling around a normal right main pulmonary artery. *J Thorac Cardiovasc Surg* 1977;74:126–129.
18. Foster-Carter AF: Bronchopulmonary abnormalities. *Br J Tuberc* 1946;40:111–124.
19. Demos NU, Teresi A: Congenital lung malformations: A unified concept and a case report. *J Thorac Cardiovasc Surg* 1975;70:260–264.
20. Buntain WL, Issacs H, Payne VC Jr, et al: Lobar emphysema cystic adenomatoid malformation, pulmonary sequestration, and bronchogenic cyst in infancy and childhood: A clinical group. *J Pediatr Surg* 1974;9:85–93.
21. Wesley JR, Heidelberger KP, Dipietro MA, et al: Diagnosis and management of congenital cystic disease of the lung in children. *J Pediatr Surg* 1986;21:202–207.
22. Haller JA, Golladay ES, Pickard LR, et al: Surgical management of lung bud anomalies: Lobar emphysema, bronchogenic cyst, cystic adenomatoid malformation, and intralobar pulmonary sequestration. *Ann Thorac Surg* 1979;28:33–43.
23. Pierce WS, Deparedes CG, Friedman S, Waldhausen JA: Concomitant congenital heart disease and lobar emphysema in infants: Incidence, diagnosis, and operative management. *Ann Surg* 1970;172:951.
24. Remy J, Ribet M, Pagnez B, et al: L'atrésie bronchique segmentaire. *Ann Radiol* 1973;16:615–618.
25. Schuster SR, Harris GBC, Williams A, et al: Bronchial atresia: A recognizable entity in the pediatric age group. *J Pediatr Surg* 1978;13:682–688.
26. Revillon Y, Brocard M, Scheinmann P, et al: Hyperclartés pulmonaires de l'enfant par sténose ou atrésie bronchique. *Chir Pédiatr* 1982;23:321–324.
27. Wiseman DH: Unilateral pseudoemphysema: A case report. *Pediatrics* 1965;35:300.
28. Eigen H, Lemen RJ, Waring WW: Congenital lobar emphysema: Long term evaluation of surgically and conservatively treated children. *Ann Rev Respir Dis* 1976;113:823–831.
29. Ekkelkamp S, Vos A: Successful surgical treatment

of a newborn with bilateral congenital lobar emphysema. *J Pediatr Surg* 1987;22:1001–1002.

30. Martinez-Frontanilla LA, Hernandez J, Haase GM, Burrington JD: Surgery of acquired lobar emphysema in the neonate. *J Pediatr Surg* 1984;19:375–379.

31. Schneider P, Schwalbe E: Die Morphologie der Missbildungen des Menschen und der Thiere. Iena: Gustav Fisher Publishers, 1912;3:817–822.

32. Baudain P, Martin G: Les malformations vasculaires du poumon de l'enfant. *Encycl Méd-Chir (Paris). Radiodiagnostic III,* 1987;32330A30.

33. Luck SR: The small or absent lung. *Curr Probl Surg* 1986;23:273–284.

34. Stocker JT: Congenital and development diseases. In Dail DH, Hammar SP, eds. *Pulmonary Pathology.* New York: Springer-Verlag, 1988;41–71.

35. Maltz DL, Nadas AS: Agenesis of the lung: Presentation of eight new cases and review of the literature. *Pediatrics* 1968;42:175–187.

36. Delarue J, Paillas J, Abelanet R, Chomette G: Les bronchopneumopathies congénitales. *Bronches* 1959;9:114.

37. Sbokos CG, McMillan IKR: Agenesis of the lung. *Br J Dis Chest* 1977;71:183–197.

38. Dyon JF, de Marliave H, Bacle B, Bensalah S: Les fistules aéro-digestives congénitales rares. *Chir Pédiatr* 1984;25:234–244.

39. Harrison MR, Heldf GP, Brusch RC, et al: Resection of distal tracheal stenosis in a baby with agenesis of the lung. *J Pediatr Surg.* 1980;15:938–943.

40. Black PR, Welch J: Pulmonary agenesis (aplasia) esophageal atresia and tracheoesophageal fistula: A different treatment strategy. *J Pediatr Surg* 1986;21:936–938.

41. Nakayama DK, Glick PL, Harrison MR, et al: Experimental pulmonary hypoplasia due to oligohydramnios and its reversal by relieving thoracic compression. *J Pediatr Surg* 1983;18:347–353.

42. Adzick NS, Harrison MR, Glick PL, et al: Experimental pulmonary hypoplasia and oligohydramnios: Relative contribution of lung fluid and fetal breathing movements. *J Pediatr Surg* 1984;19:658–665.

43. Van Dongen PWJ, Antonissen J, Jongha HW, et al: Lethal lung hypoplasia in infants after prolonged rupture of membranes. *Eur J Obstet Reprod Biol* 1987;25:287–292.

44. Droulle P, Didier F, Devaux MA, Hoeffel JC: Diagnostic échographique des images liquidiennes intrathoraciques chez le foetus (en dehors des anomalies cardiovasculaires). *Méd italique* 1986;93:519–532.

45. Castillo RA, Devoe LD, Falls G, et al: Pleural effusions and pulmonary hypoplasia. *Am J Obstet Gynecol* 1987;157:1252–1255.

46. Nimrod C, Nicholson S, Davies D, et al: Pulmonary hypoplasia testing in clinical obstetrics. *Am J Obstet Gynecol* 1988;158:277–280.

47. Songster GS, Gray DL, Crane JP: Prenatal prediction of lethal pulmonary hypoplasia using ultrasonic fetal chest circumference. *Obstet Gynecol* 1989;73:261–266.

48. Moessinger AC, Fox HE, Higgin SA, et al: Fetal breathing movements are not a reliable predictor of continued lung development in pregnancies complicated by oligohydramnios. *Lancet* 1987;1297–1300.

49. Swischuk LE, Richardson CJ, Nichols MM, Ingmann MJ: Primary pulmonary hypoplasia in the neonate. *J Pediatr* 1979;95:573–577.

50. Rossignol AM, Dyon JF, Vailloud G, et al: Artère pulmonaire gauche aberrante associée à une hypoplasie pulmonaire droite et à une communication interventriculaire. *Arch Mal Coeur* 1989;82:803–806.

51. Boulley AM, Imbert MC, Dehan M, et al: Hypoplasie pulmonaire bilatérale du nouveau-né. Etude clinique et anatomo-pathologique. A propos de 17 cas. *Arch Fr Pédiatr* 1982;39:423–428.

52. Gordon I, Helms P: Investigating the small lung: Which imaging procedure? *Arch Dis Child* 1982;57:696–701.

53. Pena SDJ, Shokeir MHK: Syndrome of camptodactyly, multiple ankyloses, facial anomalies, and pulmonary hypoplasia. *J Pediatr* 1974;85:373.

54. Dyon JF, Gout JP, Baudain P, Sarrazin R: A propos d'une association rare: Lobe azygos et anomalie d'implantation bronchique. *Chir Pediatr* 1980;21:209–213.

55. Orzem F, Angelini P, Oglietti J, et al: Horseshoe lung: Report of two cases. *Am Heart J,* 1977;93:501–505.

Malformations of the Lung Mass

Kathryn D. Anderson, MD

This is an excellent overview of congenital malformations of the lung and presents a logical classification for them. Dyon et al rightly state that it is not possible to draw a distinction between a primary anomaly of parenchyma or a bronchial obstruction occurring early in development with congenital lobar emphysema. In cases where the infant presents in severe respiratory difficulty, bronchography—which the authors advocate to define the lesions—may be hazardous, as may bronchoscopy. It is important to have an operating room immediately available if either of these studies are contemplated and I believe one should rely on the radiologist to rule out other lesions such as pulmonary artery sling. Bronchial foreign body is extremely rare in the newborn and in small infants. If the presence or absence of foreign body is uncertain, it is important to undertake bronchoscopy with the patient breathing naturally and not under positive pressure ventilation, which may well make the emphysema worse.

It is my experience that drainage of pulmonary emphysema is not possible by thoracentesis. The characteristic of congenital lobar emphysema is that the lung will not deflate even if extrapleural air is introduced. I believe, therefore, that temporary alleviation of respiratory distress is not possible by introducing extrapleural air, and emergency surgery is often the only alternative. In the differential diagnosis of this lesion, specific areas of emphysema are occasionally seen secondary to air trapping when the infant is being ventilated with high inflating pressures for other causes of respiratory distress, such as hyaline membrane disease (respiratory distress syndrome). This differential diagnosis is usually obvious, because the baby with congenital lobar emphysema prior to the onset of the air trapping is usually breathing spontaneously and does not need ventilation for other problems. In the case of respiratory distress syndrome, localized emphysema can usually be treated conservatively, because air trapping is not as severe as with the congenital form. If necessary, an endotracheal tube may be placed in the bronchus of the unaffected lung until the trapped air is reabsorbed. This does not work with the congenital type.

The discussion of agenesis and aplasia of the lung is excellent. For patients who do survive, this anomaly must be followed long term because absence of the lung on one side will cause scoliosis to develop in the spine as unequal growth of the chest occurs. Various prostheses have been proposed to act as space-occupying areas in the chest, including the most recent tissue expanders, which can gradually be increased in size as the patient grows, so long-term follow-up is clearly necessary to see if these prostheses do in fact help.

Hypoplasia of the lung is a rare condition as a single entity and, as the authors state, is often associated with other causes, such as maldevelopment of the kidneys with resulting oligohydramnios. Perhaps the commonest cause of lung hypoplasia is congenital diaphragmatic hernia in which the ipsilateral lung is markedly hypoplastic but the contralateral lung also has varying degrees of hypoplasia. This lesion is far more common than isolated hypoplasia and is far more amenable to treatment associated with hypoplastic kidneys. The authors do mention the treatment of hypoplasia, including extracorporeal membrane oxygenation. Because hypoplastic lung vasculature seems to be extremely vulnerable to hypoxia, there is often a component of persistent pulmonary hypertension associated with them, and this is probably the only component that can be successfully treated with extracorporeal oxygenation. Nonetheless, it is useful to diminish this component and may in fact allow time for the hypoplastic lungs to grow and expand after birth. In the future, it may be useful as a bridge to lung transplantation for hypoplasia incompatible with life. At the present time, this is in experimental stages only but may well have a place in the armamentarium of the surgeon in the not-too-distant future.

655 Avenue of the Americas, New York, NY 10010
Current Topics in General Thoracic Surgery:
An International Series

Chapter 8

Esophageal Atresia, Tracheoesophageal Fistula, and Complications

Arnold G. Coran, MD

The common form of esophageal atresia—namely, esophageal atresia with distal tracheoesophageal fistula—was first described in 1697 by Thomas Gibson,[1] though in 1670 William Durston[2] provided the first description of congenital esophageal atresia. Management by nonsurgical means resulted in 100% mortality over the next $2\frac{1}{2}$ centuries.

A surgical approach to this entity awaited the development of thoracic surgery as a specific discipline in the 1920s. In 1929, Vogt[3] described the various types of esophageal malformations, which provided a basis for the subsequent clinical classifications of the anomaly. In 1936, Lanman[4] first attempted a primary repair of esophageal atresia. The first survivors with the anomalies were reported independently by Leven[5] of Minneapolis and Ladd[6] of Boston in patients admitted on successive days in late 1939. Both cases were managed using a staged approach with initial gastrostomy, secondary fistula ligation or division with cervical esophagostomy, followed by the creation of an antethoracic skin tube conduit from the esophagostomy to the gastrostomy.

In 1939, Haight first attempted a primary repair without success. Following four failed attempts at achieving survival with primary repair, he finally achieved his first successful primary repair of esophageal atresia with tracheoesophageal fistula using a left extrapleural approach, as initially described by Lanman in 1940, and a single-layer anastomosis.[7] Postoperatively, the

patient developed an anastomotic leak, which was managed nonoperatively. She later developed a stricture at the anastomosis, which responded to a single dilatation. No other complication followed, and the child ate and continued to grow normally.

In 1943, Haight revised his procedure to a right extrapleural approach as he felt better exposure of the distal segment was obtained from this side.[7] He also moved to a modified two-layer, "telescoping" anastomosis in the hope of decreasing the risk of leak. Many of Haight's initial teachings continue to guide current management of the infant with congenital atresia of the esophagus.

CLASSIFICATION

Fig. 8.1 depicts the anatomic classification of the anomaly based on both the criteria described by Haight[8] and the more condensed classification of Gross.[9] Esophageal atresia with distal tracheoesophageal fistula is by far the most common type of esophageal atresia encountered. This anatomic variant accounts for between 85% and 90% of all cases.[10] Isolated esophageal atresia occurs in about 5% to 7% of infants with this anomaly and is the second most common form of this entity. Tracheoesophageal fistula without esophageal atresia is the third most common form of the defect and accounts for between 2% and 6% of all cases. The other much rarer forms of this anomaly are esophageal atresia with proximal tracheoesophageal fistula and esophageal atresia with both proximal and distal tracheoesophageal fistula. Both these latter variants occur with a frequency of less than 1%.

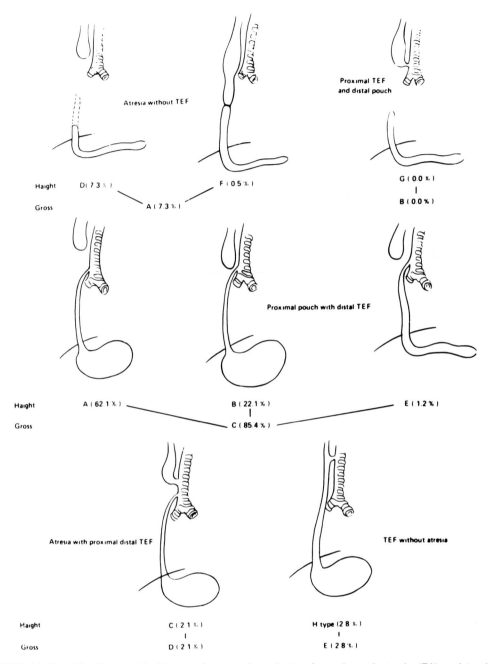

FIGURE 8.1 Classification and incidence of anatomic variants of esophageal atresia (EA) and tracheoesophageal fistula (TEF). Both the Haight and Gross schemes are demonstrated.

INCIDENCE

Haight,[8] in 1957, determined the incidence of esophageal atresia in the Washtenaw County of Michigan to be 1 in 4425 live births. This same incidence was found by Meyers[11] in Australia. The incidence reported from Finland was somewhat higher, at 1 in 3000 live births.[12]

CLINICAL FINDINGS

Pathophysiology

The clinical manifestations of the most common variant of esophageal atresia—namely, proximal atresia with distal tracheoesophageal fistula—will be discussed first. These infants develop sig-

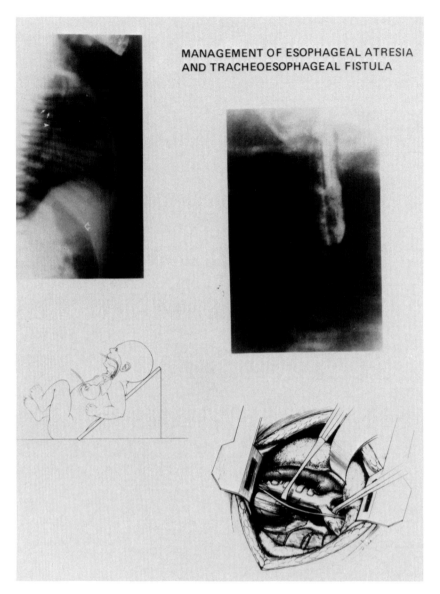

FIGURE 8.2 The management of esophageal atresia and tracheoesophageal fistula. Upper left: Lateral roentgenogram. Small arrows: air pouchogram. Arrowhead: air in distal esophagus. Open arrow: air in stomach confirming fistula. Upper right: Contrast pouchogram (recommended in all cases). Lower left: Sump suction of upper pouch, tube gastrostomy, and upright posture as initial therapeutic interventions. Lower right: Division of fistula and esophageal anastomosis via extrapleural approach.

nificant respiratory difficulty immediately after birth for several reasons. The esophageal atresia itself impedes the swallowing of saliva and results in the accumulation of fluid in the proximal esophageal pouch. This puts the infant at significant risk for the development of aspiration pneumonia.

The distal tracheoesophageal fistula produces the most serious physiological disturbance. Because most newborns have free gastroesophageal reflux, gastric juice, which is usually acid, refluxes unimpeded into the tracheobronchi tree and causes a chemical pneumonitis. A second result of the distal tracheoesophageal fistula is intestinal and abdominal distention due to large volumes of air passing from the trachea into the fistula and down into the stomach and gastrointestinal tract. Elevation of the diaphragm results from the gastric and intestinal distention, and this may seriously impair the neonate's ventilatory capacity because he uses his diaphragm as the major respiratory muscle.

Diagnosis

Polyhydramnios is quite common with this anomaly, especially when isolated esophageal atresia is present. Infants with esophageal atresia tend to drool shortly after birth and to accumulate an excessive amount of secretions in their posterior pharynx. This is often associated with the early onset of choking, coughing, and episodes of cyanosis.

The simplest way to rule out a diagnosis of esophageal atresia is to pass a nasogastric tube through the mouth or nose into the stomach. If passage of the tube meets with obstruction, then a plain roentgenogram in the frontal and lateral projections will document the atresia (Fig. 8.2). Contrast studies can then be carried out to confirm the diagnosis. Usually .5 to 1.0 mL of thin barium is injected through the tube into the upper pouch. This will outline a blind-ending smooth upper esophageal pouch (Fig. 8.2). One should look carefully at the abdomen on the plain film to determine whether gas is present. A gasless abdomen confirms the diagnosis of esophageal atresia without tracheoesophageal fistula.

Isolated tracheoesophageal fistula without atresia is much more difficult to diagnose in the newborn. A properly done esophagogram usually shows the communication (Fig. 8.3). If the x-ray study is normal, then simultaneous bronchoscopy and esophagoscopy will almost always identify the fistula.

Associated Anomalies

Patients with esophageal atresia and tracheoesophageal fistula frequently have associated anomalies. The incidence of recognizable defects associated with the esophageal malformation is between 50% and 70%.[13] The anomalies vary from minor skeletal deformities to uncorrectable cardiac defects. The most common associated anomalies are cardiac and gastrointestinal, especially imperforate anus. Most importantly, every newborn with an imperforate anus should be carefully checked for the presence of esophageal atresia and vice versa.

PREOPERATIVE TREATMENT

Pneumonitis is the most critical problem to deal with in the immediate preoperative period. Pneumonitis results both from aspiration of pharyngeal contents and from the reflux of gastric juice into the tracheobronchial tree. Preoperative

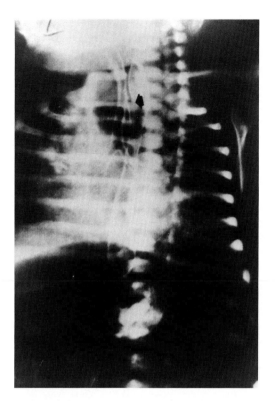

FIGURE 8.3 Arrow points to tracheoesophageal fistula. No esophageal atresia is present.

treatment involves prevention of further aspiration and reflux and treatment of any pneumonitis that may be present. This is accomplished by placing a sump catheter into the upper pouch and by performing a gastrostomy under local anesthesia. In addition, the infant is placed on broad-spectrum antibiotic coverage. The infant is kept in an upright position until definite surgery is carried out (Fig. 8.2).

SURGICAL TREATMENT

The main goal of operative therapy is to completely correct the anomaly with one operation. This necessitates division of the tracheoesophageal fistula and a primary repair of the esophageal atresia. This approach was first successfully performed in 1941 by Cameron Haight and has remained standard treatment since that time. Prematurity, significant pneumonia, or severe associated congenital anomalies all increase the risk of operation and the postoperative morbidity. In 1962, Holder et al[14] presented the concept of staging the operation in this group of patients, which involved extrapleural division of the distal tracheoesophageal fistula and placement of a gastrostomy tube. Proximal pouch suction was to prevent aspiration pneumonia. This approach allows treatment of pneumonia, prematurity, and the other anomalies to proceed before definite anastomosis of the esophagus.[15] The disadvantage of this staged approach is that the extrapleural route can no longer be used for the esophageal anastomosis. During the last 10 years this type of staging has been abandoned, and most high-risk infants with esophageal atresia and tracheoesophageal fistula are managed with decompression gastrostomy and proximal esophageal suction together with parenteral nutrition. Once the patient is stable, an extrapleural thoracotomy is carried out for division of the tracheoesophageal fistula and primary repair of the esophageal atresia (Fig. 8.2). The results with this approach have been better than those with the previously described staged operation.

Operative Technique

A right posterolateral, extrapleural thoracotomy is used unless a right-sided aortic arch is present. The chest is entered through the fourth intercostal space and the intercostal muscles are separated carefully until the pleura is visualized. Wet, cotton-tipped applicators are used to dissect the parietal pleura off the chest wall. The small amount of extra time spent in doing an extrapleural dissection is certainly worthwhile because it markedly reduces the risk of an empyema if an esophageal leak were to occur. The extrapleural dissection is continued posteriorly until the azygous vein is identified; this vein is then ligated and divided. The distal esophageal fistula usually lies immediately underneath the divided azygous vein. The fistula is then circled with a 1-0 silk tie and the crotch between the fistula and the trachea is dissected cephalad. Once the entrance of the fistula into the trachea at the level of the carina is fully visualized, the fistula is divided. Care must be taken not to remove any tracheal wall because this can result in a postoperative tracheal stricture. Rather, a small rim of esophageal wall is left at the fistula site and is used for the subsequent closure. As the fistula is divided, the tracheal end is closed with interrupted sutures of 5-0 or 6-0 silk or Prolene. Next, the upper esophageal pouch is visualized by having the anesthesiologist gently push down on the sump tube. Then the very distal end of the upper esophageal pouch is grasped with a heavy silk suture. The proximal esophagus is then dissected up the thoracic inlet by dividing the tissue between the esophagus and the trachea. Great care must be taken during this dissection so that the trachea is not accidentally entered. At this point, the surgeon assesses the feasibility of doing a primary anastomosis between the two esophageal segments. If there is too much tension, the distal esophagus is dissected further. The distal esophagus, however, should be handled and dissected as little as possible in order to prevent injury and ischemia. If further length is needed, a proximal esophagomyotomy can be performed.[16,17] This will usually give an additional length of 1 to 1.5 cm.

In general, I prefer a single-layer anastomosis of 5-0 or 6-0 silk; however, occasionally the Haight two-layer telescoping anastomosis is used. The sutures are placed through all layers of the esophageal wall and are tied within the lumen posteriorly and outside the lumen anteriorly. The anterior anastomosis is usually done over the sump tube, which is passed into the distal esophagus by the anesthesiologist.

MANAGEMENT OF THE PATIENT WITH ESOPHAGEAL ATRESIA WITHOUT TRACHEO-ESOPHAGEAL FISTULA

In this condition the distal esophageal segment is much shorter than when a distal tracheoesophageal fistula is present. For this reason, it is difficult to do a primary anastomosis. In the past, the standard approach to this anomaly has been performance of a cervical esophagostomy for salivary drainage and a feeding gastrostomy in the first days of life. When the child is 6 months to 1 year of age, a coloesophagoplasty or gastric tube interposition is usually performed. During the past 15 years, a number of institutions have reported significant success with stretching of the esophageal segments, especially the upper one, over a period of weeks in order that a subsequent primary esophageal anastomosis could be performed.[18,19] If a primary repair is contemplated, then a preliminary gastrostomy is inserted and the upper esophageal segment is stretched daily for about three weeks. After this period of stretching, roentgenograms will usually demonstrate a significant lengthening of the upper esophageal segment. At this point, a standard right extrapleural thoracotomy is performed. The approach is the same as when a tracheoesophageal fistula is present. The proximal pouch is dissected out in a routine fashion and the distal esophageal segment is dissected down to the gastroesophageal junction. Sometimes the stomach itself has to be mobilized into the chest. An esophagomyotomy is performed in the proximal segment about 1 to 1.5 cm proximal to the end of the esophagus to give additional length.

The anastomosis is then performed between the two esophageal segments using the technique described in the previous section.

TRACHEOESOPHAGEAL FISTULA WITHOUT ESOPHAGEAL ATRESIA

Although this anomaly is rare, it is frequently encountered during the work-up of infants with repeated bouts of coughing during feeding. The diagnosis is often difficult to make but the fistula can sometimes be visualized with a carefully performed barium swallow (Fig. 8.3). If the barium swallow is normal, combined bronchoscopy and esophagoscopy with the use of methylene blue instilled into the trachea can usually visualize the fistula. Once the fistula is seen at endoscopy, a ureteral or Fogarty catheter is passed through it from the trachea into the esophagus to aid in identification of the fistula at the time of surgery.

These fistulas can be easily approached through a cervical incision. A 3-cm transverse incision is made 1 to 2 cm above the clavicle over the sternocleidomastoid muscle. The right side is the preferred route to eliminate risk of damage to the thoracic duct. A nasogastric tube in the esophagus aids in identification. The sternocleidomastoid and omohyoid muscles are retracted laterally and posteriorly and the strap muscles are retracted medially and anteriorly. The middle thyroid vein is exposed and the recurrent laryngeal nerve is identified underneath it so that the nerve is kept out of harm's way. The esophagus is encircled with care again being taken not to injure the recurrent laryngeal nerve. At this point the fistula is palpated with the catheter going through it and is encircled. The fistula is then divided and both ends are closed with several interrupted sutures of 5-0 or 6-0 silk.

POSTOPERATIVE CARE

Antibiotics are continued for 10 days and intravenous fluids are maintained until gastrostomy feedings are begun. Peripheral intravenous nutrition is started on the first postoperative day. If the child is stable with no evidence of saliva leaking through the chest tube, gastrostomy feedings are sometimes begun on the fourth postoperative day. On the 10th postoperative day, a Hypaque swallow is performed and, if no leak is seen, this is followed by a barium swallow to completely visualize the anastomosis. Formula feedings are begun immediately after the x-ray films show no evidence of a leak and the chest tube is removed. The child is discharged home with the gastrostomy tube in place. The tube is subsequently removed one month postoperatively in the office.

COMPLICATIONS

There are three types of complications related to the esophageal anastomosis: leak, stricture, and recurrent fistula.[20] The incidence of leak varies from 10% to 20% depending on the type of anastomosis done and the degree of tension at the anastomosis. In general, the leak incidence is lower with a Haight-type, two-layer anastomosis than with a single-layer one. Conversely, the stricture rate is higher with a Haight than with a single-layer anastomosis and varies between 10% and 25%. The frequency of recurrent tracheoesophageal fistula is hard to determine because very few series have been reported; however, it appears to range around 10%.

The two other significant complications that are seen postoperatively are gastroesophageal reflux[21] and tracheomalacia.[22] The gastroesophageal reflux is probably secondary to extensive mobilization of the distal esophagus and can sometimes be treated with simple medical maneuvers.[23] However, a significant percentage of these infants continue to have significant reflux, which can sometimes manifest itself as a recurrent anastomotic stricture.[24] In this group of infants, a fundoplication is often necessary.

Tracheomalacia of a severe degree has been reported with increasing frequency as a complication not of the repair, but of the esophageal atresia itself. Benjamin[25] reported the presence of tracheomalacia in 20 of 80 patients (25%) with esophageal atresia and tracheoesophageal fistula. Most infants with tracheomalacia improve with time; however, a small percentage develop severe respiratory difficulty, which can result in respiratory arrest and death. Several authors have treated these latter patients with aortopexies, in which the transverse aorta is sutured to the undersurface of the sternum.[26] This has been successful in most of the patients thus far reported.

RESULTS OF OPERATION

The vast majority of children born with esophageal atresia and tracheoesophageal fistula can survive and have a normal existence. The overall survival rate ranges between 85% and 90% and for those in the low-risk category, the survival is greater than 95%.[12,27-33]

THE UNIVERSITY OF MICHIGAN EXPERIENCE

From March 1935 to September 1985, a total of 428 patients with esophageal atresia and/or tracheoesophageal fistula were admitted to the University of Michigan Medical Center. This did not include patients initially operated on at other institutions. Earlier reviews of that institution's experience were presented by Haight in 1943, 1957, and 1966,[27] by Strodel et al in 1979,[33] and by Manning et al in 1986.[31]

All cases were classified into anatomic type of anomaly based on the criteria described by both Haight and Gross. Infants were also assigned to risk groups A, B, or C as described by Waterston et al[34]: in group A birth weight was greater than 2500 grams and the patient was otherwise well; in group B birth weight was 2000 grams to 2500 grams and the patient was well, or had higher weight with moderate associated anomalies; in group C birth weight was less than 2000 grams, or it was higher with severe associated anomalies. A severe anomaly was defined as one that required operative intervention or intensive care management to sustain life. Pneumonia was omitted from consideration in the Waterston classification.

The year-to-year incidence of cases has varied somewhat, but over the course of the last 50 years a fairly constant rate of 8 to 9 new cases per year has been observed. Table 8.1 shows the distribution of patients by Waterston risk class over the last two decades. Overall survival data are also given.

Associated Anomalies

The proportion of patients with associated congenital anomalies has not changed significantly over the period of observation (Table 8.2). Cardiovascular and gastrointestinal malformations are the most commonly seen major anomalies, whereas skeletal and limb defects are the most common minor types seen. The constellation of defects referred to as the VATER or VACTERL syndrome was seen in 17.5% of patients (11/63)

TABLE 8.1 Risk Groups

Waterston Group	1966–1976		1977–1985	
	N	% Survival	N	% Survival
A	35	97.0	30	100.0
B	20	95.0	6	83.3
C	22	59.0	27	63.0
Total	**77**	**86%**	**63**	**82.5%**

TABLE 8.2 Severe Associated Anomalies

	1935–1966	1966–1976	1976–1985
Cardiovascular	44	12	10
Gastrointestinal	31	8	10
Neurological	9	1	2
Genitourinary	4	1	1
Orthopedic	0	0	0
Other	3	1	1
Total	**91**	**23**	**24**
Percentage	**31.6%**	**27.3%**	**34.0%**

in the most recent group reviewed.[35] The most frequent cardiovascular anomalies encountered included patient ductus arteriosus and ventricular or atrial septal defects. The less common cardiac anomalies encountered were tetrology of Fallot, common A-V canal, total anomalous pulmonary venous return, and single ventricle. The most frequently encountered gastrointestinal malformations were imperforate anus, duodenal atresia (with or without annular pancreas), and pyloric stenosis.

Operative Management

Primary repair of the esophagus was performed in 90.3% (371/411) of patients for the entire series. In the overall series, a staged approach was used in 9.7% (40/411). In the most current group, 3 patients underwent a staged approach. In 14 patients (5 in the last 10 years), no repair was attempted due to the severity of additional defects and their associated grave prognoses. These patients were palliated with gastrostomy and sump suction of the proximal pouch to decrease the risk of pulmonary complications.

A classic Haight two-layer telescoping anastomosis was performed in 87.5% (358/411) of the entire series. Since the time of the most recent review, however, a change was made to a single-layer technique that appears to have gained preference worldwide. Therefore, although a two-layer repair was performed in 98% of patients before 1977, this has been used in only 17% of cases (9/53) since that time.

Cases of H-type fistulas (without esophageal atresia) were considered as a separate management group. Simple division of the fistula was accomplished without complication in all cases via either a thoracotomy or cervical approach (a cervical approach was used exclusively in the recent group).

Survival

In my institution's most recent group of 63 patients, the overall survival was 82.5% (52/63). Five

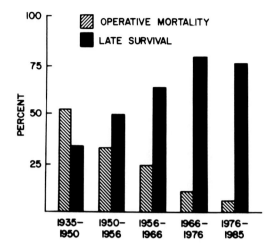

FIGURE 8.4 Trends in operative mortality and late survival over the last 50 years at the University of Michigan Medical Center.

of these patients were not operated upon due to severe associated anomalies. Survival rates by Waterston risk class are given in Table 8.1. Four deaths occurred in the immediate postoperative period, for an operative mortality rate of 6.9%. As seen in Figure 8.4, this continued the trend of decline in operative mortality seen in the past 50 years. Of the operative deaths, 2 were related to the esophageal anastomosis and 2 died of complications related to severe underlying congenital anomalies. Late deaths occurred in 2 patients, both resulting from the pulmonary complications that developed at times remote from the operative period.

Complications

Accurate data concerning the complication rates have been compiled only during the past 30 years.

During the most recent 30-year period (1956–1985), the incidence of anastomotic leak was 8.5% (19/224). As seen in Table 8.3, the rate

TABLE 8.3 Complications by Type of Anastomosis: 1956–1985

Type of Repair	Leak[a]	Stricture[b]	Recurrence
One-layer (n = 47)	8 (17.0%)	2 (4.3%)	3 (6.4%)
Two-layer (n = 177)	11 (6.2%)	41 (23.2%)	11 (6.2%)

[a] p < .03.
[b] p < .002.

was 17% for those undergoing a single-layer repair and 6.2% for those treated with a classic two-layer telescoping anastomosis. In all cases, the leak remained in the extrapleural space and was almost always asymptomatic. Ninety-five percent were treated conservatively with spontaneous resolution. One patient had incomplete disruption of the anastomosis (which was performed under tension despite upper-pouch myotomy) and underwent cervical esophagostomy, followed later by colon interposition. Two patients who developed anastomotic leaks died in the postoperative period secondary to recurrent aspiration and pneumonia.

During the same period, the incidence of recurrent fistula was 6.3% (14/224). There was no significant difference between the one-layer and two-layer anastomosis groups (Table 8.3).

The incidence of anastomotic stricture was difficult to establish precisely because most patients in the early years underwent routine postoperative esophageal sounding. For purposes of comparison, anastomotic strictures have been defined as those requiring more than two dilatations. During the past 30 years, the incidence of stricture has been 19% (43/224). There was a significant difference in stricture rate between those undergoing one-layer and two-layer repair (4.3 vs. 23.2%; see Table 8.3). All strictures responded to esophageal dilatation.

As noted by several investigators, gastroesophageal reflux (GER) is now recognized as a significant postoperative problem in patients undergoing repair of esophageal atresia.[12,23,24,36] The rate of GER was not documented in prior reports of this series. In the present update the incidence of symptomatic GER is 37.9% (22/58). Seventy-seven percent of these 22 patients have undergone fundoplication at a median age of 4 months. In the recent group, less frequently occurring complications include tracheomalacia in 10.3% of patients (6/58), three of whom required an aortopexy, and esophageal foreign body impaction in 12.1% (7/58).

SUMMARY

Changing referral patterns in my region have led to an increased proportion of neonates with severe associated congenital anomalies or significant prematurity undergoing treatment at my institution. I have seen more Waterston group C patients in the past decade than in the previous decade (41% vs. 26%). In spite of this, operative mortality has continued to decline in recent years. Continued advances in the perioperative intensive care management of high-risk neonates account for much of this decrease in operative mortality.

My institution's basic scheme for the perioperative management (from diagnosis to repair) has not changed significantly in the past 20 years and is summarized in Figure 8.2. The importance of urgent gastrostomy tube placement for decompression continues to be stressed. This allows fistula division and repair of the esophageal atresia to be performed on an elective basis after further preoperative preparation and evaluation for associated anomalies has been accomplished. It also allows for early enteral feeding after the repair.

Although my colleagues and I have always attempted to perform a primary repair in the patient with congenital esophageal atresia, some surgeons prefer to routinely approach certain neonates in a staged fashion. We have found this to be necessary only rarely and in very selected infants. Factors that should influence one's decision in favor of a staged approach have been emphasized by others.[15,32] These include prematurity, established pneumonia, severe associated anomalies, widely separated proximal and distal segments (precluding primary anastomosis) and deterioration of the patient in the operating room. Most recent studies have found that with current intensive care management, primary repair in the high-risk infant carries no more morbidity or mortality, and probably less, than does a staged approach. A 1981 review by Hicks and Mansfield[28] in which all high-risk infants were routinely staged showed an operative mortality of 27% and an overall survival of 45%. Comparable figures in my institution's most current group are 18.2% and 63% for Waterston group C risk patients undergoing primary repair.

The choice between a retropleural and transpleural operative approach has become a matter of debate. The 1964 survey of the Surgical Section of the American Academy of Pediatrics reported by Holder et al[10] showed that in patients who developed anastomotic leaks, survival was better for those who had undergone retropleural dissection (60% vs. 32%). Even excluding those who developed leaks, they found improved survival with a retropleural approach. Other authors have echoed this preference, emphasizing the greater margin of safety afforded by the retropleural technique, particularly in cases in which a leak develops (10% to 20% of most series).[32,33] Two series, however, note that the choice of exposure did not affect overall mortality.[28,30] With a retropleural approach, the leak becomes an easily managed esophagocutaneous fistula, which in most instances closes spontaneously (95% in my series), whereas if a transpleural approach has been used, a leak becomes a potentially life-threatening empyema, which often requires operative management.

The type of anastomosis used for the esophageal repair has undergone a transition over the past 25 years. Haight used a single-layer technique in his earliest cases, but he soon adopted his classic two-layer telescoping method. In the 1964 survey by Holder et al,[10] nearly half of those polled used a single-layer technique. That report noted a significantly higher leak rate but a lower incidence of stricture with a single-layer repair. More recently, Hicks and Mansfield[28] found a 17% and 18% leak rate with one-layer and two-layer anastomoses, respectively, and reported strictures occurring three times more often with a two-layer repair. Louhimo and Lindahl[30] noted a similar incidence of leak with the two types of anastomoses but no difference in the stricture rate when all patients underwent routine postoperative dilatation. They favor the single-layer technique, however, because it requires less distal mobilization (thus preserving the vascular supply to this segment). Although the single-layer anastomosis has resulted in a slight increase in leak rate, it has also resulted in significantly fewer strictures. It must be kept in mind, however, that there is a strong association between gastroesophageal reflux and persistent stricture, as pointed out by Pieretti et al.[24] The importance of early recognition and management of GER in these patients was further emphasized by Ashcraft et al.[21] In fact, three of the four patients with significant strictures seen at my institution in the last nine years had reflux. That gastroesophageal reflux is common in infants following repair of esophageal atresia is emphasized by the incidence seen in our most current group (37.9%). Our tendency toward more aggressive management of postoperative gastroesophageal reflux over the past decade is evidenced by the 77% fundoplication rate for symptomatic reflux. This has undoubtedly contributed to our decreased incidence of stricture formation.

In summary, in the last half century at the University of Michigan, we have seen congenital esophageal atresia transformed from an anomaly with 100% mortality to one with an expected survival exceeding 80%. This has come about largely through advances in both the operative and, more importantly, the perioperative management of the high-risk neonate. A plateau has probably been reached, so further improvement in the outcome of these infants will primarily depend on improvement in management of other severe anomalies that may occur simultaneously.

REFERENCES

1. Gibson T: *The Anatomy of Humane Bodies Epitomized.* 6th ed. London: Awnsham & Churchill; 1703.
2. Durston W: A narrative of monstrous birth in Plym-

outh October 22, 1670; Together with the anatomical observation taken thereupon by William Durston, Doctor in Physick, and communication to Dr. Tim Clerk. *Philos Trans T Soc* 1670;V:2096.

3. Vogt EC: Congenital esophageal atresia. *AJR* 1929;22:463.

4. Lanman TH: Congenital atresia of the esophagus: A study of 32 cases. *Arch Surg* 1940;41:1060.

5. Leven NL: Congenital atresia of the esophagus with tracheoesophageal fistula: Report of successful extrapleural ligation of fistulous communication and cervical esophagostomy. *J Thorac Surg* 1941;10:648.

6. Ladd WE: The surgical treatment of esophageal atresia and tracheoesophageal fistulas. *N Engl J Med* 1944;230:625.

7. Haight C, Towsley HA: Congenital atresia of the esophagus with tracheoesophageal fistula. Extrapleural ligation of fistula and end-to-end anastomosis of esophageal segments. *Surg Gynecol Obstet* 1943;76:672.

8. Haight C: Some observations on esophageal atresias and tracheoesophageal fistulas of congenital origin. *J Thorac Surg* 1957;34:141–172.

9. Gross RE: *Surgery of infancy and childhood.* Philadelphia, Penn: WB Saunders Co; 1953.

10. Holder TM, Cloud DT, Lewis JE Jr, et al: Esophageal atresia and tracheoesophageal fistula. A survey of its members by the Surgical Section of the American Academy of Pediatrics. *Pediatrics* 1964;34:542.

11. Myers NA: Oesophageal atresia with distal tracheoesophageal fistula in identical twins. *J Pediatr Surg* 1978;13:361–362.

12. Sulamaa M, Grinpenberg L, Alvenainen EK: Prognosis and treatment of congenital atresia of the esophagus. *Acta Chir Scand* 1951;102:141–157.

13. Waterston DJ, Bonham-Carter RE, Aberdeen E: Oesophageal atresia, tracheoesophageal fistula—A study of survival in 218 infants. *Lancet* 1962;1:819.

14. Holder TM, McDonald VG Jr, Woolley MM: The premature or critically ill infant with esophageal atresia: Increased success with a staged approach. *J Thorac Cardiovasc Surg* 1962;44:344.

15. Abrahamson J, Shandling B: Esophageal atresia in the underweight baby: A challenge. *J Pediatr Surg* 1972;7:608–613.

16. Livaditis A: End-to-end anastomosis in esophageal atresia: A clinical and experimental study. *Scand J Thorac Cardiovasc Surg* (suppl 2).

17. Livaditis A, Radberg L, Odensjo G, et al: Esophageal end-to-end anastomosis. *Scand J Thorac Cardiovasc Surg* 1972;6:206.

18. Howard R, Myers NA: Esophageal atresia: A technique for elongating the upper pouch. *Surgery* 1965;58:725–727.

19. Mahour GH, Woolley MM, Gwinn JL: Elongation of the upper pouch and delayed anatomic reconstruction in esophageal atresia. *J Pediatr Surg* 1974;9:373–383.

20. Kafrouni G, Baick CH, Woolley MM: Recurrent tracheoesophageal fistula: A diagnostic problem. *Surgery* 1970;68:889–894.

21. Ashcraft KW, Goodwin C, Amoury RA, et al: Early recognition and aggressive treatment of gastroesophageal reflux following repair of esophageal atresia. *J Pediatr Surg* 1977;12:317.

22. Filler RM, Rossello PJ, Lebowitz RL: Life-threatening anoxic spells caused by tracheal compression after repair of esophageal atresia: Correction by surgery. *J Pediatr Surg* 1976;11:739.

23. Skinner DB, Belsey RH, Hendrix TR, Zuidema GD: Gastroesophageal reflux and hiatal hernia. Boston, Mass: Little, Brown, and Co: 1972:Chap 7.

24. Pieretti R, Shandling B, Stephens CA: Resistant esophageal stenosis associated with reflux after repair of esophageal atresia. *J Pediatr Surg* 1974; 9:355–357.

25. Benjamin B, Cohen D, Glasson M: Tracheomalacia in association with congenital tracheoesophageal fistula. *Surgery* 1976;79:504–508.

26. Schwartz MZ, Filler RM: Tracheal compression as a cause of apnea following repair of tracheoesophageal fistula: Treatment by aortopexy. *J Pediatr Surg* 1980;15:842–848.

27. Haight C: Congenital esophageal atresia and tracheoesophageal fistula. In: *Pediatric Surgery.* 2nd ed. Chicago, Ill: Year Book Medical Publishers, 1969.

28. Hicks LM, Mansfield PB: Esophageal atresia and tracheoesophageal fistula: Review of thirteen years' experience. *J Thorac Cardiovasc Surg* 1981;81:358.

29. Holder TM, Ashcraft KW: Developments in the care of patients with esophageal atresia and tracheoesophageal fistula. *Surg Clin North Am* 1981;61:1051.

30. Louhimo I, Lindahl H: Esophageal atresia: Primary results of 500 consecutive treated patients. *J Pediatr Surg* 1983;18:217.

31. Manning PB, Morgan RA, Coran AG, et al: Fifty years' experience with esophageal atresia and tracheoesophageal fistula. *Ann Surg* 1986;204:446–451.

32. Myers NA, Aberdeen E: Congenital esophageal atresia and tracheoesophageal fistula. In: *Pediatric Surgery.* 3rd ed. Chicago, Ill: Year Book Medical Publishers, 1979.

33. Strodel WE, Coran AG, Kirsh MM, et al: Esophageal atresia: A 41-year experience. *Arch Surg* 1979; 114:523–527.

34. Waterston DJ, Bonham-Carter RE, Aberdeen E: Congenital tracheo-oesophageal fistula in association with oesophageal atresia. *Lancet* 1963;2:550–555.

35. Heyman MB, Berquist WE, Fonkalsrud EW, Lewin KJ, Ament ME: Esophageal muscular ring and the VACTERL association: A case report. *Pediatrics* 1981;67:638.

36. Orringer MB, Kirsh MM, Sloan H: Long-term esophageal function following repair of esophageal atresia. *Ann Surg* 1977;186:436.

Esophageal Atresia, Tracheoesophageal Fistula, and Complications

Thomas M. Holder, MD

A. G. Coran's chapter accurately and admirably presents the current status of the care of infants with esophageal atresia (EA) and tracheoesophageal fistula (TEF) based on the University of Michigan experience, which includes Cameron Haight's first successful primary repair. A few of Coran's points warrant comment.

Current experience at my institution based on 111 consecutive patients treated over the past 15 years reveals a higher incidence of proximal pouch TEF (with or without distal fistula) than reported by Coran. It is important, therefore, for any infant who on the esophageal contrast study demonstrates media in the trachea to undergo bronchoscopy. Eight proximal TEFs and one laryngotracheoesophageal cleft were thus visualized.

The patients with long-gap atresia (usually atresia without TEF but also a few patients with distal fistula) still present a major problem in a satisfactory esophageal reconstruction or replacement. In addition to colon interposition or use of the reverse gastric tube, Spitz has recently popularized bringing the stomach up through the bed of the esophagus, without thoracotomy, for cervical esophagogastrostomy.[1] Determining how this approach will compare with other forms of reconstruction will have to await longer-term evaluation.

I particularly agree with Coran's last statement, "Further improvement in the outcome of these infants will primarily depend on improvement in the management of other severe anomalies that may occur simultaneously." Recognition and treatment of concomitant disease has been a major component of the approach to the

care of those infants at my institution for the past 15 years.

Since the early 1960s it has been apparent that large, healthy babies with EA/TEF did well and that very small babies with major associated anomalies did poorly.[2,3] As experience increased, it was apparent that major anomalies were a more important factor in outcome than was size per se. By the mid-1970s my colleagues and I had adopted an approach directed toward the identification and treatment of the concomitant disease as well as correction of the EA/TEF[4] (Table D8.1).

The healthy babies, irrespective of size, were treated by primary repair. During the early years a gastrostomy was done during the same anesthetic, whereas in recent years the gastrostomy frequently has been omitted. There were no deaths in this group.

For those infants with atelectasis and pneumonia treatment by upper pouch suction, antibiotics, and decompression gastrostomy was effective in clearing the lungs in a matter of a few days. Repair was then undertaken, which was successful in all patients in this group.

The ill infants with known or suspected major anomalies, sepsis, IRDS, or marked prematurity were selected for delayed repair. They were treated by upper pouch suction, antibiotics, decompression gastrostomy, and a central venous catheter for total parenteral nutrition. The most urgent problem, which was often the concomitant disease, was treated first. Twenty patients required operation for associated anomalies before repair of their EA/TEF. There was one death (Table D8.2). It is to be noted that none of these infants was treated by staging with gastrostomy and division of the TEF. Three patients did have their TEF divided at the time of thoracotomy for a more urgent cardiac problem. This was particularly beneficial in those infants who

TABLE D8.1 EA/TEF Therapeutic Approach (111 Patients)

Condition

Healthy baby $\xrightarrow{\hspace{1cm}56\hspace{1cm}}$ Primary repair

Pneumonia-atelectasis $\xrightarrow{\hspace{0.5cm}18\hspace{0.5cm}}$ Gastrostomy $\longrightarrow$ Repair

Ill baby (small preemie, major anomaly, IRDS, sepsis) $\xrightarrow{\hspace{0.5cm}37\hspace{0.5cm}}$ Gastrostomy & TPN catheter $\longrightarrow$ Rx Most urgent problem $\longrightarrow$ De-layed repair
individualize

TABLE D8.2 Prerepair Operation for Life-Threatening Associated Anomalies in 111 Patients with EA/TEF

	No. of Patients	Died	Survived
Systemtic-pulmonary shunt	2	1	1
Patent ductus arterio-sus: ligation	5	0	5
Imperforate anus: colostomy	5	0	5
Duodenal obstruction	5	0	5
Gastroschisis: repair	1	0	1
Tracheoesophageal cleft: tracheostomy	1	0	1
Subglottic stenosis: tracheostomy	1	0	1
Total	**20**	**1**	**19**

also had IRDS requiring ventilator support. As soon as the patient's postoperative condition permitted or the nonoperative problem resolved, repair of the EA/TEF was undertaken. All deaths were in this group of ill infants.

Four patients, critically ill with associated anomalies died, without repair, and two infants' postoperative deaths were related to the EA/TEF repair. Two other patients died long after repair (more than 2 ½ months) because of an associated anomaly but during the original hospitalization. Thus 98% of patients operated upon survived repair, 95% of the entire group (including those who died early of an associated anomaly) survived the repair, and 93% of the entire group left the hospital alive (Table D8.3). This approach has been helpful in improving survival of infants with EA/TEF.

REFERENCES

1. Spitz L: Gastric transposition via the mediastinal route for infants with long-gap esophageal atresia. *J Pediatr Surg* 1984;19:149–154.
2. Waterston DJ, Bonham-Carter RE, Aberdeen EL: Oesophageal atresia, tracheoesophageal fistula—A study of survival in 218 infants. *Lancet* 1962;1:819.
3. Holder TM, McDonald VG Jr, Woolley MM: The premature or critically ill infant with esophageal atresia: Increased success with a staged approach. *J Thorac Cardiovasc Surg* 1962;44:344–358.
4. Holder TM, Ashcraft KW, Sharp RJ, Amoury RA: Care of infants with esophageal atresia, tracheoesophageal fistula and associated anomalies. *J Thorac Cardiovasc Surg* 1987;94:828–835.

TABLE D8.3 Neonatal Deaths by Waterston Risk Groups in 111 Patients with EA/TEF

	Group A (42 patients)	Group B (26 patients)	Group C (43 patients)	Totals
Preoperative deaths	0	0	4	4
Postrepair deaths	0	0	2	2
Survived repair (%)	100	100	95	98
Survived (all patients; %)	100	100	86	95

Chapter 9

Foregut Duplications

Juan C. De Agustín, MD, PhD and Juan G. Utrilla, MD

The term *duplications*, first proposed by Ladd in 1937, can be defined as cystic or tubular structures that are lined with intestinal epithelium, have a smooth muscle wall, and share a common blood supply.[1] They can be connected to the adjacent gut through the lumen or by a common muscle wall. Multiple duplications may occur in a single patient.[2] Thus duplications of the foregut could connect the esophagus, as a tubular structure, with the pancreatic ducts or duodenum, or even more distally. More frequently, however, they are cystic, enteric-lined structures, enclosed in a common muscular wall adjacent to the gut.

EMBRYOLOGY

In the cephalic portion of the embryo, the primitive gut forms a blind-ending tube: the foregut. It lies caudal to the pharyngeal tube and pouches and extends as far caudally as the liver and pancreatic duct outgrowth. Caudal to this structure the midgut begins.[3]

The blood supply of the foregut comes from the celiac artery.

The endoderm forms the epithelial lining of the digestive and tracheobronchial tract. The muscular and peritoneal components of the wall of these structures are derived from the splanchnic mesoderm. Thus a variety of epithelium-lined duplications occur in the mediastinum, and classification of foregut duplications can be done according to their pathology and to their location: bronchogenic, enteric (neuroenteric), and esophageal duplication cysts.

Often they are connected with abdominal structures and in some instances are attached to the spine. As in the posterior mediastinum, in-traspinal enterogenous cysts have been reported with and without vertebral anomalies. To explain the morphogenesis of enteric cysts within the spinal canal, it is necessary to postulate that the endoderm becomes intercalated not merely in the notochord but farther dorsally, into the neuroectoderm. Some of the endodermal cells might well become detached from the endodermal tube as the latter is drawn away by the descent of the foregut.[4]

The ends of the duplicated intestinal tract may either remain open or be closed off from the original communications.[2]

It is also known that mediastinal duplications have occurred in patients who had intestinal intraabdominal duplications.

Mediastinal duplications can be satisfactorily explained on the basis of embryological and clinical studies, though for duplications of the stomach and duodenum no one theory is totally satisfactory.[1,5]

Bronchogenic cysts develop from abnormal budding of the ventral portion of the foregut. The laryngotracheal groove appears on the ventral wall of the primitive foregut in the 3-mm embryo (third week of intrauterine life). This groove later transforms into a tube, separated from the foregut by a spur of mesenchyma, and represents the respiratory diverticulum. In the 10-mm embryo this tube divides into two buds, which further divide and grow. If abnormal budding occurs before this stage, it results in paraesophageal cysts. Otherwise, if the abnormal budding remains attached to the primitive tracheobronchial tree, the cysts will be found along the trachea, bronchus, or pulmonary parenchyma or in sites where the development is arrested. Finally, cysts can also be pinched off from all these structures and migrate some distance, so that they are found in the neck, pericardium, and vertebral, and subpleural areas.[6] Bronchogenic cysts will be described in Chapter 6 more extensively.

Enterogenous cysts arise from abnormal development of the dorsal portion of the foregut. As the esophageal tube is formed after proliferation and later vacuolization of epithelial elements of the dorsal foregut, the incomplete vacuolization results in an esophageal cyst. Enteric cysts occur when dorsal mesoderm splits in the middle, and the endoderm herniates through it. Thus the resulting cyst may be attached to the dorsal ectoderm and can result in the appearance of vertebral and neural tube defects.[6]

Other cysts appearing in the mediastinum, with no typical histologic appearance of bronchogenic cysts, could be considered of foregut origin. They can be located in relation to the tracheobronchial tree and esophagus showing a similar symptomatology, but their epithelial lining cells have been lost because of infection that invariably is present. They can represent up to 20% of mediastinal foregut cysts.[7]

Persistent embryonic diverticulum or incomplete vacuolization in the fifth to eighth week of gestation can be responsible for the small intramural duplications that are found all along the gastrointestinal tract.

A septum that divides the esophagus, stomach, or duodenum in two parallel tubes might be the cause of the tubular duplications lying close to the gut, sharing a common muscular wall.[6]

Finally, duplications may represent reparative efforts gone wrong.[2] We have observed two autopsies in which duplications were associated with other malformations. In the first case polysplenia was associated with duplication of the stomach and intestine, pancreatic heterotopia in gastric mucosa, bilateral diaphragmatic hernia, congenital heart disease, and cryptorchidism. In the second patient, a supernumerary adrenal gland was associated with bicephalus and duplication of the spine, heart, lungs, esophagus, liver, stomach, and intestine.

CLINICAL PRESENTATION

Thoracic foregut duplications are usually posterior mediastinal, expanding, space-occupying lesions. They can be present at any age[8] as a cause of severe respiratory distress in the newborn or respiratory or gastrointestinal complaints in the older child.[9]

Enterogenous cystic malformations account for approximately 15% to 20% of foregut duplications located in the thorax, usually in the posterior mediastinum[7,10] and represent 14% of all digestive duplications in our institution.[11] Twenty-two percent occur adjacent to the upper third of the esophagus.[12] The lesions encountered in the lower third are asymptomatic in 35% of the patients.

Enterogenous cysts can be subdivided into two categories: enteric and esophageal duplication cysts.[8] Enteric cysts appearing in the mediastinum have the morphology of normal thick-walled bowel. They may be lined by any type of alimentary tract epithelium, including ciliated epithelium covered with a longitudinal and circular muscle with myenteric plexuses. Gastric mucosa can be observed in duplicated gut elsewhere. Other locations observed are the neck[13] and spinal canal,[14] and in these cases communication with the esophagus may be present. Respiratory symptoms, a mediastinal mass, and vertebral anomaly form a triad present in 70% of patients with neuroenteric cysts.[8]

Esophageal cysts are frequently intramural and contain a ciliated epithelial lining but no intestinal mucosa. However, cartilage, muscle, and, in a high proportion of cases, vertebral anomalies are observed.

Symptoms are almost always present, due to compression of the esophagus or respiratory tree and to ulceration of the cyst. Fever may be related to ulceration and surrounding inflammation.

Compression appears because the epithelium continues to secrete and the mass grows as it fills. This results in respiratory (50%–90% of reported cases) or gastrointestinal symptoms (10%–15% of cases); see Table 9.1. Respiratory symptoms include stridor, cough, hemoptysis, and chest pain. Atelectasia and pneumonia can occur. Esophageal compression causes cervical, retrosternal, or epigastric pain, vomiting, hematemesis, gagging, and dysphagia.[8,15–23]

The presence of ectopic gastric mucosa causes peptic ulceration with retrosternal pain, erosion into the tracheobronchial tree, and hemorrhage.

We have not observed malignancy in enterogenous cysts, but in our institution, cancer has been detected in two adult patients with bronchogenic cysts (7% of all foregut cysts detected in adulthood).

Connection with the alimentary canal is one of the most interesting aspects of these malformations. Thoracoabdominal duplications can end blindly or be connected with the lumen of the jejunum or a major pancreatic duct.[2] We have observed a duplicated esophagus that penetrated the diaphragm, connecting the carina with the biliary tree (Fig. 9.1).[24] Biliary reflux into the duplicated structure was observed during bronchoscopy.

Associated anomalies are frequently encountered in neuroenteric cysts and are related to their embryological development. These include anomalies in the fusion of the vertebral body (spina bifida, hemivertebrae, fused verte-

TABLE 9.1 Foregut Cysts

Case No.	Age	Sex	Type of Cyst	Shape	Size	Location	Symptoms	Complications
1	22 mo	male	enteric	cystic	3 × 3 cm	paraesophageal	respiratory	
2	4 mo	female	enteric	cystic	3 × 4 cm	posterior mediastinum	respiratory	atelectasis RUL aspiration
3	2 yr	female	esophageal	cystic	4 × 1.5 cm	paraesophageal	vomiting	
4	1 mo	male	esophageal	tubular	15 × 4 cm	tracheoesophageal fistulas	respiratory	aspiration
5	7 yr	male	enteric	cystic	10 × 4 cm	left hilar	respiratory	recurrent pneumonia
6	3 mo	male	enteric	cystic	2 × 4 cm	mediastinum	respiratory	
7	3 yr	male	neuroen-teric	cystic	C-6 to T-1	spinal canal	abdominal pain paraparesis	

RUL = right upper lobe.

brae) with an overall incidence of 80%.[8] True communication with the esophagus is rarely seen.[23] Although we have not observed any additional gastrointestinal duplications in our patients, there is a reported incidence of 12%.[8]

DIAGNOSIS

A preoperative diagnosis of foregut cysts can be made in 70% of patients from the clinical picture and basic diagnostic studies.[7,25] The precise etiology is provided only by operative excision and pathological study of the resected tissue.

Plain chest roentgenograms and computed tomography (CT) scans are the two most valuable diagnostic studies. Magnetic resonance imaging (MRI) and ultrasonography may also be helpful in delineating the mass. Barium swallow and bronchography can also be of diagnostic aid in certain circumstances (Fig. 9.1A). Technetium pertechnetate scanning must be done when pain is present because of the frequent finding of gastric mucosa which may be responsible for peptic ulceration. Although myelography has been recommended when respiratory symptoms and vertebral abnormality appear together, CT scan and MRI may be more specific.[13] Finally, arteriography may be required to exclude pulmonary sequestration or vascular compression.

The diagnosis is suggested on chest roentgenograms when there is a radiopaque mass of variable size, appearing with a smooth margin, projecting from the mediastinum (Fig. 9.2). On occasion emphysema may be present because of bronchial compression. Mediastinal masses generally do not demonstrate an air-fluid level.

CT scan has been proved to be better than MRI in evaluating mediastinal and hilar lung masses.[26] On CT scan duplication masses can be

seen as cystic lesions of low density, frequently surrounded by grayish areas corresponding to inflammatory reaction.[27] More dark areas next to the cyst may be areas of hyperinflation. When a cyst is infected it has small areas of low density within a mass. This finding is characteristic of microabscess formation (Fig. 9.3).

MRI and the CT scan are methods of choice for studying duplications cysts of the spinal canal, because they can show the character of the mass and may be able to distinguish cystic from solid tumors. Sagittal MRI clearly visualizes extension of the cyst.[12,14] Also, MRI has proved to be of value in assessment of the location and size of cervical esophageal cysts as well as its effects on neighboring anatomic structures. In this way MRI helps in operative planning.[13]

Esophageal duplication cysts may also be located at the cervical level, usually causing acute respiratory distress in infants[28] or, less frequently, feeding difficulty and irritability or rapidly growing neck masses due to infection.[13] Other causes of neck masses must be considered in the differential diagnosis: cystic hygroma, branchial cyst, abscess, thyroglossal duct cyst, and cervical thymic cyst. Esophagogram and MRI add specificity to the diagnosis and delineate the course of the esophagus or a communication with the cyst.[13]

Alternative diagnoses for thoracic masses include pneumonia, empyema, pneumatocele, congenital lobe emphysema, and hypoplastic lung and may be responsible for delayed treatment. A clue to diagnosis is the failure of resolution of the inflammation. Pericardial and thymic cysts are easily diagnosed by CT scan or MRI findings.[2] Lymphoma, fibroma, hemangioma, and neurogenic tumors must also be excluded.

Thoracic duct cyst is a rare entity that

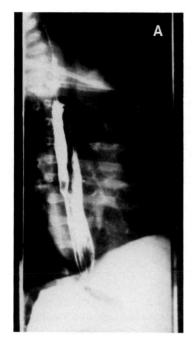
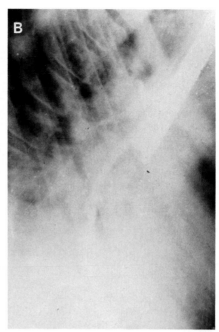
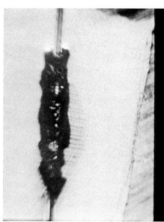
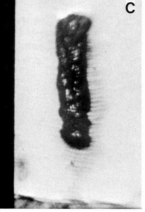
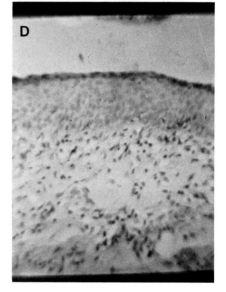

FIGURE 9.1 **A.** Lateral view of an esophagogram of a duplicated esophagus showing a double filled structure in the posterior mediastinum. **B.** The tracheoesophageal fistula is seen with radiological contrast introduced through the rigid bronchoscope. **C.** At surgical intervention a tubular structure connected the carina with the biliary tree. Biliary reflux was observed during the bronchoscopy of the duplicated structure. **D.** Histological image of the duplicated esophagus showing a stratified epithelium.

should be included in the differential diagnosis of mediastinal masses. Chest discomfort after a meal, CT scan, and needle aspiration may establish the diagnosis. Surgery is unnecessary if the lesion is asymptomatic (20%).[29]

TREATMENT

Cancer in the mucosa of a duplicated structure may develop with time.[30] The long-term risk of malignancy is 40% when a mediastinal mass is

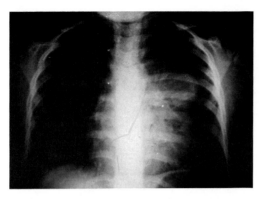

FIGURE 9.2 This plain anteroposterior chest roentgenogram was taken from a patient who had an enteric cyst of the mediastinum and shows the characteristic smoothly rounded mass.

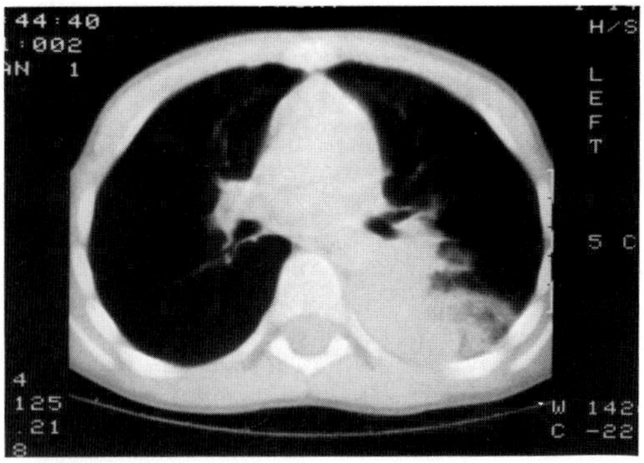

FIGURE 9.3 CT scan of an infected cyst in a 4-year-old patient. The posterior left mass of soft tissue density has small areas of hypodensity characteristic of microabscess formation.

detected in childhood,[8] so operative treatment is indicated in the face of a mass and is clearly needed when symptomatology is present (Table 9.2).

Optimal timing for operation depends on the severity of symptoms. Therefore, when hemorrhage by erosion into the lung, bronchus, or esophagus is present, emergency thoracotomy must be undertaken. Partial pulmonary resection or pneumonectomy has been lifesaving in cases of potentially fatal hemorrhage into the bronchial tree.[8]

Cervical foregut duplications require a careful surgical approach. The delicate neurovascular structures can be easily dissected away, except in cases when inflammation has developed.[13,15] A low transverse incision gives an excellent exposure of all structures and good cosmetic results.

Thoracic duplication cysts of foregut origin require an aggressive treatment, with total excision, in order to prevent cancer development or recurrence of symptoms.[31] Nevertheless, the benign nature of the lesion dictates that vital structures be preserved. Lateral thoracotomy is a reasonable approach in all cases.[32]

Conventional anesthesia is carried out with special care during the induction phase, particularly in stridorous patients. When a communication with the bronchial tree is suspected, a double-lumen Carlens endotracheal tube has been advocated in order to obtain a better exposure of the lesion and adequate ventilation.[25] In our institution we do not use such a tube in children because of the small diameter of the bronchi. An uncuffed endotracheal tube is preferable when possible and can be selectively guided through a small, flexible bronchoscope.

TABLE 9.2 Surgical Treatment

Case No.	Nature of Structures at Operation	Surgical Procedure
1	Well encapsulated, adherent to esophagus, pulmonary vein, aorta, and left bronchus	Total excision with partial excision of esophageal wall
2	Adhesions and RUL atelectasis	Total excision with RUL lobectomy
3	Paraesophageal	Total excision
4	Tracheoesophageal biliary fistulas	Total excision by thoracolaparotomy
5	Strong adhesions to LLL and abscesses	Total excision with LLL lobectomy
6	Posterior mediastinum and bronchial adhesions	Unroofing with partial excision, de-epithelialization, and bronchial suture
7	Extradural without thoracic communication or vertebral anomaly	Total excision through laminectomy from C-5 to T-2

RUL = right upper lobe; LLL = left lower lobe.

We also routinely use epidural anesthesia in thoracotomy, through a thoracic epidural catheter inserted in the operating room prior to the skin incision. This maneuver reduces the need for analgesics during anesthesia and provides a better postoperative recovery phase.

The skin incision is made horizontally, beginning in the anterior axillary line 2.5 to 7.5 cm inferior to the nipple and continued posteriorly behind the angle of the scapula. If the mass is located in the superior mediastinum, the fourth intercostal space is chosen; if the mass is elsewhere, the thorax is entered through the fifth intercostal space. A lower intercostal space can be selected if the mass is located in the lower third of the esophagus. Transdiaphragmatic extension of enterogenous cysts must be looked for; if present, a thoracoabdominal approach is required. In this case an initial thoracotomy incision through the seventh intercostal space can be extended anteriorly if necessary.

We have observed in some of our patients strong pleural adhesions, secondary to the inflammatory process. Such adhesions make access to the mass difficult, and sharp dissection is necessary until the lung can be retracted and the esophagus exposed (Table 9.2).

Once the mass has been identified the diagnosis of foregut duplication can be confirmed. Aspiration of the cyst should be performed if its large size makes mobilization and removal difficult or causes serious respiratory embarrassment. A purse-string suture is placed in the wall of the cyst, and the aspiration needle is inserted through it.

Except in rare cases, enteric cysts are readily dissected away from the esophagus (Fig. 9.4). To preserve vital structures, peeling the mucosal lining of the cysts with a wet swab can easily be done, leaving the nonmucosal portion of the wall.

Sometimes cysts are firmly attached to the anterior surface of the vertebral body by a fibrous band. In such cases, the band can be safely left after the excision of the cyst.[4] When communication with the spinal canal is suspected or a spinal extension cyst is proved, it must be managed cooperatively with the neurosurgeon. We have not observed such a communication in our patients (Table 9.1). A laminectomy is always indicated in order to decompress the intraspinal elements. The timing of the laminectomy and the thoracotomy is debatable, as they can be done during the same or separate operations. However, the most symptomatic component should be removed first.

A single drainage tube is inserted two intercostal spaces below the thoracotomy, in the mid-axillary line, and attached to underwater-seal si-

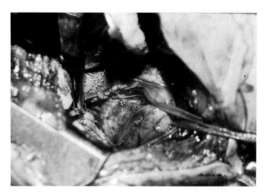

FIGURE 9.4 Intraoperative photograph showing the esophagus retracted with a cotton tape. This maneuver permits precise visualization of an enterogenous cyst, which is then easily dissected away using a wet swab.

phon drainage. Suction is rarely necessary and can be dangerous in small children and infants.

Antibiotic coverage is mandatory in every case. We use intravenous cefazolin, half of the full-day dose (25–50 mg/kg) 30 min preoperatively and eight regular postoperative doses or until the thoracotomy drain has been removed.

Of special interest is that a lung abscess in children as an underlying congenital malformation is frequent. If no symptoms are present, antibiotic coverage, physical therapy, and postural drainage must be started before surgical removal. Segmentectomy or lobectomy can be performed electively. Bronchoscopy or guided-needle aspiration may be useful as diagnostic and treatment measures. Tube drainage or emergent thoracotomy may be required because of the severity of the symptoms.

Mortality is low and varies among different series. We had no mortality in our patient group, and complications are specified in Table 9.1. Scherer and Grosfeld evaluated 62 reported cases related to sepsis and aspiration and reported a mortality of 8% for mediastinal enterogenous duplications.[8] Two cases occurred before operation as a result of hemorrhage from heterotopic gastric mucosa and sudden respiratory obstruction. In the same study the rate of complications was 8% and consisted of wound infection and aspiration. The low incidence of complications and the potential mortality of operative delay justify prompt surgical excision of these lesions.

ACKNOWLEDGMENTS

Thanks to Dr. Colon from the Department of Anesthesia and Dr. Isla from the Division of Neurosurgery at La Paz Children's Hospital in Madrid for their assistance and contribution in the sections related to their specialties.

REFERENCES

1. Ravitch MM: Duplications of the gastrointestinal tract. In: Welch KJ, Randolf JG, Ravitch MM, et al, eds. *Pediatric Surgery*. Chicago, Ill: Year Book Medical Publishers, Inc, 1986;2:911–913.
2. Ravitch MM: Mediastinal cysts and tumors. In: Welch KJ, Randolf JG, Ravitch MM, et al, eds. *Pediatric Surgery*. Chicago, Ill: Year Book Medical Publishers, Inc, 1986;1:606–609.
3. Langman J: Alimentary tract. In: Sadler TW, ed. *Langman's Medical Embryology*. 5th ed. Baltimore, Md: Williams & Wilkins, 1985;226–235.
4. Rahaney K, Barclay GPT: Enterogenous cyst and congenital diverticula of the alimentary canal with abnormalities of the vertebral column and spinal cord. *J Path Bact* 1959;77:457–462.
5. Wieczorek RL, Seidman I, Ranson JHO, Ruoff M: Congenital duplication of the stomach: Case report and review of the English literature. *Am J Gastroenterol* 1984;79:597–602.
6. Gray SW, Skandalakis JE: *Embryology for Surgeons*. Philadelphia, Penn: WB Saunders Co, 1972.
7. Sirivella S, Ford WB, Zikria EA, et al: Foregut cysts of the mediastinum: Results in 20 consecutive surgically treated cases. *J Thorac Cardiovasc Surg* 1985;90:776–782.
8. Scherer LR, Grosfeld JL: Congenital esophageal stenosis, esophageal duplication, neuroenteric cyst and esophageal diverticulum. In: Ashcraft KW, Holder TM, eds. *Pediatric Esophageal Surgery*. Orlando, Fla: Grune & Stratton, Inc, 1986;61.
9. Haller JA, Shermeta DW, Donahoo JS, White JJ: Life-threatening respiratory distress from mediastinal masses in infants. *Ann Thorac Surg* 1975;19:364–370.
10. Wychulis AR, Payne WS, Clagett OT, Woolner LB: Surgical treatment of mediastinal tumors: A 40-year experience. *J Thorac Cardiovasc Surg* 1971;62:379–392.
11. Mariño JM, Martinez-Urrutia MJ, Santamaría P, et al: Duplicaciones digestivas. *Ann Esp Pediatr* 1986;24:298–302.
12. Aoki S, Machida T, Sasaki Y, et al: Enterogenous cysts of cervical spine: Clinical and radiological aspects (including CT and MRI). *Neuroradiology* 1987;29:291–293.
13. Rhee RS, Ray CG III, Kravetz MH, et al: Case report: Cervical esophageal duplication cyst: MR imaging. *J Comp Assist Tomgraph* 1988;12:693–695.
14. Miyagi K, Mukawa J, Mekaru S, et al: Enterogenous cyst in the cervical spinal canal: Case report. *J Neurosurg* 1988;68:292–296.
15. Gans SL, Lackey DA, Zukerbraun L: Duplication of the cervial esophagus in infants and children. *Surgery* 1968;63:849–852.
16. Grosfeld JL, O'Neill JA, Clatworthy HW: Enteric duplication in infancy and childhood: An 18-year review. *Ann Surg* 1970;172:83–90.
17. Favara BE, Franciosi RA, Akers DR: Enteric duplications: Thirty-seven cases: A vascular theory of pathogenesis. *Am J Dis Child* 1971;122:501–506.
18. Ahmed S, Jolleys A, Dark JF: Thoracic enteric cysts and diverticulae. *Br J Surg* 1972;59:963–967.
19. Pokorny WJ, Sherman JO, Idriss FS: Mediastinal masses in infants and children. *J Thorac Cardiovasc Surg* 1974;68:869–875.
20. Deiraniya AK: Congenital oesophageal stenosis due to tracheobronchial remnants. *Thorax* 1974; 29:720–725.
21. Bower RJ, Sieber WK, Kiesewetter WB: Alimentary tract duplications in children. *Ann Surg* 1978;188:669–674.
22. Cohen SR, Geller GA, Birns JW, et al: Foregut cysts in infants and children: Diagnosis and management. Ann Otol Rhinol Laryngol 1982;91:622–627.
23. Superina RA, Ein SH, Humphreys RP: Cystic duplications of the esophagus and neuroenteric cysts. *J Pediatr Surg* 1984;19:527–530.
24. Cuadros J, Aransay A, Nistal M, Monereo J: Fistula traqueobiliar congénita. *Ann Esp Pediatr* 1974; 7:256–262.
25. Di Lorenzo M, Collin PP, Vaillancourt R, and Duranceau A: Bronchogenic cysts. *J Pediatr Surg* 1989;24:988–991.
26. Levitt RG, Glazer HS, Roper CL, et al: Magnetic resonance imaging of mediastinal and hilar masses: Comparison with CT. *AJR* 1985;145:9–14.
27. Jost RG, Sagel SS, Stanley RJ, Levitt RG: Computed tomography of the thorax. *Radiology* 1978;126:125–136.
28. Robinson RJ, Pavlina PM, Scherer LR, and Grosfeld JL: Multiple esophageal duplication cysts. *J Thorac Cardiovasc Surg* 1987;94:144–147.
29. Moretin LB, Allen TE: Thoracic duct cyst: Diagnosis with needle aspiration. *Radiology* 161:437–438, 1986.
30. Krous HF, Sexauer CL: Embryonal rhabdomyosarcoma arising with a congenital bronchogenic cyst in a child. *J Pediatr Surg* 1981;16:506–508.
31. Miller DC, Walter JP, Guthaner DF, Mark JBD: Recurrent mediastinal bronchogenic cyst. *Chest* 1978;74:218–220.
32. Cooper DKC, de Leval M: Mediastinal masses. In: Nixon HH, ed. *Operative Surgery: Fundamental International techniques: Pediatric Surgery*. 3rd ed. London: Butterworth & Co (Publishers) Ltd, 1978;282–293.

Foregut Duplications

James A. O'Neill, Jr., MD

De Agustin and Utrilla review the origin of the term *intestinal duplication* and clearly describe the currently held theories regarding the embryology of these lesions. The authors particularly address those lesions that result during the period of foregut differentiation and elaboration. Although the authors indicate that the term *duplication* was first proposed by Ladd in 1937, my review of the literature indicates that the term was first used by Fitz in a paper written in 1884.[1] However, Ladd did describe the currently accepted classification of intestinal duplications based on their location along lines of embryologic blood supply. In 1952 Gross et al reported a large series of duplications and described the two basic forms, cystic and tubular duplications, including those that communicate and those that do not communicate with the main intestinal lumen.[2] The authors of Chapter 9 also explain why some duplications are connected to the spinal canal and what that pattern of presentation is.

With specific reference to foregut duplications, the authors particularly analyze a group of epithelial-lined duplications occurring in the mediastinum and emphasize a common etiologic mechanism along with a classification based on an analysis of the lining of the anomaly. As some others before have done, De Agustín and Utrilla discuss these entodermal plate or lung bud anomalies capturing a wide variety of diagnoses including bronchogenic cysts, neurenteric cysts, esophageal duplications, lobar emphysema, cystic adenomatoid malformation, and intralobar pulmonary sequestration.

Current information suggests that the primitive respiratory system first appears as a longitudinal groove in the foregut just beyond the pharyngeal pouches. During the fourth week of fetal development, the groove develops into a ridge that will eventually form the trachea, bronchi, and lung buds. During the period of tracheobronchial development, bronchogenic cysts may originate from the embryonic lung bud tissue, but it is of interest that they may be lined with either respiratory or squamous epithelium, which is probably the result of the anomaly forming during a time when the primitive cells have more than one potential for development. For this reason, esophageal duplication cysts may be seen located adjacent to bronchi and vice versa. In another sense, they may be considered to represent ectopic cysts formed from foregut cells that became displaced prior to the period of final differentiation. Esophageal duplication cysts that lie adjacent to or within the wall of the esophagus therefore represent anomalies that form adjacent to the foregut structures of origin. In the case of duplication cysts that occur within the mediastinum but communicate below the diaphragm, the presumption would be that the anomalies began at the primitive junction point between the foregut and midgut derivatives. That foregut duplications are frequently associated with other congenital malformations is probably based on the fact that duplications have their beginning very early in the developmental process. The incidence of associated malformations in a series recently reported by my colleagues and I was 12%.[3] Most of these were gastrointestinal.

The authors also properly emphasize the fact that occasional patients have more than one duplication; in our series this occurred in 5 of 96 patients. They also point out the totipotential nature of the primitive lining cells, as many patients have ectopic gastric and/or pancreatic mucosa present within the duplications. In our series of 101 duplications, gastric mucosa was found in 21 instances and pancreatic glandular tissue in 5. Ileal and esophageal duplications were the most likely to have gastric mucosa, which indicates a potential for ulceration and bleeding in those patients. In our series 8 of 24 patients had ectopic gastric mucosa. With regard to clinical presen-

Current Topics in General Thoracic Surgery:
An International Series

121

tation, the authors indicate that enterogenous cystic malformations account for approximately 15% to 20% of foregut duplications located in the thorax, and our experience is similar. The authors' 7 cases are somewhat unusual in that all of the patients were symptomatic. In our experience, the vast majority of such patients are asymptomatic, and the lesions are discovered incidentally when roentgenograms are taken for another reason. In fact, some of their cystic lesions were only 3 cm or so in diameter and yet caused respiratory symptomatology. Our experience and that reported by most others would be contrary to this. Something we have not seen and which is distinctly unusual is a unique case reported by these authors in which a duplicated esophagus connected the carina with the biliary tree. The authors describe communication of an esophageal duplication below the diaphragm with the jejunum and pancreatic duct, and we have also seen gastric connections of such lesions. Although vertebral anomalies were noted in 80% of the author's cases, this incidence is much higher than the 20% incidence in foregut lesions we encountered.

With regard to diagnosis, it should be pointed out that frequently the precise nature of an incidentally discovered mediastinal mass is unclear. Additionally, the presence of a small lesion may be difficult to determine despite the fact that wheezing or some other vague respiratory symptom may be present. The authors correctly point out that a precise preoperative diagnosis can be made only 70% of the time, but recent advances have certainly increased diagnostic accuracy. The authors describe a variety of diagnostic modalities. In order to simplify matters, we have approached patients with foregut duplications in the following fashion. First, plain roentgenograms of the chest may demonstrate a mediastinal mass either with or without vertebral malformations. Then we prefer to obtain a computed tomographic (CT) scan both with and without contrast enhancement. In cases where vertebral anomalies are encountered and neuroenteric cysts are suspected, either a CT myelogram or magnetic resonance imaging is then performed. Abdominal ultrasound is also performed in order to rule out a possible associated abdominal duplication. In the case of suspected sequestrations of the lung, aortography is the most accurate way to pin down the diagnosis, but occasionally, computer reconstruction of an enhanced CT scan will demonstrate the abnormal systemic vasculature. Although we used these studies more often in the past, contrast esophagography, bronchography, and endoscopy are now reserved for those rare cases where a duplication is suspected to communicate either with the gastrointestinal tract or the biliary tree. With regard to mediastinal masses in general, however, the goal of preoperative diagnostic studies is not so much to pin down the precise diagnosis as it is to sort out those patients who will benefit from operation from those who will not, such as patients with lymphoma or treatable infections.

The authors make several recommendations regarding therapy. They categorize patients according to whether they require emergency or elective operation, and certainly, most patients can be treated electively. They make the logical suggestion that in the case of lesions that communicate with the tracheobronchial tree that a Carlen's double-lumen endotracheal tube should be used. This is a good suggestion, and it is not generally stressed in the literature. It is of interest that the authors stress a high frequency of inflammatory pleural adhesions surrounding the lesions they encounter. The overwhelming majority of patients we have seen have not had this, but it is certainly a potential in any patient who has ectopic gastric mucosa present within a duplication, because this may result in ulceration and severe surrounding inflammation. In such cases, they describe peeling away mucosa with a wet swab when it is apparent that total resection of the wall would compromise the normal attached structures. It seems that this should be a rare necessity but one worthy of remembering.

One point of disagreement relates to the management of neurenteric cysts. De Agustín and Utrilla describe leaving fibrous bands to the spinal canal alone. We find it difficult to predict what will be within the attachments of duplication cysts to the thoracic spinal canal, so we have preferred to excise these in toto. We have encountered intraspinal components of thoracic esophageal duplications and prefer to perform thoracotomy and laminectomy for total removal at the same operation.

The authors indicate that they prefer to manage tube thoracotomy drainage following thoracotomy in patients with foregut duplications without suction as they believe it to be dangerous. We have never found this to be the case.

The authors encountered sufficient inflammatory reaction with either atelectasis or abscess formation from long-standing inflammatory reaction that two of their seven patients required lobectomy. This would indicate that their patients had long-standing symptomatology, which has not been our experience.

Despite minor differences in opinion over approach to diagnosis and treatment, the authors' series of foregut duplications is exceedingly interesting and clearly illustrative of the spectrum of anomalies and their effects that pediatric surgeons are likely to encounter.

REFERENCES

1. Fitz RH: Persistent omphalo-mesenteric remains; Their importance in the causation of intestinal du-plication, cyst formation, and obstruction. *Am J Med Sci* 1884;88:30–57.
2. Gross RE, Holcomb GW Jr, Farber S: Duplications of the alimentary tract. *Pediatrics* 1952;9:449–468.
3. Holcomb GW III, Gheissari A, O'Neill JA, et al: Surgical management of alimentary tract duplications. *Ann Surg* 1989;209:167–174.

PART III

Acquired Esophageal Lesions

Chapter 10

The Treatment of Gastroesophageal Reflux and Its Complications in the Child

Jean Paul Chappuis, MD

HISTORICAL BACKGROUND

Malpositions of the stomach and esophageal lesions have been reported since the early 19th century. Billard in 1833 described the case of a child who vomited constantly and died shortly afterward. Autopsy findings led him to declare that "congenital inflammation of the stomach can impair everyday activities and lead to death." In 1853, Follin recommended the use of an esophageal probe equipped with an ivory ball at its tip "which would serve to palpate and localize the site of a stenosis and determine its nature according to its consistence." The first endoscopy was realized by Seligne in 1832, with a rigid 8-cm long tube and a laryngeal mirror.

The first radiographic image of hiatus hernia was obtained by Kohler in 1917. In 1926, Akerlund proposed its first anatomical classification.

Because they lacked investigative methods adapted to the age of their patients, pediatricians were unable to establish a relationship between the gastroesophageal reflux (GER) and a malformation of the gastroesophageal region until much later (Neuhauser and Berenberg, 1947[1]). Surgery, such as it was conceived for adults at the time, appeared to be the only therapeutic means to overcome this association of vomiting and cardial malposition of the gastroesophageal junction.

It was Carre[2] and Roviralta[3] who ardently advocated postural conservative treatment, which reduces the degree of reflux and, in many cases, results in successful treatment of the symptoms.

The appearance of different methods of exploration over the last 20 years (radiology, endoscopy, 24-hour acidimetry, manometry, scintigraphy) has allowed a better understanding of the pathophysiology of the cardiac region and has made it possible to draw a distinction between those patients who can be cured with a simple medicopostural treatment and those for whom the only solution is surgery.

Interventions in the child all derive from those indicated for adults by Nissen, Hill, Boerema,[9] Lortat-Jacob, Toupet, and Belsey. They have been adapted to the requirements of pediatric surgery, in particular by Nihoul-Fekete et al,[4] Boix Ochoa and Casasa,[5] and Jaubert de Beaujeu et al.[6]

At present, studies bear on the complications of the gastroesophageal reflux, especially respiratory complications.

REVIEW OF THE PHYSIOLOGY AND PATHOPHYSIOLOGY OF THE CARDIOESOPHAGEAL REGION

For a proper understanding of the principles that guide paraclinical examinations and therapeutic decisions when confronted with a child presenting with a GER, one should bear in mind the elements that constitute the physiological antireflux system and the main pathophysiological consequences of a declared GER.

The Antireflux Barrier

The antireflux barrier is made up of elements that may be functional or anatomical, static or dynamic, congenital or acquired, which, together or separately, contribute to prevent GER.

The anatomical elements are as follows:

1. The normal anatomy of the cardioesophageal region. The abdominal part of the esophagus and the angle of His represent the two cornerstones of this anatomy. Should they disappear or be lacking, GER will inevitably occur. The muscular hiatus, the phrenoesophageal membrane, and the gastrohepatic and gastrophrenic ligaments are complementary elements.

2. The arrangement of the muscular fibers of the lower esophagus is also primordial and consists of (a) a deep circular layer whose contraction strangles like a lasso the esophageal lumen and (b) a superficial longitudinal layer arranged in a spiral on the lower esophagus and extending over the gastric fundus toward the greater curvature—the "Helvetius necktie"—which closes the angle of His.

3. All cardioesophageal malpositions have in common certain anatomical modifications: disappearance of the abdominal segment of the esophagus, opening of the angle of His, and loosening of the hiatal orifice.

The physiological elements consist of the following:

1. The proper tonus of the abdominal part of the lower esophagus, which is subjected to positive intraabdominal and intragastric pressure and to negative thoracic pressure. This part collapses all the more readily when it is unusually long.

2. The esophageal clearance—that is, the capacity of the esophagus to empty its contents by means of reflex peristalsis.

These means of physiological defense are not yet functional in the newborn. Boix Ochoa[7] has clearly shown that there is a postnatal maturation period for this lower esophageal sphincter corresponding to the first six or seven weeks of life. During this period, the antireflux barrier is ineffective and the GER is physiological.

After the sixth postnatal month, there is a certain right to GER without complications, in particular during the postprandial period. It is accepted that the GER time should not exceed 4% of the daily 24 hours. Also after the sixth postnatal month, the GER can become pathological if one or more elements of the antireflux system disappear or are negated by an antagonistic mechanism, such as (1) increased intragastric pressure caused by disturbed peristalsis, pyloric obstruction (phrenopyloric syndrome of Roviralta, associated hypertrophic stenosis of the pylorus, and cardiac malposition of the gastroesophageal junction), duodenal obstruction preventing evacuation, or neurological disorders of central origin; (2) abdominal hyperpressure caused by a tumor, ascites, intestinal ileus, constipation, or urethral valves; and (3) hypertension of the gastric wall at the level of the fundus.

Consequences of Gastroesophageal Reflux

In the upper digestive tract GER can cause vomiting, esophagitis, and esophageal stenosis. Pulmonary and otorhinolaryngeal consequences include rhinopharyngitis, otitis, and bronchopneumopathies. General effects include anemia, height and weight abnormalities, and failure to thrive.

The acidity of the gastric liquid, through denaturation and activation of pepsin, destroys the esophageal mucosa. An associated intragastric biliary reflux makes the gastric content more corrosive through activation of gastric secretions by the biliary salts as much as by the alkaline nature of the reflux.

The esophagus, once invaded by the reflux, can defend itself only by (1) the resistance of its mucosa (but it is the most fragile of all the digestive mucosae, ill-protected by its secretions, and its resistance varies greatly from one person to another); and (2) esophageal clearance by peristalsis, which is decreased by esophagitis, leading very quickly to a vicious circle of complications.

Finally, pulmonary complications are dependent on multiple factors, the two most important being aspiration especially nocturnal, of the reflux liquid, and broncho-constrictor reflexes originating from the esophagus, affecting the tracheobronchial tract.

CLINICAL CONSIDERATIONS

The clinical symptomatology has four aspects, which I shall summarize briefly.

Digestive Symptoms

Signs related to digestion are the most common (90%) and include abnormally frequent regurgitations occurring at the slightest change of position, often associated with vomiting, the degree and frequency of which may represent a veritable handicap for the child and his family. Digestive-2 hemorrhage is indicative of peptic esophagitis and may be noted in the form of sanguinous streaks in the vomitus, or it may give rise to hypochromic anemia. Merycism may be present independent of any psychopathological context.

Dysphagia, which is all the more difficult to assess in the young child, in the infant takes on the form of difficulties of deglutition and crying when at the breast.

General Symptoms

Digestive disorders may result in poor weight gain and later, delayed growth, as well as microcytic hypochromic anemia.

Respiratory Symptoms

GER is frequently associated (10% to 60% of cases, according to the series) with relapsing, nonseasonal, bronchopneumonia in the child after 2 years of age, whether such afflictions do or do not include an obstructive component.

The association of asthma and GER is commonly observed, but the role played by GER in triggering attacks or in perpetuating the asthma is unclear.

Finally, in the infant, GER may be responsible for paroxysmal disorders: sudden attacks of cyanosis, hypotonia, convulsions, or apnea with loss of consciousness, probably due to asphyxiation.

Neurological Symptoms

Certain clinical signs seem, a priori, to have little connection with GER, though they are in fact related. These signs are bouts of fidgeting or tears, sleep disorders, recurring loss of consciousness with normal EEG, and Sandifer's syndrome, in which an attitude of torticollis is associated with facial and cranial asymmetry. For some, this torticollis is the sign of an antalgic reaction to esophageal pain; for others, it is a reaction to a reflex intended to block a pharyngeal reflux.

PARACLINICAL EXAMINATIONS

Certain paraclinical examinations enable GER to be displayed and its causes, degree of severity, and consequences to be determined (Navarro et al[8]).

The diagnosis of GER can be determined by esophagogastroduodenal barium study, which allows the reflux to be demonstrated in 75% of cases, the cardial malposition of the gastroesophageal junction to be identified (Figs. 10.1, 10.2, 10.3), and the gastric emptying and the antropyloric dynamics to be assessed. A 24-hour acidimetry is also useful: its sensitivity in detecting GER exceeds 90%; it provides information on the duration of the reflux, its acidity, and circadian variations (night, day), according to the positions or activities of the child. It also allows the reflux and serious discomfort or respiratory disorders to be correlated.

Peptic esophagitis can be visualized and quantified by endoscopy. The use of flexible

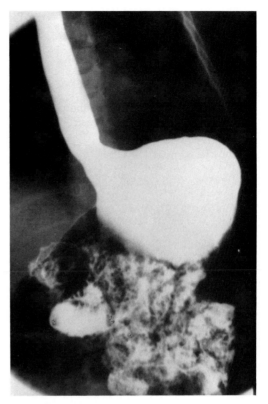

FIGURE 10.1 Gaping cardia.

tubes and the avoidance of anesthesia, or after simple premedication, make endoscopy easy. It is repeated in order to follow the evolution of peptic lesions or to assess the efficacy of a treatment, and it allows bile reflux to be detected.

The relation between GER and respiratory symptoms can be established by means of scintigraphy, with images centered on the pulmonary regions; upper esophageal manometry, which can reveal diminished tonus of the upper esophageal sphincter, and, of course, nocturnal acidimetry.

Failure of medical treatment can be confirmed by acidimetry during treatment and by endoscopy.

MEDICAL TREATMENT

The vast majority of children with GER undergo a trial of medical treatment consisting of three parts: postural treatment, hygienic and dietetic measures, and medicinal treatment.

With regard to postural treatment, acidimetric studies have proved that a 30° angle of ventral orthostatism is the most efficacious for preventing reflux and facilitating gastric emptying.

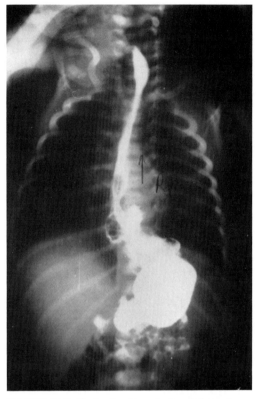

FIGURE 10.2 Mediastinal hernia (frontal view).

Hygienic-dietetic measures include fractionation of meals, thickening meals with pectinate or cellulose products, and reduction of fats.

Medicinal treatment consists of (1) substances that protect the esophageal mucosa—that is, antacids (alumina or magnesium hydroxide, organic polysaccharidic gel, dimeticone, and alginate) and inhibitors of gastric acid secretion (cimetidine and ranitidine)—and (2) modifiers of the tonus of the lower esophageal sphincter, such as metoclopramide, domperidone, and bethanechol, which increase the pressure of the lower esophageal sphincter and improve gastric emptying.

SURGICAL INDICATIONS

Surgical treatment may be considered in various situations, including failure of medical treatment (or incapacity of the parents to carry out the correct medical treatment). Surgery can be proposed without hesitation for large anatomical malformations: large right hernia (Fig. 10.4) or permanent or intermittent mediastinal hernia (Figs. 10.4, 10.5, 10.6). Although they are rarely accompanied by a pathogenic GER, such malfor-

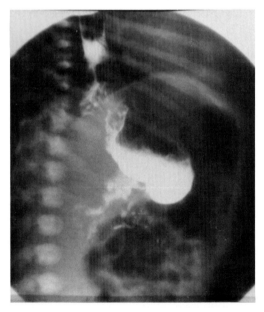

FIGURE 10.3 Intermittent mediastinal hernia.

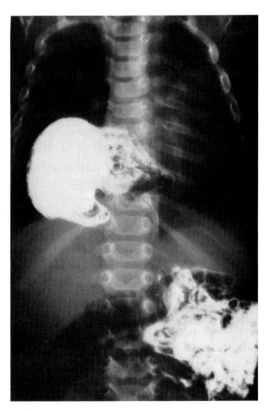

FIGURE 10.4 Large right hernia.

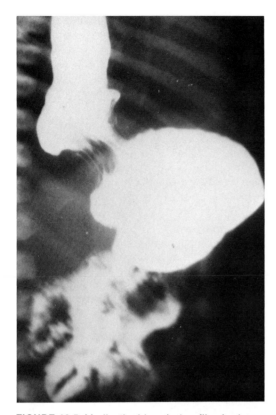

FIGURE 10.5 Mediastinal hernia (profile view).

mations are serious enough to require surgical repair.

In patients with the phrenopyloric syndrome of Roviralta,[3] the association of a hypertrophic stenosis of the pylorus and a mediastinal hernia requires at the same operative time extramucosal pylorotomy and hiatal repositioning.

Peptic stenoses (Fig. 10.7) diagnosed by eso-phagogastroduodenal study and endoscopy require, in addition to an operation for antireflux, preoperative, perioperative, or postoperative dilatations, which almost always avoid the need for esophagoplasty.

In cases of serious vomiting with overall consequences, surgery may be necessary.

Certain associations also demand surgical intervention: namely, Sandifer's syndrome, mental retardation (certain encephalopaths vomit regularly, thus making it impossible to feed them by mouth and very difficult to nurse), and Down's syndrome.

Two difficult situations may be encountered. One is the case of the infant who has been treated medically for GER since the neonatal period and who has reached the age of walking. Should the medicopostural treatment be continued, or

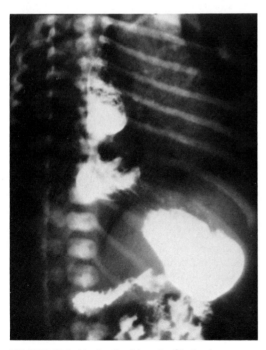

FIGURE 10.6 Mediastinal hernia (¾ view).

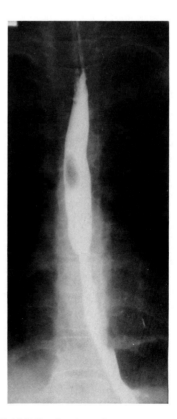

FIGURE 10.7 Peptic stenosis.

should surgical treatment be envisaged? We believe that if the malposition of the gastroesophageal junction is evident, and if acidimetry indicates the persistence of abnormal GER, then surgical treatment is justified. Respiratory complications of GER may also necessitate surgical intervention, if (1) 24-hour acidimetry, especially overnight, and scintigraphy disclose a relationship between reflux and respiratory accidents; (2) improvement of respiratory signs under GER medical treatment and their aggravation on cessation of treatment implicate digestive pathology as the cause; or (3) according to the attending physician, the particular case of the infant with GER and apnea is a clear indication.

SURGICAL TECHNIQUES

Pediatric surgeons have adapted to the child the techniques used for adults:

Simple Gastropexy (Boerema and Germs)

Through a short laparotomy, after producing a sufficiently long intraabdominal esophagus, the anterior wall of the stomach is drawn forward and fixed to the anterior abdominal wall.[9] This procedure does not restore the normal anatomy, and we are of the opinion of Boix Ochoa, who remarked that "the possible successful outcome from this technique is equivalent to the result obtained from this condition's natural tendency to cure itself."[5]

Nissen's Operation

Nissen's operation consists of a complete "muffing" of the abdominal esophagus by the gastric fundus. It is the best known of the antireflux procedures. I believe it is indicated in the adult whose physiological antireflux system has been damaged and has no chance of recovery. The Nissen procedure replaces the physiological antireflux system by a local hyperpressure mechanism capable of producing the same effects. The main drawback of this technique is that, physiologically speaking, it is not suitable for children. Further, it carries a morbidity greater than that of other techniques (postoperative occlusions, frequent dumping syndromes, deep-rooted stenoses, etc.).

Our Technique: Hiatal Reposition with Anterior Valve

The technique used by myself and my colleagues is adapted from Thal's method and is very similar to those described by Ashcraft and Holder[10] and Boix Ochoa.[5] This technique is based on two principles that appear to us to be fundamental:

Reconstitution of normal anatomy so as to allow the physiological antireflux system to recover its normal function.

Simple reinforcement of this antireflux system by a procedure that modifies neither its physiology nor its possibilities for growth.

1. Positioning. The child is placed in dorsal decubitus position with a block raising the lower part of the thorax. Two nasogastric probes are inserted under anesthesia so as to fit exactly the esophageal lumen and facilitate dissection of the esophagus.

2. Approach. The incision consists of a short median supraumbilical laparotomy, starting from the tip of the xyphoid as far as 2 to 3 cm above the umbilicus. The hiatal region is approached by retracting the left lobe of the liver after sectioning the suspensory ligament. Particular caution must be taken when dividing the right extremity of this ligament so as not to damage the suprahepatic veins. The left lobe is held back under a compress using a semirigid retractor. Another compress protects the spleen and also allows the left angle of the colon and the small intestine to be retracted with a second semirigid retractor. These two retractors are held in place by an assistant. A self-retaining retractor secures the edges of the laparotomy.

An atraumatic clamp then allows the stomach to be drawn downward and thereby discloses the hiatal region.

3. Lowering of the inferior esophagus. After sectioning of the upper portion of the lesser omentum, the peritoneum of the hiatal orifice is incised along its right edge and then along its anterior surface. A dissecting tampon allows the posterior surface of the lower esophagus to be progressively freed and thus gives access to its left edge, where the posterior parietal surface is incised. A curved clamp enables a tape to be passed around the esophagus; the gastric traction clip can then be removed. The freeing of the esophagus is continued in the mediastinum until 3 to 5 cm (according to the child's age) of esophagus can be lowered to an intraabdominal position (ie, below the muscular hiatal orifice) (Fig. 10.8A). Freeing the lower esophagus may be rendered difficult by the presence of a periesophageal inflammation, adherence of the esophagus to fibers of the hiatus and, especially, of the pillars, thickening of the parietal peritoneum, or local adenopathies.

The pneumogastric nerves should be localized and preserved; the right one should be left

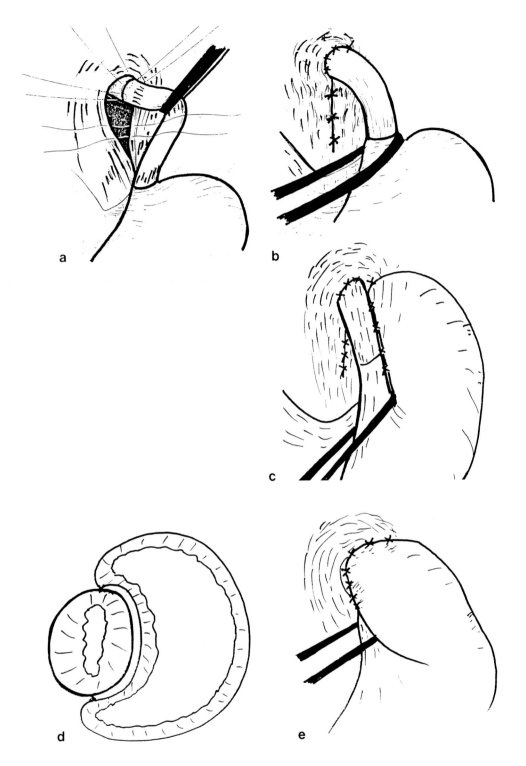

FIGURE 10.8 A. The lower esophagus has been freed up and pulled down through the hiatus. **B.** The diaphragmatic pillars have been sutured together, and the esophagus has been sutured to the hiatal orifice. **C.** The angle of His has been restored. **D.** This view in cross-section shows the fundus sutured to the esophagus. **E.** The fundus has been sutured to the hiatus and down the right edge of the esophagus.

in contact with the posterior surface of the esophagus.

Particular attention should be given to the pleural culs-de-sac, which are pushed back by the dissecting tampon. Any pleural opening should be identified and repaired immediately.

4. Repairing of the hiatal orifice. The hiatal orifice is generally very loose, and the diaphragmatic pillars are often hypoplasic, especially on the right. The muscular fibers of this orifice should be clearly visible and completely free of their peritoneal covering. The two diaphragmatic pillars are brought together behind the esophagus by two or three separate Vicryl 2-0 or 3-0 sutures (Fig. 10.8A). When the pillars are brought together, they should not compress the esophagus. Between the esophageal wall and the tightened hiatal orifice, it should be possible to easily insert a 5-mm diameter instrument (the esophagus itself still contains the two esophageal probes.

5. Suturing the esophagus around the hiatal orifice. The esophagus is sutured around the muscular hiatal orifice by means of separate Vicryl 4-0 stitches, each stitch firmly securing the esophageal wall and a muscular strip generally; four to six stitches are sufficient. Care must be taken to draw the esophagus downward and to push the hiatal orifice upward during the stitching procedure, so as to maintain the greatest possible length of abdominal esophagus (Fig. 10.8B).

6. Restoring the angle of His. The angle of His is reconstructed by suturing the gastric fundus to the left edge of the abdominal esophagus—the first stitch picking up the gastric wall at the level of the first short splenic vessel—and by suturing the hiatal orifice to the left of the esophagus. Then a series of stitches bring together, face to face, the gastric fundus and the esophagus (four to six Vicryl 4-0 stitches; Fig. 10.8C).

7. Fashioning an antireflux valve. The gastric fundus is stitched along the edge of the hiatal orifice by means of four to six Vicryl 4-0 stitches, thus progressively bringing the gastric fundus around to the front of the abdominal hiatus. It is then sutured on the right edge of the esophagus with a line of four to five stitches which is parallel to those of the angle of His (Figs. 10.8D & E).

8. No further maneuvers are carried out on the pylorus unless there is an obvious obstruction (hypertrophic stenosis of the pylorus, considerable antral dyskinesia requiring extramu-

cosal pylorotomy or a minimal pyloroplasty). One of the two probes is then removed. Hemostasis of the hiatal region is checked, and the left hepatic lobe is brought down in front of the operative site. The laparotomy is closed in three planes by Vicryl: 5-0 on the peritoneum, 3-0 on the aponeurosis, and 5-0 on the subcutaneous tissue. The cutaneous edges are brought together with an intradermal suture using colorless resorbable material.

9. Operative follow-up care is simple: For 24 hours, the child remains lying on the back, while retaining the nasogastric probe. At 24 or 48 hours, the probe is removed and the child can begin to drink a few milliliters of sugared water. From the third day, feeding is progressively resumed and the child can leave the hospital between the sixth and eighth postoperative day. Once feeding is restored, we prescribe a mixed regimen over four weeks to avoid dysphagic disorders related to the postoperative edema, and regular administration of esophageal protective drugs (eg, dimeticone gel).

10. The child is reviewed in consultation one month after his or her discharge. If the symptoms have disappeared all treatment is stopped, and a normal dietary regimen can be resumed. The operative result is assessed at three months by contrast radiography and/or acidimetry. The result is satisfactory if the examinations are normal after three to five years (Fig. 10.9).

RESULTS

Between 1968 and 1987, 179 children were operated on with our technique. The indications are given in Table 10.1. The results are considered very good in 95%. A clinical, radiological (Fig.

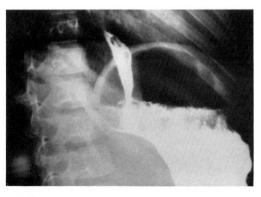

FIGURE 10.9 Fourth postoperative year roentgenogram.

TABLE 10.1 Indications for Surgical Treatment

Condition	Number of Cases	%
Large anatomical malformation	24	13.41%
Peptic stenosis	6	3.35
Syndrome of Roviralta	4	2.24
Failure of medical treatment for		
vomiting	71	39.67
respiratory disorders	26	14.53
apnea	2	1.11
esophagitis	36	20.11
hypertrophy	1	0.56
Encephalopathy	9	5.02
Total	**179**	**100.00%**

10.4), and endoscopic check-up was done in 135 children with a minimum follow-up of one year.

There were two postoperative deaths at 24 hours: one because of obstruction of the nasotracheal tube in a 30-day-old infant operated on for a serious esophagitis that was resistant to medical treatment, and the other because of acute febrile respiratory impairment in a 14-year-old boy presenting with Cornelia-Delange nanism and peptic stenosis of the esophagus.

Twelve patients had intestinal obstruction: six by adhesions, and six by ileoileal intussusceptions between the fourth and eighth postoperative day. All these obstructions occurred before 1981. Since then, we remove the nasogastric probe at an early stage and rapidly restore normal feeding. This contributes to the reestablishment of peristalsis and avoidance of adhesions. We have also discouraged the postoperative semirecumbent position.

The results vary according to the type of operative indication. An excellent result is obtained in 100% of cases if the indication was for serious anatomical malformation, vomiting, or peptic stenosis. Nevertheless, 5% still have a very slight radiologically demonstrated gastroesophageal reflux, but such cases are asymptomatic.

For indications related to respiratory problems, although the GER may have disappeared, elimination of respiratory signs is obtained in only 65% of cases. The other children are only improved, either by a reduced frequency of bronchopneumonia or by a reduced need for medication, in particular in the case of asthma.

Inferior results are obtained in encephalopaths, in whom the suppression of GER is obtained in only 50%. Our present procedure for this type of patient is to adopt a Nissen-type antireflux operation, as recovery of a normal physiology is, in such cases, impossible. Consideration should be given to combining the antireflux procedure with a gastrostomy or a feeding jejunostomy if the neurological disorders prevent oral alimentation.

CONCLUSION

A child is not a small adult, but rather a developing being. To ignore the normal physiology of the antireflux barrier and to replace it with a set-up suitable only for adults is, in our opinion, a mistake. In the vast majority of cases, surgery is indicated only after failure of medicopostural treatment. The intervention should reconstitute a normal anatomy in the cardioesophageal region, leaving intact all the elements of the antireflux system and affording them the possibility of adaptation and growth.

REFERENCES

1. Neuhauser E, Berenberg W: Cardio-oesophageal relaxation as a cause of vomiting in infants. *Radiology* 1947;48:480.
2. Carre IJ: Postural treatment of children with partial thoracic stomach ("hiatus hernia"). *Arch Dis Child* 1960;35:569.
3. Roviralta E: El lactande vomitator. Barcelona: Jané Ed, 1950.
4. Nihoul-Fekete C, Lortat-Jacob S, Jehannin B, Pellerin D: Résultat de l'intervention de reposition Nissen-pyloroplastie et indications chirurgicales dans le traitement du reflux gastro-oesophagien et de la hernie hiatale du nourrisson et de l'enfant. *Chirurgie* 1983;109:875–881.
5. Boix-Ochoa J, Casasa JM: Une chirurgie physiologique pour les anomalies du secteur cardio-hiatal. *Chir Pédiatr* 1983;24:117–121.
6. Jaubert de Beaujeu M, Campo-Paysaa A, Mollard P: Hernies hiatales et malpositions cardiotubérositaires du nouveau-né, du nourrisson et de l'enfant: Indications chirurgicales et résultats des 217 cas opérés. *Lyon Médical* 1970;223:1217–1223.
7. Boix-Ochoa J, Canals J: Maturation of the lower oesophagus. *J Pediatr Surg* 1976;11:749–756.
8. Navarro J, Cargill G, Fourcaude P: *Pathologie de l'oesophage. le reflux gastro-oesophagien: Gastroentérologie pédiatrique.* Paris: Flammarion Ed, 1987;109–128.
9. Boerema I, Germs R: Fixation of the lesser curvature of the stomach to the anterior wall after reposition of the hernia through the oesophageal hiatus. *Arch Chir Neerl* 1955;7:35110.
10. Ashcraft W, Holder T, Amouty M, Sharp RJ: The Thal fundoplication for gastroesophageal reflux in children. *J Pediatr Surg* 1984;19:480–483.

The Treatment of Gastroesophageal Reflux and Its Complications in the Child

J. Boix-Ochoa, MD and J. M. Casasa, MD

Chappuis presents the treatment of gastroesophageal reflux and its complications in childhood, based on the physiology and physiopathology of the cardiohiatal zone. He stresses those factors and functions that are most significant, some of which act as an esophageal reflux barrier for the gastric content and some of which favor its appearance.

For many years we have insisted on this concept of gastric esophageal pathology in the child, and we can congratulate ourselves that Chappuis agrees and has based his surgical technique on the basic principles we published.

PATHOLOGY AND TREATMENT

One of the most significant aspects in understanding the evolution of this pathology with age is to accept that gastroesophageal reflux tends spontaneously toward cure. The antireflux mechanisms mature with age, so that 50% of our patients diagnosed in the first months of life are not only free of symptoms at one year but radiologically appear cured. We have applied only postural treatment to these patients. The seated position with an inclination between 30° and 45° opposes gastroesophageal reflux by gravity and favors clearance. It is also convenient to thicken the feedings, give smaller amounts more frequently, and, on occasion, administer drugs that facilitate gastric clearance, particularly in those cases in which radiology or gammagrams show disturbance of gastric motility. Reflux is eliminated, and with it the cause of the vomiting. This allows for a gradual reinforcement of the car-

diohiatal region: the stomach remains in place, the lower esophagus does not rise, and the hiatus tightens around the esophagus. After a few months without vomiting the reflux may disappear. As mentioned by Chappuis, we carried out an investigation on the maturation of gastroesophageal reflux by completing 4020 manometric studies of the lower esophagus in 680 newborns and infants from 1 day to 6 months of age, in which we observed that an adequate high-pressure zone was obtained between the fifth and seventh week of life. Gastroesophageal reflux seen before this age can be physiological but it should not be ignored. Roentgenographic examinations in the first weeks of life show normality in the cardiohiatal region in most cases. A good example is hypertrophic stenosis of the pylorus, which in spite of introducing an important factor that favors gastric retention and, consequently, reflux—namely, obstruction of the pyloric channel—it is detected in only 10% of cases.

We believe that all gastroesophageal reflux diagnosed in the first weeks of life should receive postural treatment, with radiological evaluation at six months—not at one year, as we advise in cases diagnosed from the second month onward. If the reflux is physiological, it will be completely cured at six months.

GASTROESOPHAGEAL REFLUX AND RESPIRATORY MANIFESTATIONS

We must be cautious in accepting a relationship between radiological reflux and repeated respiratory manifestations. The data are confusing on this subject. In fact, if gastroesophageal reflux were responsible for serious respiratory illness, it is difficult to explain why, in the more than 2500 patients we have studied, it is not consistently the respiratory complications that attract attention. Indeed, gastroesophageal reflux diagnosed in children with respiratory illness generally has not caused prior digestive symptoms. In children without a history of vomiting and in whom after 2 or 3 years of age radiological gastroesophageal reflux may be discovered, reflux may be blamed for the respiratory problems. We disagree with this. We studied 35 children referred from the department of respirology with the clinical picture of atopic asthma. We carried out four tests: radiology, acidimetry, study of gastric chemistry, and esophageal gammagram (to see if there was reflux of contrast and aspiration into the respiratory tree; this was never observed). Four cases were selected for operation. One developed a severe asthmatic crisis on the 10th postoperative day. The four improved in the months following operation, though it is possible that this improvement might have happened without surgery.

Our opinion about this subject is shared by the majority of European services. In a survey taken four years ago of 37 important centers for pediatric surgery, we learned that in 75% of these centers only 5% of interventions for gastroesophageal reflux were carried out for respiratory manifestations. This opinion is in contrast with that of American surgeons, who more often favor surgical repair. We do not deny that in some cases gastroesophageal reflux can be the cause of respiratory problems, but we doubt that the high percentage published in which this is claimed can resist a rigorous scientific examination.

MEDICAL TREATMENT

Conservative treatment is very effective in the infant, to the point that we have not operated on any child younger than 1 year for many years. However, precise conditions must be stated.

1. The treatment must be strictly followed, 24 hours a day, for months. The child will stop vomiting in a few days. This can result in a relaxation on the part of the parents as well as the pediatrician, who then allows the child to sleep lying down. This is a major error because although the vomiting may not recur, the esophagus can slowly become affected, and a serious esophagitis can appear some months later.

2. The semi-seated position is the most comfortable and, as demonstrated by acidimetry, achieves esophageal clearance most rapidly. We do not favor the prone position. A child

cannot be maintained prone 24 hours a day without serious behavioral problems as this is the time when he or she is developing relationships with those around him. Furthermore, the acidimetry demonstrates that in the prone position, although reflux is less in quantity, it lasts longer and is therefore more dangerous.

3. If with correct postural treatment vomiting persists, other causes must be investigated: overfeeding; tonsil, ear, or renal infections; digestive intolerance; disturbance of esophageal gastric motility; hypertrophic stenosis of the pylorus, and so on. It should be remembered that reflux can also appear secondary to repeated episodes of vomiting for other reasons.

4. Caution should be employed in the administration of drugs to help overcome gastroesophageal reflux. The infant has a weak neurovegetative system, which can be affected by minimal doses of drugs. For example, alkalines or inhibitors of acid secretion should not be administered without the patient being investigated for hyperacidity. We accept the use of preparations that regulate intestinal motility, thus favoring gastric clearance, such as domperidone and, recently, cisapride.

SURGICAL TREATMENT

Chappuis has appropriately selected his patients for surgical intervention. Apart from the large hiatal hernias that clearly need repair, simple reflux should not be forgotten even though the child receiving postural treatment has stopped vomiting. A silent gastroesophageal reflux still merits concern. Its persistence can affect the esophagus and lead to an esophagitis, hemorrhage, or stenosis. For this reason it is important to carry out a radiological study between 12 and 14 months of age in all cases of gastroesophageal reflux diagnosed in the first months of life, even if symptoms have subsided. If the reflux persists, harmful effects in the esophagus must be sought. We use two tests: 24-hour acidimetry, which gives the number of reflux episodes and the time they remain in the esophagus, and study of the acidity of gastric juice which gives us very precious information as to the danger of this reflux: by means of the study of basil acid output and monoamine oxidase by stimulation with pentagastrin we can measure maximum acid secretions. In 10% to 15% of cases its presence alone is indication for surgical intervention.

We will not discuss the details of the technique proposed by Chappuis that differ from our own, as the basic philosophy is the same; however, we would like to stress the importance of the superior gastropexy that we employ. In this step, three fixing stitches from the greater gastric curvature to the diaphragmatic dome maintains the stomach in its place and favors maintenance of the angle of His.

In Roviralta's phrenopyloric syndrome, hypertrophic stenosis of the pylorus markedly favors reflux. Pyloromyotomy is sufficient to achieve good gastric clearance.

Once the pylorus has been operated on, these infants must continue with postural treatment for reflux in the same way as the infants who have normal pyloric sphincters.

Chapter 11

Indications For and Means of Surgical Treatment of Corrosive Esophagitis in Children

Jean de Ville de Goyet, MD, Didier Moulin, MD, and Jean-Bernard Otte, MD

INTRODUCTION

Serious forms of corrosive esophagitis frequently lead to major sequelae (extensive stenosis, shortening of the esophagus, and gastroesophageal reflux) with a high risk of malignant degeneration. Medical treatment consisting of repeated dilatation has long prevailed, but is characterized by high morbidity and unsatisfactory results. The experience gained over the last three decades and progress made in pediatric surgery and emergency care enabled the development of a modern therapeutic strategy.

Medical treatment in the acute phase is based on the clinical and endoscopic findings. Management of those forms with good prognosis is simplified, whereas more intensive treatment is imposed on the prognostically doubtful cases.

The place of surgery is currently well defined. Elective esophagoplasty, not indicated for emergencies except in the event of complications, is the treatment of choice for major sequelae and is performed as early as the second or third month after the accident. It may also be indicated for treatment of limited stenosis resistant to dilatation.

EPIDEMIOLOGY

The availability of concentrated acid and alkaline solutions for household use results in the frequency of corrosive esophagitis.[1] In children the

lesions are almost always accidental and usually less serious than in adults (who more often deliberately ingest large amounts of caustic agents). Appropriate licensing and increasing public awareness has begun to reduce the incidence and severity of the accidents.

In 1970 in the United States there were 13 000 recorded cases of caustic ingestion, 100 of these being fatal; hospitalization was necessary in 87% of the patients. The number of patients in 1982 was 30% lower; in addition, no fatal cases were reported, and the rate of hospitalization dropped to 35%.

Nevertheless, the ingestion of caustic agents continues to be a frequent household accident. Unsatisfactory results occur in 15% to 30% of medically treated patients. The development of esophageal stenosis must be expected in two-thirds of children with severe burns.

PHYSICAL PATHOLOGY

Several factors influence the distribution and severity of the lesions, but strict correlations cannot yet be established. The amount of ingested caustic agent and duration of contact are important but nearly always impossible to evaluate. Animal experiments have shown that concentrated caustics cause extremely serious lesions instantaneously. For weakly concentrated chemicals, duration of contact is more important.[1,2]

Information elicited from the patient or the patient's family, physical examination, and endoscopy will allow one to determine the area of the burned mucosa and the characteristics of the caustic involved—that is, its nature (acid or base), form (solid, liquid, or powder) and concentration.

Distribution of the lesions depends on the physical form of the caustic (liquid or solid, granules or powder). Easily swallowed liquids extend the burn from the mouth to the stomach. Adherence to the mucosa prolongs the contact, especially when the viscosity is high, as is concentrated caustic soda. In contrast, adherence of solids to the oropharyngeal mucosa slows swallowing. Burns of the lips and mouth prevent complete deglutition and cause active expulsion, so that a smaller amount is actually swallowed. Finally, even if it is swallowed, the distribution of solids is less uniform along the esophagus.

The nature and concentration of the caustic will determine the type of tissue damage. During contact with tissue, concentrated acids provoke coagulation necrosis and a superficial eschar. This eschar plays a protective role, preventing deeper penetration. Deep and extensive lesions are seen only after massive ingestion. In contrast, liquefactive necrosis and extensive tissue diffusion is typical after ingestion of alkali. These burns are deep or transmural and associated vascular thromboses are responsible for secondary extension by causing ischemia and the resultant necrosis. Such lesions may be produced by small amounts of concentrated alkaline substances and are responsible for most of the serious sequelae seen in children.[2]

CLINICAL DESCRIPTION

Caustic lesions may be scattered across the buccal, oropharyngeal, laryngotracheal, esophageal, and gastric regions. They may be limited to one area or may be multifocal. Esophageal lesions may occasionally be observed in the absence of any oropharyngeal lesion. The symptoms are rather varied and often nonspecific. Physical examination and eliciting all the symptoms have not produced information that is truly predictive for either the lesions' severity or prognosis, though several correlations have been made.

We retrospectively reviewed the records of 51 children admitted to the emergency room between January 1977 and April 1989. All had been hospitalized within 12 hours of the accident and presented objective lesions. The caustics involved, the initial symptoms, and the distribution, severity, and evolution of the lesions were analyzed for possible correlations or prognostic values[3] (P. Vergauwen and D. Moulin, unpublished data, 1990).

The mean age of this group of 51 patients (24 girls and 27 boys) was 24 months (range, 10 months to 9 years). Thirty-six had swallowed an alkali (liquid in 19 cases), and the others had ingested various types of acids. Ten children showed no particular symptoms. The other 41 presented a wide range of symptoms, such as irritability and crying, ptyalism, vomiting, dysphagia, coughing, or respiratory distress. All patients were examined by endoscopy within 48 hours to identify the oropharyngeal, laryngotracheal, and gastroesophageal lesions. The acute esophageal lesions were graded 1 (simple mucosal inflammation), 2 (necrosis limited to one esophageal segment), or 3 (necrosis extending over the entire esophagus). Thirty-two patients had multifocal lesions. These lesions were located in the mouth (48 cases), esophagus (29 cases), larynx (18 cases), pharynx (12 cases), stomach (9 cases), and, finally, lungs (3 cases). Eight patients showed respiratory distress at the time of admission and seven of them had laryngeal burns; five required urgent intubation. In these eight children, an oropharyngeal burn with considerable edema was the cause of the distress. Six of them had associated esophageal lesions: four grade 2 and two grade 3. The endoscopic examinations performed on the 43 other patients without respiratory distress on admission revealed 10 cases of supraglottic laryngeal burns. Three of these children had grade 2 esophageal lesions, and four had grade 3 esophageal lesions. Conversely, 27 of the 33 children who were free of laryngeal lesions were also free of serious esophageal lesions. Of the remaining six children, four had grade 2 lesions and two had grade 3 lesions.

If we compare these two groups—the group with laryngeal involvement (with or without symptoms) and the group free of laryngeal lesions—a significant difference in the frequency of esophageal sequelae can be seen (Table 11.1). This confirms that laryngeal involvement is an indicator of severity.

Study of the correlations among the initial symptoms, severity of the lesions, and the sequelae leads to three other observations: (1) The

TABLE 11.1 Negative Prognostic Value of Laryngeal Burn

	No Laryngeal Burn ($n = 33$)	Laryngeal Burn ($n = 18$)	
Esophageal lesions	16 (48%)	14 (78%)	$p < .05$
Burn grade 1	10	1	$p < .01$
Burn grades 2 + 3	6	13	
Esophageal sequelae	5 (9%)	11 (33%)	$p < .001$

absence of symptoms does not exclude the existence of caustic lesions but, if lesions are found, they are often minor and have a good prognosis. In our series, of 10 asymptomatic patients 5 had grade 1 esophageal lesions, 4 had isolated lesions of the tongue, and 1 had isolated lesions of the pharynx. None of them developed sequelae. (2) Pain, crying, ptyalism, and dysphagia were always associated with lesions of the mouth but were not in themselves indicative of other lesions. (3) The incidence of acute esophageal and laryngeal lesions and of esophageal sequelae was significantly increased when there had been spontaneous or induced vomiting (Table 11.2), probably by prolonging caustic contact.

The prognosis for esophageal lesions per se is directly related to the grade of the acute lesions on one hand and type of caustic on the other. Twenty-nine patients had acute esophagitis initially. Sixteen of them had sequelae (major sequelae in 12 and minor in 4). No sequelae were observed in children with grade 1 esophagitis, whereas all 8 patients with grade 3 esophagitis developed major sequelae. Finally, 4 of the 11 children with grade 2 esophagitis developed major sequelae, 4 developed minor sequelae, and 3 healed without sequelae.

We also have compared the effects of the nature and type of caustic agent. Eighteen patients had ingested potassium hydroxide in powder form and 17 other patients had ingested sodium hydroxide in liquid form. The incidence and severity of esophageal lesions were significantly higher in the second group (Table 11.3). Comparison of the acute lesions produced by acids (15 cases) or bases (36 cases) does not reveal any significant differences in the topography (Table 11.3). However, the prognosis (sequelae = later development of lesions requiring dilatation or surgery) is significantly worse after ingestion of sodium hydroxide (p < .01).

These observations are in accordance with the results published by several authors, though comparison is difficult because of differences in treatment protocols, clinical criteria, selection methods, and populations.[4–7]

TABLE 11.2 Negative Influence of Vomiting

	Vomiting (n = 19)	No Vomiting (n = 32)	
Esophageal burn	16 (84%)	13 (40%)	p < .01
Burn grade 1	0	10	} p < .001
Burn grades 2 + 3	16	3	
Esophageal sequelae	14 (74%)	2 (6%)	p < .001

TABLE 11.3 Prognostic Value of the Nature of the Ingested Caustic

	Sodium Hydroxide (NaOH) (n = 17)	Potassium Hydroxide (KOH) (n = 19)	Acids (n = 15)
Esophageal burn	15 (88%)*	5 (27%)	7 (47%)
Burn grade 1	4	3	2
Burn grades 2 + 3	11	2	5
Esophageal sequelae	10 (59%)**	2 (11%)	2 (13%)

p given only when significant.
* NaOH vs Acids: p < .02; NaOH vs KOH: p < .001
** NaOH vs Acids: p < .01; NaOH vs KOH: p < .01

TREATMENT

Emergency Care

Any child suspected of having ingested a caustic substance must be referred immediately for emergency care and must be thoroughly examined. A thorough oral and laryngotracheal examination must be carried out immediately. Although it is often difficult to determine the exact amount of ingested agent, efforts should be made to do so and the substance itself must be identified. The circumstances of the accident must be elicited, especially the presence or absence of spontaneous vomiting.

An intravenous infusion, laboratory workup, and chest roentgenograms are needed if there are definite symptoms or an obvious lesion. Endoscopy is performed under general anesthesia within 48 hours of the accident to grade the esophageal damage and to determine the extent of the stomach lesions. A nasogastric tube should be inserted under endoscopic monitoring if grade 2 or 3 esophageal lesions are encountered.

Later treatment will depend on the lesions found. In the case of minor lesions (grade 1), oral nutrition is allowed and the child is discharged from the hospital when he or she eats normally. In severer cases (grade 2 or 3 or when there are laryngotracheal lesions), the medical treatment should include parenteral feeding, antacid treatment, and antibiotics. Children with severe epiglottic or laryngotracheal lesions must be admitted to the intensive care unit. We do not perform gastrostomy but use a small gastric tube to allow feeding to start during the first week. This gastric tube is also useful if the patient develops a stricture, because it will facilitate the insertion of a guide wire for dilatation, thus reducing the risk of perforation.

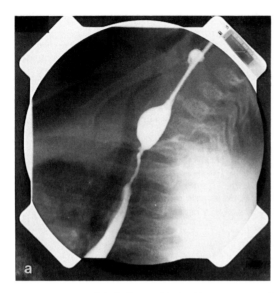 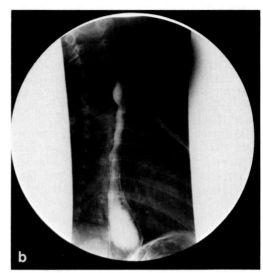

FIGURE 11.1 Limited but narrow stricture **(a)** before and **(b)** after dilations.

Until 1980, we used small doses of corticosteroids without noting any particularly beneficial effect. This observation has been borne out in most of the large series reported in the literature.[6,7] Steroids, which are useless in the case of grade 1 lesions, are very probably ineffective in treating grade 3 lesions. The question of their usefulness in grade 2 lesions remains. open, but the disadvantages linked to the use of steroids—increased vulnerability to infection and depression of healing processes—are of concern. Today, we use steroids only to treat edema or burns of the laryngotracheal area.

The therapeutic role of parenteral nutrition, recommended by some authors[8] remains difficult to ascertain. We have used intravenous feeding systematically, and the incidence of secondary stenosis in our patients is equal to that in the large series in the literature.

Finally, some authors have proposed the use of an esophageal mold for endoluminal calibration to prevent the development of multiple, extensive areas of stenosis.[9,10] Anatomical and histological examination of surgical specimens has never convinced us that simply keeping open the esophageal lumen after transmural destruction

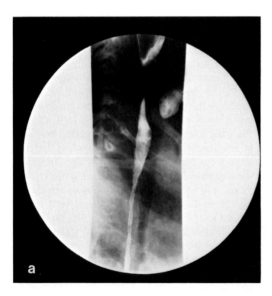 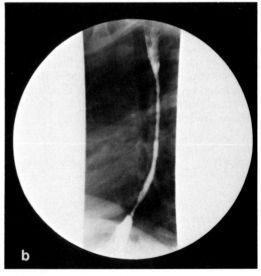

FIGURE 11.2 Extensive stricture of cervical and intrathoracic esophagus.

would prevent stenosis and fibrosis. The efficacy of the esophageal mold remains anecdotal and its usefulness has not been proved.

Reevaluating the Lesions and Prognosis

Patients with severe lesions are assessed radiologically after 3 to 4 weeks of treatment. If the sequelae are minimal or moderate, endoscopy with calibration of the esophagus is performed.[11-14] In the case of a limited stricture, a course of dilatation is started and the endoscopic and radiological exams are repeated later (Fig. 11.1). When the lesions are severe and extensive from the beginning, we prefer to terminate medical treatment in favor of early surgical repair (Fig. 11.2). Repeated dilation carries a high risk of iatrogenic complications that are sometimes fatal. Dilations are often necessary for many years. Moreover, multiple stenoses often lead to brachyesophagus and associated gastroesophageal reflux.

The treatment problems and persistence of symptomatic sequelae convinced us, like other authors, as early as 1979 that early surgical repair might be preferable.[15] A period of three to six weeks after the accident is sufficient for correctly reevaluating the lesions. When the condition continues to deteriorate and the lesions are extensive, continuing conservative treatment is senseless. Early surgery avoids later repeated hospitalizations and reduces effects on the child's psychological development and scholastic performance.

SURGICAL TREATMENT
Acute Stage

Children usually swallow small amounts of caustic substances. One seldom comes across complete necrosis of the esophagus with mediastinitis and perforating lesions of the stomach wall, as is seen in adults. The adult aggressive surgical approach (emergency exploratory laparotomy and esophagogastrectomy) should not be applied to children.[16] We believe that exploratory surgery should be reserved for patients with obvious signs of peritoneal irritation and esophageal or gastric perforation. A gastrostomy may prove useful at a later stage, but we do not perform it early. As a rule, the acute phase should be treated medically.

Later Stage (Sequelae)

Extensive, tight stenotic lesions usually require surgery, either right away or after failure of other treatment. It consists inevitably of replacement esophagoplasty. Short stenoses resistant to dilatation can usually be corrected by segmental resection followed by end-to-end anastomosis, though some authors prefer myotomy, stricture plasty, or even esophagoplasty in the most severe cases.

Some special aspects are worth emphasizing: it is essential to preserve the superior esophageal sphincter and the first part of the cervical esophagus to permit normal swallowing (Fig. 11.3). If a stenosis develops later at this level, it can usually be dilated. In the event of a major

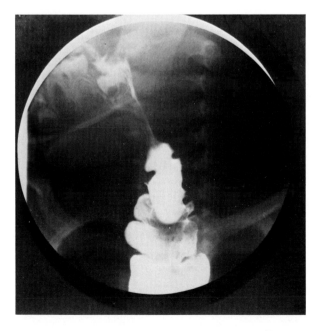

FIGURE 11.3 Esophagocoloplasty: upper anastomosis.

lesion of the hypopharynx, with stricture of the pharyngoesophageal junction and upper esophagus, an extensive reconstruction must be considered, and the functional prognosis is poor.

Excision of the damaged esophagus is mandatory to prevent later malignant transformation as well as the risk of development of cysts or abscesses, which occur when the esophagus is not removed. Indeed, when the esophagus is preserved, inflammation, stasis and infection, and peptic reflux will cause chronic irritation and increase the risk of cancer.[17-19] The chance of a malignant transformation in such individuals might be 1000 times the natural risk. Carcinoma developing in a healed caustic stenosis has a better prognosis because it originates in dense, fibrous scar tissue, which slows the neoplastic transmural infiltration and regional extension. However, the existence of old morphological changes and dysphagia must not be permitted to delay the diagnosis. If unexpected relapse of stenosis or abnormal resistance to dilation is observed, the diagnosis of carcinoma must be suspected. When the esophagus is not removed at the time of esophagoplasty, cancer will develop with few symptoms and the diagnosis will be late. For all these reasons, excision of the burned esophagus is recommended. The progress made in anesthesia and esophageal surgery permits excision and reconstruction in one single procedure.

Esophagocoloplasty is the most widely used technique.[20-24] Closed-chest esophagectomy has recently been recommended.[25,26] However, we prefer not to perform this operation beyond the acute phase because of the risk of tracheal or vascular lesions related to the tight adhesions encountered when the initial lesion is transmural. During the last 15 years, we have used the one-step technique learned from R. Belsey[27] and have performed it through a left thoracotomy with the use of the transverse colon on a left colic artery pedicle.

The graft must be able to reach the upper neck without tension. Perioperative dilatation of the cervical esophagus and upper esophageal sphincter is carried out, if necessary, before performing the esophagocolic anastomosis. After esophagectomy, the graft is placed in the posterior mediastinum. The mediastinal pleura is closed over the graft to exclude it from the pleural space. This permits optimal alignment of the graft with minimal cervicothoracic, intrathoracic, or thoracoabdominal bends, thereby guaranteeing better function subsequently (Fig. 11.4). The hiatal orifice is enlarged and the graft sutured to the edge of the diaphragm. We place the colon behind the stomach and perform the cologastric anastomosis on the inferior and posterior aspect of the stomach to avoid reflux (Fig. 11.5). A pyloromyotomy is routinely done.

The described technique was performed in 16 children for lye stricture. Ten of these children had been admitted to the emergency room of our hospital and are part of the reported series of 51 patients discussed previously; the remaining six patients were referred at a later stage. The indications for surgery were based on the existence

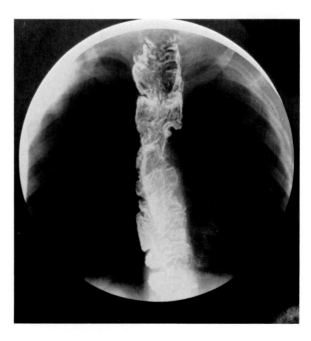

FIGURE 11.4 Esophagocoloplasty: intrathoracic alignment.

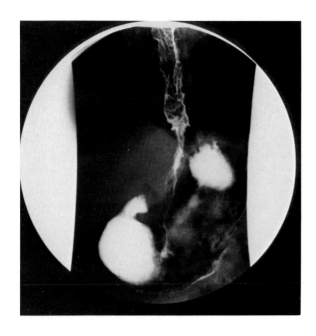

FIGURE 11.5 Esophagocoloplasty: intraabdominal positioning and cologastric anastomosis.

of lesions that were severe and extensive or resistant to dilatation. Half of these cases had acquired a short esophagus combined with gastroesophageal reflux. The decision to operate was made one to nine months after the accident. The ablation of the esophagus and coloplasty were performed at the same time (except in one case, because of associated mediastinitis). There were no deaths. Twisting of the graft was corrected early and successfully in one case; in another case, we observed a postoperative perforation in a dysgenic area of colonic muscle layer requiring excision of the graft and repeated plastic surgery (Gastric-tube).

The long-term results for 14 of the patients are excellent, despite the fact that transient dilation of the cervical esophagus was required in 5 of them. The development of stasis and dilatation of the graft with areas of excessive tortuosity in one child needed surgical revision seven years after the initial surgery with a good result. One other child has persisting problems with swallowing and recurrent respiratory infections, subsequent to extremely severe lesions with extensive involvement of the epiglottis, larynx, and pharynx. Gastric stasis was seen in none, though one patient has gastrocolic reflux without peptic complications. One child suffered temporarily from moderate dumping syndrome.

CONCLUSION

Ingestion of a caustic agent remains a serious household accident. No therapy has proved effective in preventing the sequelae. The intensity of medical treatment in the acute phase must be adapted to each individual case.

In the case of minor or benign lesions, simple medical treatment is successful. Patients with grade 2 or 3 lesions must receive the appropriate medical treatment systematically for 2 to 3 weeks before being reevaluated.

In the case of small, isolated stenotic lesions, dilatation should be performed. When the lesions are resistant to dilatation or severe from the beginning, surgical correction should be recommended. Esophagoplasty and excision of the burned esophagus, as one step, constitute the ideal procedure. This approach minimizes the length of hospitalization and morbidity and offers the best chance for rehabilitation.

REFERENCES

1. Leape L, Ashcraft KW, Scarpelli DG, Holder TM: Hazard to health: Liquid lye. *N Engl J Med* 1971;284:578.
2. Ashcraft KW, Padula RT: The effect of dilute corrosives on the esophagus. *Pediatrics* 1974;53:226.
3. Moulin D, Bertrand JM, Buts JP, et al: Upper airway lesions in children after accidental ingestion of caustic substances. *J Pediatr* 1985;100:408.
4. Gaudreault P, Parent M, McGuiggan M, et al: Predictability of esophageal injury from signs and symptoms: A study of caustic ingestion in 378 children. *Pediatrics* 1983;71:767.
5. Crain E, Gershel JC, Mezey AP: Caustic ingestions: Symptoms as predictors of esophageal injury. *AJDC* 1984;138:863.
6. Hawkins DB, Demeter MJ, Barnett TE: Caustic ingestion: Controversies in management: A review of 214 cases. *Laryngoscope* 1980;90:98.
7. Kirsh MM, Peterson A, Brown JW, et al: Treatment of caustic injuries of the esophagus: A ten-year experience. *Ann Surg* 1978;188:675.

8. Di Costanzo J, Noirclerc M, Jouglard J, et al: New therapeutic approach to corrosive burns of the upper gastrointestinal tract. *Gut* 1980;21:370.

9. Hill JL, Norberg HP, Smith MD, et al: Clinical technique and success of the esophageal stent to prevent corrosive strictures. *J Pediatr Surg* 1976;11:443.

10. Harouchi A, Fehri M: La prévention des sténoses caustiques de l'oesophage par moule endooesophagien. *Chir Pédiatr* 1984;25:317.

11. Oakes DD, Sherck JP, Mark JB: Lye ingestion: Clinical patterns and therapeutic implications. *J Thorac Cardiovasc Surg* 1982;83:194.

12. Imre J, Kopp M: Arguments against long-term conservative treatment of oesophageal strictures due to corrosive burns. *Thorax* 1972;27:594.

13. Camboulives J, Gregoire A, Garcin M, et al: Lésions caustiques de l'oesophage chez l'enfant. *Ann Anesth Franç* 1977;4:341.

14. Goldman LP, Weigert JM: Corrosive substance ingestion: A review. *Am J Gastroenterol* 1984;79:85.

15. Otte JB, de Ville de Goyet J, Kestens PJ, et al: Modification de la stratégie thérapeutique dans les oesophagites caustiques graves chez l'enfant: Plaidoyer pour l'intervention chirurgicale précoce dans les formes diffuses. *Acta Gastro-ent Belg* 1982;45:527–535.

16. Ray JR, Myers WO, Lawton BL, et al: The natural history of liquid lye ingestion. *Arch Surg* 1974;109:436.

17. Lansing PB, Ferrante WA, Ochsner JL: Carcinoma of the esophagus at the site of lye stricture. *Am J Surg* 1969;118:108.

18. Kay EB, Cross FS: Chronic esophagitis: A possible factor in the production of carcinoma of the esophagus. *AMA Arch Int Med* 1956;98(4):475.

19. Appelqvist P, Salmo M: Lye corrosion carcinoma of the esophagus. *Cancer* 1980;45:2655.

20. Stone MM, Mahour GH, Weitzman JJ, et al: Esophageal replacement with colon interposition in children. *Ann Surg* 1986;203:346.

21. Soulier Y, Valayer J, Melin Y, et al: Les oesophagoplasties coliques en chirurgie pédiatrique: Etude d'une série de 30 cas. *Ann Chir* 1979;33:257.

22. Kelly JP, Shackelford GD, Roper CL: Esophageal replacement with colon in children: Functional results and long-term growth. *Ann Thorac Surg* 1983;36:634.

23. Neville WE, Najem AZ: Colon replacement of the esophagus for congenital and benign disease. *Ann Thorac Surg* 1983;36:626.

24. Nendren WH; Hendren WG: Colon interpositron for esophagus in children. *J Pediatr Surg* 1985;20:829.

25. Aigrain Y, Weisgerber G, Boureau M: Sténose caustique organisée chez l'enfant. *Nouvelle Presse Médicale* 1984;13:2810.

26. Rodgers BM, Ryckman FC, Talbert JL: Blunt transmediastinal total esophagectomy with simultaneous substernal colon interposition for esophageal caustic strictures in children. *J Pediatr Surg* 1981;16:184.

27. Belsey R: Reconstruction of the esophagus with left colon. *J Thor Card Vasc Surg* 1965;49(1):33.

Indications For and Means of Surgical Treatment of Corrosive Esophagitis in Children

David P. Mitchell, MD, FRCS(C)

EPIDEMIOLOGY

Before 1927, when the U.S. Congress introduced the first consumer protection legislation requiring bottles of lye to be labeled as poisonous, accidental burns of the esophagus were extremely common in children.

Since this historic legislation was enacted at the urging of endoscopist Chevalier Jackson, extensive packaging protection has been introduced resulting in the incidence of these injuries being drastically reduced. However, many still store these caustics and acids in unsuitable containers, and lye is often diluted with water in such kitchen receptacles as teacups. The milk-like solution produced has caused many accidental burns of the esophagus. In addition, adult suicides are still attempted on a regular basis with lye, bleach, and plumbing acids.

TYPES OF CORROSIVES

Acids

These include sulphuric acid, hydrochloric acid, nitric acid, and bleach, which breaks down into hydrochloric acid. Acids are liquid and tend to pass quickly to the stomach, often doing little damage to the mouth and esophagus. They produce a coagulation type of necrosis, usually without damage to the underlying muscular layers.

Alkalis

These are strong basic substances and include ammonium, potassium, and sodium hydroxide.

Published 1991 by Elsevier Science Publishing Co., Inc.
655 Avenue of the Americas, New York, NY 10010
*Current Topics in General Thoracic Surgery:
An International Series*

Generally in powder form, they are retained in and therefore tend to produce burns in the mouth and esophagus. Such caustics produce a liquefactive type of necrosis and penetrate the deeper muscular layers more easily. Some of the more common alkalis are Drano, Gillete's Lye, and Liquid Plumber.

Diagnoses

It is very important to establish the type and quantity of caustic ingested. When in doubt, consultation with a poison control center can be useful. Frequently, parents are frightened by the incident and are unsure of many of the details. Suicide attempts may exaggerate the quantities consumed. A careful physical examination is important, looking for evidence of mouth burns, laryngeal edema, respiratory distress, mediastinitis, peritonitis, and so on.

TREATMENT

In order to demonstrate difference of opinions on this topic, I have chosen to present in brief form the management policy at my institution, which the reader will recognize as less aggressive than that of de Ville de Goyet, Moulin, and Otte.

First Aid

Vomiting should not be induced because a substance that burns going down can burn coming back. Sips of clear water can be given in an attempt to neutralize the corrosive.

Initial Medical Management

If it is determined that the corrosive ingested was an acid, therapeutic doses of cimetidine should be administered intravenously. Sips of clear liquids can be given by mouth, but no food should be permitted until the extent of the burn has been established.

Batteries in the esophagus or stomach should be considered an emergency and removed within one or two hours.

Antibiotics

Research has suggested that antibiotics may reduce the granulation response. Penicillin is recommended at 100 mg/kg/day when extensive burns are suspected.

Steroids

In the 1950s and 1960s research suggested that granulation and scar tissue were reduced when steroids were administered shortly after the ingestion of caustic. It was the impression of the clinicians at the Hospital for Sick Children in Toronto that early scar tissue was reduced but that the scarring was simply delayed and possibly enhanced by the use of steroids. It is now our practice to use steroids only in the presence of developing respiratory distress.

Endoscopic Diagnosis

The early signs of sloughing or granulation do not appear until four days after the injury. Therefore we do not perform an endoscopy on these children until that time.

STRICTURE MANAGEMENT

In the event that a circumferential burn of the esophagus longer than 1 cm is discovered at the time of endoscopy, stricturing is inevitable and stringing of the esophagus with gastrostomy is performed. Three weeks later, retrograde dilation of the esophagus is initiated.

A reversed gastric tube or colon transfer with microvascular anastomosis is considered when dilation fails to produce a resolution of the problem. In my experience, colon transfer should be considered when there is a significant cervical stricture, as reversed gastric tubes do not reach into this area.

In the event that no significant sloughing is encountered, the patient is released from the hospital with appropriate dietary instructions (liquids, soft food, etc.). Instructions are also given to watch for signs of stricture development. These patients are seen three weeks after ingestion, and if there is any question about the ability to swallow, a barium examination with or without further esophagoscopy is performed.

PART IV

Tracheobronchial Obstruction

Chapter 12

Tracheal Stenosis

Dale G. Johnson, MD

BACKGROUND

Most tracheal stenoses in infants and children are acquired through long-term intubation and involve the upper airway. Congenital lesions are less frequent and usually involve the lower trachea.

Treatment for high tracheal lesions is often delayed or staged following tracheostomy. Low lesions can seldom be bypassed with a tracheostomy and require more urgent treatment. A variety of techniques for dilating, splinting, ablating, resecting, and grafting have been and still are applied in appropriate circumstances. This chapter reviews past experience and current management alternatives.

CLINICAL PRESENTATION

Infants symptomatic from a fixed stenosis of the airway usually present with noisy respiration and variable degrees of respiratory distress. Cyanotic episodes and chest wall retractions may occur with exertion. Raspy, stridorous breathing is usually inspiratory and expiratory in timing.

Less than half of the infants with congenital stenosis of the trachea are symptomatic at birth. Acquired postintubation strictures also may appear either late or require prompt tracheostomy after failed extubation.

MANAGEMENT OF SPECIFIC ACQUIRED STENOSES

Postintubation Injury

In severe cases, intubation injury to the infant's airway involves both the larynx and the upper trachea. Inflatable cuffs are not used around in-

fant tubes, in contrast to adult management, and the site of tracheal injury is therefore higher. Maximal tube contact is at the cricoid, the only complete ring of cartilage and the smallest diameter in the normal infant trachea.

Reports between 1965 and 1976 recorded a postintubation subglottic stenosis incidence ranging from 1.6% to 6.7%.[1] This alarming frequency resulted in protocols for avoiding tight-fitting endotracheal tubes, acceptance of a small air leak, better stabilization of tubes, control of infection, and minimizing intubation times. Subsequent reduction in incidence of intubation injury has been gratifying. This complication is unlikely to disappear, however, as long as infants require management with endotracheal tubes.

Oblique Resection with Anastomosis

Resection of a stenotic segment with direct anastomosis of normal trachea proximal and distal to the lesion, though standard treatment for adults, is seldom possible for the high acquired lesions in infants. Grillo has reported success with oblique resection of the cricoid at the upper margin in older children (14 years) and adults, but there are no reports with this approach in infants.[2] Concerns about interference with subsequent growth of the larynx or injury to the recurrent nerves, which enter the larynx along the back of the posterior cricoid lamina, have restricted application of the oblique resection technique. This same dangerous proximity of the recurrent nerves to the posterior cricoid plate has eliminated any consideration of complete circumferential resection of the cricoid.

Dilation

Dilation, by bronchoscope or by a variety of dilators, was once a mainstay of treatment for upper airway stenosis.[3] As one would expect, dilation is often effective for mild stenoses or membranous obstructing webs, and very disappointing for the more extensive fibrous strictures.

Some infants have suffered scores of dilations over periods of months and years with minimal progressive improvement.

Therapeutic dilation of airway stenosis has been revived, however, with the development of high-pressure precision balloon dilators (Greuntzig) and their successful use in blood vessels and in the gastrointestinal tract. Enthusiasts recommend balloon dilation as initial therapy for most stenotic lesions of the airway, whether congenital or acquired.[4] Radiographic monitoring of incremental dilation plus the application of pure radial distending forces at the stricture site would seem to make this the safest form of dilatation. Successful cases have included both acquired and congenital lesions, but experience is still small and the stenoses have been localized. It seems unlikely that dilation will ever have much effect on lesions associated with complete cartilage rings, but balloon dilatation should be considered for segmental stenoses, particularly if they are acquired.

Steroid Injection

Intralesional injection with steroids has been advocated as a means of softening the scar and improving the effectiveness of dilation. There are no controlled studies proving effectiveness of intralesional or systemic steroids, but numerous clinical reports claim benefit from steroids used in conjunction with dilation,[5] dilation and stenting,[6] or endoscopic resection.[7]

Intraluminal Stenting

Dilation and intraluminal stenting has a relatively long history in the management of subglottic stenosis, and it is still considered by some as the method of choice.[8] The Montgomery T-tube of Silastic,[9] the keel stent of Silastic or Portex,[10] the Evans "Swiss roll" of Silastic,[10] and the Aboulker stent of Teflon[11] have all been used with success in specific circumstances according to the preferences of different surgeons (Fig. 12.1). Standard endotracheal tubes have been used as short-term stents, even though this type of stenting simulates the very mechanism of injury that caused the stenosis in the first place. Formation of granulation tissue around the indwelling stent remains a problem, and successes and failures have been reported with all methods. Recommendations for duration of stenting vary from 3 weeks to 13 months; morbidity with the stent in place can be significant.

Localized Intraluminal Scar Resection

Localized resection of scar is another approach to treatment. Cold-knife excision following direct exposure of the larynx and upper trachea, endoscopic electrosurgical resection,[12] cryotherapy and resection,[13] and more recently the endolaryngeal laser excisions[14] have all been advocated as treatment alternatives. Most have been effective and appropriate for less severe laryngeal stenoses, but the failure rate goes up when the stenotic lesion is thick enough to extend beyond the cricoid into the upper trachea.

Laryngotracheal Split with Interposition Grafting

Interposition grafting procedures are designed to increase the diameter of the cricoid and upper trachea. Composite pedicle grafts of hyoid or free grafts using hyoid, thyroid cartilage, or costal cartilage have all been advocated.

For anterior subglottic stenosis, Cotton and Evans[15] favor a costal cartilage graft, placed with

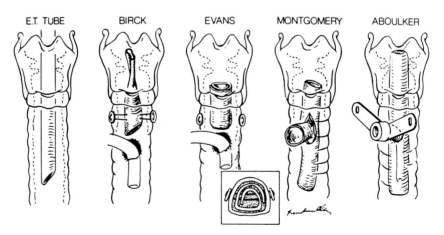

FIGURE 12.1 Stents used for treating subglottic stenosis of the larynx and upper trachea.

the perichondrium facing the tracheal lumen. The incision starts in the upper two or three tracheal cartilages and extends through the anterior cricoid and the lower thyroid cartilage. The edges of the graft are notched to prevent inward displacement toward the lumen. Interrupted sutures are preferred, using an absorbable, monofilament material to minimize subsequent granuloma formation.

More severe strictures require anterior and posterior division of the cricoid cartilage. Care must be taken not to injure the esophagus or the recurrent nerves on the lateral aspect of the posterior cricoid surface. Cartilage grafts are then interposed in both defects to distract the two C-segments of cricoid cartilage and increase the lumenal size in a horizontal dimension (Fig. 12.2).

Tracheostomy Site Obstructions

Intraluminal Granuloma

Granulation tissue may grow around a tracheostomy tube at the stomal level. Polypoid extension of granuloma into the tracheal lumen always follows the cephalad aspect of the curved tube, and this potentially obstructing mass may be missed if decannulation is accomplished without prior endoscopic evaluation.

Minor granulations can be cauterized with a silver nitrate stick. Electrosurgical cauterization or direct excision, after anesthetic infiltration, are also effective for more exuberant growths. Intraluminal polypoid granuloma can be retrieved with a curved instrument passed through the stoma; excision is then accomplished at the skin level. A more precise alternative involves endoscopic excision using an infant urethral resectoscope at the time of endoscopic evaluation for decannulation (Fig. 12.3).[16]

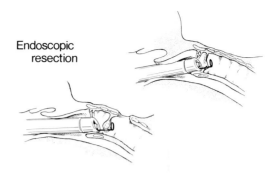

FIGURE 12.3 Endoscopic excision of intraluminal granuloma or subglottic web of scar, using infant urethral resectoscope.[16]

Stenotic Scar and Cartilaginous Deformity

Stenosis at the tracheostomy site is usually a complication of improper tracheostomy technique. Cartilage should never be excised from an infant's trachea. Closure by contraction of a cartilage-deficient stoma results in compromise of the anterior tracheal lumen. A too-short incision is likely to cause inward deformity of the upper tracheal ring, and lateral pressure from a tight tube may cause necrosis of the incised cartilage ends (Fig. 12.4c).

Some tracheostomy site stenoses can be managed by incision and splinting with an interposition cartilage graft. Severe strictures are better handled by segmental resection with end-to-end anastomosis.

Balloon Cuff Stenoses

Tracheal strictures associated with pressure from the balloon cuffs on tracheostomy or endotracheal tubes are usually seen in the cervical or high thoracic trachea (Fig. 12.4a,b). Such cuff

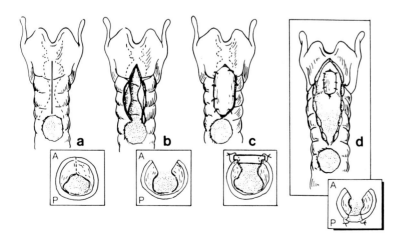

FIGURE 12.2 Laryngotracheoplasty operations interposing costal cartilage grafts in the anterior tracheal wall **(a,b,c)**. The severe, circumferential stenoses require interposition of cartilage both anteriorly and posteriorly at the cricoid level **(d)**.[15]

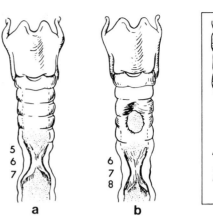

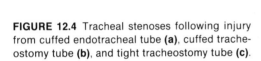

FIGURE 12.4 Tracheal stenoses following injury from cuffed endotracheal tube **(a)**, cuffed tracheostomy tube **(b)**, and tight tracheostomy tube **(c)**.

cuff strictures fortunately have become rare since the introduction of large-volume, low-pressure cuffs. This type of injury stimulated the development of tracheal resection techniques. Resection with direct anastomosis is accepted as the treatment of choice.[17]

Stenosis Following External Trauma or Inhalation Injury

Accidental injury, though the leading cause of death in children, causes airway stenosis infrequently. An unrecognized tear of the trachea or bronchus can result in stenosis, and direct crush or penetration of the larynx or trachea occasionally follows accidents with skateboards, motorbikes, snowmobiles, all-terrain vehicles, and the like. Treatment is determined by the extent and location of the lesion according to methods discussed in other sections of this chapter. Severe inhalation burn is the most challenging injury to the airway; reconstruction may be complex and results discouraging.[18]

MANAGEMENT OF CONGENITAL TRACHEAL STENOSIS

Historical Perspective

In 1941 Wolman reported 11 cases of congenital tracheal stenosis, including one of his own, documented since 1832.[19] One child (1927) with dyspnea for the first seven years of life improved after tracheostomy. All others died. Benjamin et al reported 21 cases of congenital tracheal stenosis seen in Sydney, Australia, between 1971 and 1980.[20] Despite nine deaths in that series, the authors emphasized that 12 of the 21 patients survived after mostly conservative treatment (excepting one pneumonectomy and one tracheopexy), and they concluded "there appears to be little place for surgical resection of the

stenosis . . ." Case reports of successful resection (congenital tracheal stenoses) in babies started to appear after 1980,[21–27] and aggressive surgical treatment of symptomatic lesions is the accepted standard at present. The anatomic variations in these reported successful resections are illustrated in Figure 12.5.

Clinical Investigation

High-contrast radiographs, preferably magnified, plus fluoroscopy in two projections will give fairly accurate information about an infant's airway. Bronchograms were avoided in the past because of their danger to the patient, but this situation has changed. The new nonosmotic soluble contrast media provide superior imaging with a good margin of safety for all but critically compromised infants. Bronchoscopy is the definitive study, but the scope should not be passed through a tight stenosis unless this is part of the plan for definitive repair at the same time. Injudicious bronchoscopic manipulation may precipitate acute obstruction.

Important supplementary studies include the esophagram to provide indirect evidence of compression from a vascular malformation, computed axial tomography to measure the extent of airway narrowing, and inspiratory-expiratory flow volume curves for functional correlations. Echocardiography and angiography may be indicated for suspected vascular ring anomalies.

Patterns of Congenital Tracheal Stenosis

Three Basic Types

Three basic variations in the pattern of congenital tracheal stenosis were described by Cantrell and Guild in 1964 after review of 24 acceptably documented cases from the literature[28] (Fig. 12.6). These patterns have subsequently been

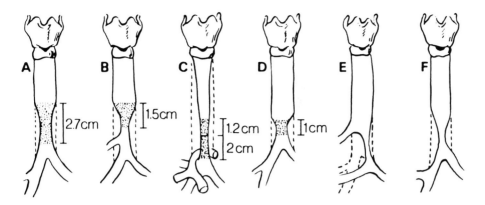

FIGURE 12.5 Reported patterns of tracheal stenosis successfully resected in infants since 1980.[21,22,23,24,25,26,27]

confirmed by Landing and are described as "(1) diffuse 'generalized hypoplasia' (approximately 30 percent of tracheal stenosis), (2) funnel-like stenosis, as in the sling left pulmonary artery syndrome (approximately 20 percent of cases?), and (3) segmental stenosis (approximately 50 percent of tracheal stenosis.) Segmental stenosis is approximately evenly distributed in the subcricoid area, in the central trachea, and above the carina."[29]

Vascular Compression and the Ring-Sling Complex

Tracheal compression associated with congenital anomalies of the aortic arch is well recognized as a cause of stridor, cyanotic attacks, repeated

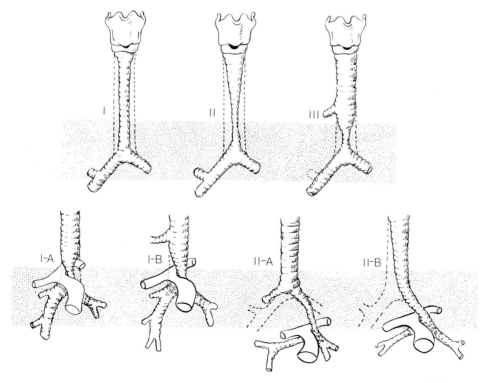

FIGURE 12.6 Top row: Three types of tracheal stenosis described by Cantrell and Guild: generalized hypoplasia, funnel-like stenosis, and segmental stenosis.[28] Bottom row: Group Ia, Ib and group IIa, IIb of the left pulmonary artery ring-sling anatomy reviewed by Wells et al.[33]

upper respiratory infections, and dysphagia. Anomalous origin of the innominate artery on the aortic arch may lead to airway compression as the vessel crosses the trachea. A right aortic arch and a left descending aorta give rise to anterior tracheal compression from the left subclavian and carotid arteries.[30] These anomalies usually cause tracheomalacia rather than tracheal stenoses and may be handled by vascular suspension procedures if symptoms are severe.

An anomalous left pulmonary artery (PA) may arise from the right pulmonary artery, as was first noted in the literature by Glaevecke in 1897, and pass to the left lung between the trachea and esophagus. Berdon et al published a review in 1984 and emphasized the reported mortality of 50% in these "PA sling" patients. They separated their patients into two groups—tracheal compression symptoms were relieved by division and reanastomosis of the vessel in group I patients and not in group II. Further analysis of five group II patients collected from four different institutions revealed in all cases a coexistent long-segment tracheal stenosis due to complete cartilage "O" rings of trachea. They coined the term ring-sling syndrome.[31] Surgical experience has since confirmed their opinion that repair of the vascular anomaly alone may not improve respiratory symptoms. When primary tracheal pathology can be identified preoperatively, simultaneous repair of the vascular and tracheal anatomy is recommended.[32]

Further details concerning variations in the tracheobronchial anatomy of PA sling patients have been supplied by Wells et al based on five cases from Los Angeles Children's Hospital and 30 cases capable of being evaluated from the literature[33] (Fig. 12.6).

Indications for Surgery

Variations in degree of tracheal stenosis obviously exist, and not all congenital or acquired stenoses require surgical treatment. Indications for resection or tracheoplastic reconstruction are expanding, however, as recent experience has shown that one can correct lesions previously thought to be uncorrectable. Indications for operation will vary with the functional status of the patient, the anatomic location and extent of the lesion, and the experience and ability of the surgical team.

Technical Aspects of Reconstruction

Support of Respiration

Preoperative equipment planning should involve additional sterile breathing circuits, a backup anesthesia machine, and possibly a high-frequency jet ventilating device. Most segmental resections can be handled safely and efficiently by temporary intubation of the distal trachea or bronchi across the operative field while the sutures are preplaced for the anastomosis. Jet ventilation has been recommended for tight stenoses to avoid the necessity of a hazardous forceful dilation before induction of anesthesia.[34] Fine catheters are threaded through the stenosis and maintained in place for jet ventilation before and during the resection.[35] Louhimo and Leijala[36] recommend cardiopulmonary bypass for tracheal resection as a safer approach in infants even though they recognize that most successful resections published to date have been accomplished without bypass.

Incisions

Standard incisions used for tracheal reconstruction are shown in Fig. 12.7. Most postintubation tracheal strictures, along with the higher congenital strictures which are segmental, can be managed by an anterior cervical approach. The lower congenital stenoses usually require either a sternotomy or an upper sternal extension of the low cervical collar incision. Segmental stenoses near or below the carina may be better handled through a posterolateral thoracotomy.[37]

Segmental Resection for Localized Stenoses

Segmental resection of a short stenosis (less than three to five rings) with end-to-end anastomosis is accepted by most tracheal surgeons as the treatment of choice. This presupposes the anastomosis will be constructed with normal tracheal tissue at the proximal and distal ends. More extensive congenital lesions and some tracheal burn stenoses are better managed with tracheoplastic techniques.

The largest series of tracheal resections in children (20 patients) has been reported by Grillo.[38] His technical recommendations, based upon a total experience with 279 adults and children, have been published recently[39] and are paraphrased in part as follows:

The anterior surface of the trachea can be exposed as necessary from cricoid to carina, but great care should be given to preserve the lateral blood vessels. Initial circumferential dissection (maximum 1 to 2 cm length to preserve tracheal blood supply) should be started at a point just below the stenosis, where tissues are more normal. Any posterolateral dissection must be right on the tracheal wall to avoid recurrent laryngeal nerve injury.

Division of the trachea is commenced close

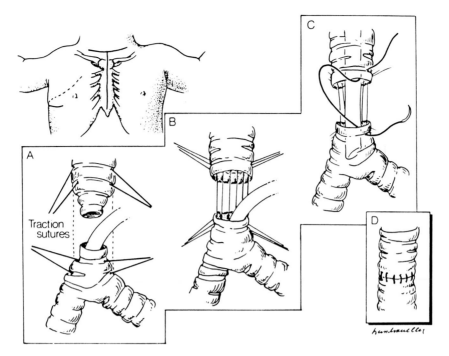

FIGURE 12.7 Technique for resection of segmental tracheal stenosis, described in text. Depending upon location of the stenosis, the approach may be through a transverse cervical, an upper sternotomy, a right posterolateral incision, or a combination of these. **A.** Placement of traction sutures. **B.** Resection of stenosis and placement of posterior sutures with distal intubation. **C.** Transanastomatic intubation for anterior sutures. **D.** Completed anastomosis.

to the stenosis to allow a conservative resection, but good cartilaginous rings should be present at the point of final division, both proximally and distally. Removal of insufficient amounts of trachea may lead to prompt recurrence of stenosis. Both ends of the stenosis must be resected back to normal tissue and normal lumen size.

The posterior four to five sutures are preplaced first, with the knots outside, while ventilation is maintained through a separate anesthesia circuit connected to the distal trachea. The translaryngeal endotracheal tube is then advanced across the gap (after removing the distal tube) and additional sutures are preplaced around the circumference of the anastomosis (Fig. 12.7).

Suture material should be absorbable (synthetic composition) to minimize the chance of intraluminal granuloma formation after operation. Formation of granulation tissue at the anastomosis, according to Grillo, must now be classified as due to an error in technique. Traction sutures, placed in the midlateral trachea on either side and at least 1 cm proximal and distal to the anastomosis, may be tied together at completion of the anastomosis to relieve tension on the suture line.

Grillo recommends a heavy restraining suture between the chin and the anterior chest wall to maintain head and neck flexion postoperatively. We prefer a prosthetic brace for children.

Laryngeal release procedures (thyrohyoid[40] or suprahyoid[41]) should be reserved as a last resort for severe length problems. Fixation of the larynx, postoperative dysphagia, and aspiration have been associated with both procedures, but more so with the thyrohyoid release. Pediatric surgical experience has favored one of the tracheoplasty techniques without resection for long stenoses in children that would otherwise require a laryngeal release to accomplish successfully.

Tracheostomy should be avoided for lower tracheal strictures. It delays definitive diagnosis and treatment, compromises humidification of gases, introduces wound contamination at the time of reconstruction, and may limit mobilization of the trachea.

Tracheoplastic Techniques for Extensive Stenoses

Many congenital stenoses and some cases of long-segment acquired stenosis cannot be managed by resection with reanastomosis of normal trachea. A variety of tracheoplastic techniques have been applied to this challenge.

In 1982, Kimura et al reported successful reconstruction in a 12-month-old infant born with subtotal tracheal stenosis and complete tracheal rings.[42] They used a modification of Cotton and Evans'[15] interposition costal cartilage grafting technique. That same year Ein et al reported success with a 7-month-old infant treated by posterior tracheal incision and interposition of the anterior esophageal wall. This infant also had a similar total tracheal stenosis with complete rings.[43] This patient developed symptoms of diffuse tracheomalacia, however, and died seven months later following tracheostomy complications.

Additional reports of successful tracheoplasty for long segment stenosis have since included five infants from Chicago, Illinois (pericardial patch),[44] one from Denver, Colorado (costal cartilage),[45] five from Galveston, Texas (costal cartilage or dura),[46] three additional patients from Kobe, Japan (costal cartilage),[47] and three from Toronto, Canada (esophagus, tantalum mesh and skin, pericardium and stent).[48] The anatomic variations described in these reports are

illustrated in Figure 12.8. The basic technique for tracheoplasty is illustrated in Figure 12.9.

Posterior incision of tracheal rings with sutured interposition of the esophagus resulted in long-term survival for only one of three such patients reported from Toronto. The interposition cartilage grafts in the anterior tracheal wall have required endotracheal stenting from 3 weeks to many months, and reports suggest the postoperative course is far from trouble free. The initial case of Tsugawa et al, however (the first reported survivor following surgical reconstruction of total tracheal stenosis), is now more than 7 years old and is said to be free of airway disease. Yearly bronchoscopies have demonstrated growth in the tracheal lumen.[47]

The pericardial patch graft at present appears to be a simpler technique, with results equal or superior to other methods for managing total tracheal stenosis. Control of gas exchange during the operation is facilitated by cardiopulmonary bypass, even though advocates of the cartilage graft have used distal intubation or jet ventilation. Idriss et al suggest that postoperative tracheomalacia-like symptoms can be minimized by suspending the graft from the innominate ar-

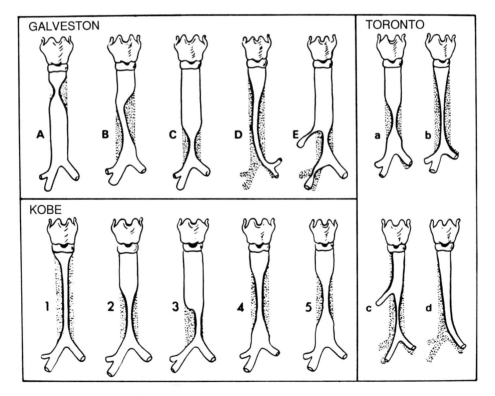

FIGURE 12.8 Variations in tracheal stricture anatomy: reported successful cases of tracheoplasty in infants.[46,47,48]

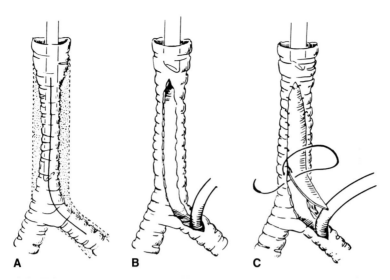

FIGURE 12.9 Generalization of basic technique for anterior tracheoplasty.

tery, which in turn should be suspended by suture to the chest wall during sternal closure.[44]

Tracheal Prosthetic Replacements

Prosthetic segments of silicone trachea have been used for short periods in adults,[49] but no one has reported experience with tracheal replacement in children.

SUMMARY

No single reconstructive technique applies to all defects of the airway. Acquired postintubation subglottic stenosis is the most common upper airway obstructive lesion in infants and children. Most of these lesions, however, can be managed with fairly simple dilations or by endoscopic resections. The advanced subglottic stenoses are usually managed by open laryngotracheoplasty involving some type of interposition graft and stent. Resection with direct anastomosis in the proximal trachea is not commonly applied to children because of concern about injury to the innervation and growth of the larynx.

Segmental stenosis of the cervical and thoracic trachea is best handled by resection and direct anastomosis if fewer than three to five tracheal rings are involved. Longer lengths of stenotic airway have been treated with tracheoplastic techniques utilizing interposition of cartilage, pericardium, periosteum, and myoosseous flaps. Success has been reported with all of the tracheoplastic techniques. Regional anatomy and location of the stenosis affect the choice of one autologous tissue patch over another, and none has clearly proven superiority. Prosthetic supports and substitute patches have been tried experimentally, but clinical experience and success are very limited.

REFERENCES

1. Parkin JL, Stevens MH, Jung AL: Acquired and congenital subglottic stenosis in the infant. *Ann Otol Rhinol Laryngol* 1976;85:573–581.
2. Grillo HC: Primary reconstruction of airway after resection of subglottic laryngeal and upper tracheal stenosis. *Ann Thorac Surg* 1982;33:3–18.
3. Schofield J: Conservative treatment of subglottic stenosis of the larynx. *Arch Otolaryngol* 1972;95:457–459.
4. Brown SB, Hedlund GL, Glasier CM, et al: Tracheobronchial stenosis in infants: Successful balloon dilation therapy. *Radiology* 1987;164:475–478.
5. Gnanapragasam A: Intralesional steroids in conservative management of subglottic stenosis of the larynx. *Int Surg* 1979;64:63–67.
6. Birck HG: Endoscopic repair of laryngeal stenosis. *Trans Am Acad Ophthalmol Otolaryngol* 1970;74:140–143.
7. O'Neill JA Jr: Experience with iatrogenic laryngeal and tracheal stenoses. *J Pediatr Surg* 1984;19:235–238.
8. Othersen HB Jr: The technique of intraluminal stenting and steroid administration in the treatment of tracheal stenosis in children. *J Pediatr Surg* 1974;9:683–689.
9. Montgomery WW: The surgical management of supraglottic and subglottic stenosis. *Ann Otol Rhinol Laryngol* 1968;77:534–546.
10. Evans JNG: Laryngotracheoplasty. *Otolaryngol Clin North Am* 1977;10:119–123.
11. Aboulker P, Sterkers JM, Demaldent JE: Modifications apportees a l'intervention de Rethi, interet dans les stenoses laryngo-tracheales et tracheales. *Ann Otol Laryngol (Paris)* 1966;83:98–106.

12. Downing TP, Johnson DG: Excision of subglottic stenosis with the urethral resectoscope. *J Pediatr Surg* 1979;14:252–257.

13. Rodgers BM, Moazam F, Talbert JL: Endotracheal cryotherapy in the treatment of refractory airway strictures. *Ann Thorac Surg* 1983;35:52–57.

14. Kouffman JA, Thompson JN, Kohut RI: Endoscopic management of subglottic stenosis with the CO_2 surgical laser. *Otolaryngol Head Neck Surg* 1981; 89:215–220.

15. Cotton RT, Evans JNG: Laryngotracheal reconstruction in children: Five-year follow-up. *Ann Otol Rhinol Laryngol* 1981;90:516–520.

16. Johnson DG, Stewart DR: Management of acquired tracheal obstructions in infancy. *J Pediatr Surg* 1975;10:709–717.

17. Grillo HC: Surgical treatment of postintubation tracheal injuries. *J Thorac Cardiovasc Surg* 1979;78:860–875.

18. Majeski JA, Schreiber JT, Cotton R, MacMillan BG: Tracheoplasty for tracheal stenosis in the pediatric burned patient. *J Trauma* 1980;20:81–86.

19. Wolman IJ: Congenital stenosis of the trachea. *AJDC* 1941;61:1263–1271.

20. Benjamin B, Pitkin J, Cohen D: Congenital tracheal stenosis. *Ann Otol* 1981;90:364–371.

21. Harrison MR, Heldt GP, Brasch RC, et al: Resection of distal tracheal stenosis in a baby with agenesis of the lung. *J Pediatr Surg* 1980;15:938–943.

22. Mansfield PB: Tracheal resection in infancy. *J Pediatr Surg* 1980;15:79–81.

23. Mattingly WT Jr, Belin RP, Todd EP: Surgical repair of congenital tracheal stenosis in an infant. *J Thorac Cardiovasc Surg* 1981;81:738–740.

24. Weber TR, Eigen H, Scott PH, et al: Resection of congenital tracheal stenosis involving the carina. *J Thorac Cardiovasc Surg* 1982;84:200–203.

25. Nakayama DK, Harrison MR, de Lorimier AA, et al: Reconstructive surgery for obstructing lesions of the intrathoracic trachea in infants and small children. *J Pediatr Surg* 1982;17:854–868.

26. Minato N, Itoh K, Ohkawa Y, et al: Surgical treatment of congenital distal tracheal stenosis involving the carina. *Ann Thorac Surg* 1986;42:326–328.

27. Healy GB, Schuster SR, Jonas RA, McGill TJI: Correction of segmental tracheal stenosis in children. *Ann Otol Rhinol Laryngol* 1988;97:444–447.

28. Cantrell Jr, Guild HG: Congenital stenosis of the trachea. *Am J Surg* 1964;108:297–305.

29. Landing BH: Congenital malformations and genetic disorders of the respiratory tract (larynx, trachea, bronchi, and lungs). *Am Rev Resp Dis* 1979;120:151–185.

30. Smith RJH, Smith MCF, Glossop LP, et al: Congenital vascular anomalies causing tracheoesophageal compression. *Arch Otolaryngol* 1984;110:82–87.

31. Berdon WE, Baker DH, Wung JT, et al: Complete cartilage-ring tracheal stenosis associated with anomalous left pulmonary artery: The ring-sling complex. *Radiology* 1984;152:57–64.

32. Hickey MSJ, Wood AE: Pulmonary artery sling with tracheal stenosis: One-stage repair. *Ann Thorac Surg* 1987;44:416–417.

33. Wells TR, Gwinn JL, Landing BH, Stanley P: Reconsideration of the anatomy of sling left pulmonary artery: The association of one form with bridging bronchus and imperforate anus: Anatomic and diagnostic aspects. *J Pediatr Surg* 1988;23:892–898.

34. Neuman GG, Asher AS, Stern SB, et al: High-frequency jet ventilation for tracheal resection in a child. *Anesth Analg* 1984;63:1039–1040.

35. Schur MS, Maccioli GA, Azizkhan RG, Wood RE: High-frequency jet ventilation in the management of congenital tracheal stenosis. *Anesthesiology* 1988;68:952–955.

36. Louhimo I, Leijala M: Cardiopulmonary bypass in tracheal surgery in infants and small children. *Prog Pediatr Surg* 1987;21:58–63.

37. Grillo HC: Surgical approaches to the trachea. *Surg Gynecol Obstet* 1969;129:347–352.

38. Grillo HC, Zannini P: Management of obstructive tracheal disease in children. *J Pediatr Surg* 1984; 19:414–416.

39. Grillo HC, Mathisen DJ: Surgical management of tracheal strictures. *Surg Clin North Am* 1988;68:511–524.

40. Dedo HH, Fishman NH: Laryngeal release and sleeve resection for tracheal stenosis. *Ann Otol Rhinol Laryngol* 1969;78:285–296.

41. Montgomery WW: Suprahyoid release for tracheal stenosis. *Arch Otolaryngol* 1974;99:225–260.

42. Kimura K, Mukohara M, Tsugawa C, et al: Tracheoplasty for congenital stenosis of the entire trachea. *J Pediatr Surg* 1982;17:869–871.

43. Ein SH, Friedberg J, Williams WG, et al: Tracheoplasty: A new operation for complete congenital tracheal stenosis. *J Pediatr Surg* 1982;17:872–878.

44. Idriss F, DeLeon SY, Ilbawi MN, et al: Tracheoplasty with pericardial patch for extensive tracheal stenosis in infants and children. *J Thorac Cardiovasc Surg* 1984;88:527–536.

45. Campbell DN, Lilly JR: Surgery for total congenital tracheal stenosis. *J Pediatr Surg* 1986;21:934–935.

46. Lobe TE, Hayden K, Nicolas D, Richardson CJ: Successful management of congenital tracheal stenosis in infancy. *J Pediatr Surg* 1987;22:1137–1142.

47. Tsugawa C, Kimura K, Muraji T, et al: Congenital stenosis involving a long segment of the trachea: Further experience in reconstructive surgery. *J Pediatr Surg* 1988;23:471–475.

48. Loeff DS, Filler RM, Vinograd SH, et al: Congenital tracheal stenosis: A review of 22 patients from 1965 to 1987. *J Pediatr Surg* 1988;23:744–748.

49. Neville WE, Bolanowski PJP, Soltanzadeh H: Prosthetic reconstruction of the trachea and carina. *J Thorac Cardiovasc Surg* 1976;72:525–538.

Tracheal Stenosis

D. Branscheid, MD, S. Krysa, MD, and I. Vogt-Moykopf, MD

The primary diagnostic techniques for tracheal anomalies are radiographic examination and bronchoscopy. The location of the lesion, its linear extent, extratracheal involvement, and (most important to the surgeon) the amount of airway involved by the process can be established. Esophagography is useful to define involvement by intrinsic compression or invasion.

Crucial for the management of all problems of the trachea is the ability to control the airway. Stenosis may present as an emergency obstructive airway problem. Endotracheal intubation may be impossible, even dangerous, since it may lead to complete airway obstruction, mostly in patients with high lesions. Maneuvers—such as elevation of the head of the patient, administration of oxygen, and sedation—may allow control of the airway to be accomplished in a quasi-elective manner. Control is best performed in the operation room, where an assortment of rigid bronchoscopes, dilators, biopsy forceps and instruments to carry out emergency tracheostomy are available.

Strictures of the trachea may result from a number of different causes. Congenital stenoses and posttraumatic strictures are rare. The most common type is still the result of iatrogenic disease, mostly following intubation for long-time ventilatory support. Infections and amyloid disease are described as unusual causes in addition to the rare ideopathic lesion.

Most patients with postintubation stenosis show signs of upper airway obstruction. Shortness of breath is initially seen, with subsequent progression even at rest with wheezing and stridor. Episodes of pneumonitis give an additional hint. A very late sign is the occurrence of stenosis. One must be aware that in any patient de-

veloping signs of upper airway obstruction an organic lesion of the trachea has to be considered, particularly if the patient has been subjected to intubation for assisted ventilation in the recent past. Many of our patients had been diagnosed as asthma despite reported previous intubation.

Our experience is based on 14 children aged from 2.5 months to 16 years, with a mean age of 3 years. All patients showed postintubation stenosis, except for one congenital lesion. The surgical approach correlated to the location and extent of the stenosis. We saw 8 stenoses in the upper third and 3 each in the middle and the lower thirds of the trachea. All lesions in the upper third could be reached through a collar approach, and included one small lesion (1 cm) at the middle of the trachea.

Segmental resection with end-to-end anastomosis seems to be the treatment of choice if the lesion is not excessively long and does not involve other anatomic structures (subglottic larynx). In children, it is easier to mobilize the trachea than in adults. When approaching both main stem bronchi, the dissection is kept very close to the trachea to avoid injury to the recurrent laryngeal nerves. By mobilizing the pulmonary ligament and circumferentially dissecting the pericardium around the vessels, we were able to perform tension-free anastomosis in our patients. A laryngeal release procedure was reserved as a last resort for length problems. In one patient with a 5 cm defect we resected the trachea, including the carina, and anastomosed the trachea to the right main stem bronchus and the left main stem bronchus to the bronchus intermedius. By means of this procedure, established in adult surgery, we feel prepared to repair extensive stenotic lesions. For surgical repair of stenosis of the antero-lateral aspect of the subglottic larynx and the upper trachea, partial removal is required. In circumferential stenosis, the scar overlying the injured mucosa may be removed from the anterior surface of the posterior cricoid plate. In these cases we feel temporary tracheostomy is necessary.

We have had good results in our operative treatment of postintubation stenosis. There was no operative death. 13 patients showed good and satisfactory long term result. Only 1 patient, with a keloid scar, showed restenosis in the anastomosed area and required endoscopic laser resection.

CONCLUSION

If conservative management, dilation, and endoscopic laser resection do not succeed in the management of stenotic lesions, prompt surgical intervention is indicated, especially for postintubation stenosis. Even stenoses of considerable length can be reconstructed satisfactorily. In none of our cases was innervation or tracheal and laryngeal growth impaired, not even after extensive mobilization.

Chapter 13

Tracheomalacia

Robert M. Filler, MD, FRCS(C)

INTRODUCTION

Collapse of a trachea because of a structural abnormality of its wall (tracheomalacia) is an uncommon but important cause of respiratory symptoms in children. Tracheomalacia is often associated with another defect such as esophageal atresia, vascular ring, or paratracheal tumor.[1] In the adult, the most common cause of tracheomalacia is obstructive lung disease.[2]

Neonates with severe bronchopulmonary dysplasia often develop tracheomalacia in association with diffuse airway pathology that involves all the large and small airways. The clinical problems in these cases are quite different from those seen in pure tracheomalacia and are not discussed in this chapter.

PATHOPHYSIOLOGY

The size of the tracheal lumen depends on the rigidity of its wall and the difference between the intraluminal and extraluminal forces that act upon it. Because of these relationships, the lumen of the normal, somewhat flexible intrathoracic trachea increases during inspiration and decreases during expiration in response to a decrease and then an increase in intrathoracic pressure. In the patient with an abnormally soft trachea, the changes in tracheal caliber caused by ventilation are magnified so that in the most severe cases complete collapse of the trachea may occur, even during unlabored expiration. When higher intrathoracic pressures are generated, such as during a cough or in clinical situations in which lung compliance is reduced, obstruction to the outflow of air is even greater. Because inspiratory efforts cause the trachea to enlarge, obstruction to air inflow does not occur in tracheomalacia. Tracheomalacia in the cervical trachea rarely produces airway obstruction during quiet or forceful respiration because the pressure inside and outside of the cervical trachea is equal (ie, atmospheric) when the glottis is open. The dynamics of airway collapse have been discussed in detail by Wittenborg et al.[3]

In addition to changes in airway size that occur in response to variations in intrathoracic pressure, an abnormally soft trachea can be compressed by adjacent intrathoracic structures, especially the esophagus posteriorly and the ascending aorta and aortic arch anteriorly. The aortic size and position is relatively constant, but the esophageal size increases with swallowing, gastroesophageal reflux, and in the presence of obstructive lesions of the lower esophagus, so that patients with tracheomalacia often have their most severe symptoms during or shortly after eating (Fig. 13.1).

PATHOLOGY AND PATHOGENESIS

A variety of structural abnormalities can produce tracheomalacia. However, the most common type encountered in childhood is usually found in children also born with esophageal atresia. This defect was first described by Wailoo and Emery in 1979.[4] These workers studied an unselected sequential series of tracheas obtained from 53 deceased infants and children born with esophageal atresia and tracheoesophageal fistula. Their evaluations showed that 75% of cases had a segment of trachea in which cartilaginous rings were fragmented and/or had an elliptical rather than C shape. In addition, the membranous portion of this segment of trachea was extremely wide and floppy. The net result was a trachea whose lumen could be readily compromised because of the ease in which anterior and posterior walls could appose. These pathological findings correspond precisely to those seen at

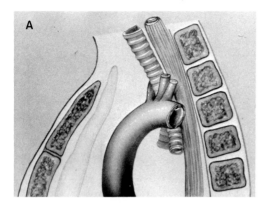

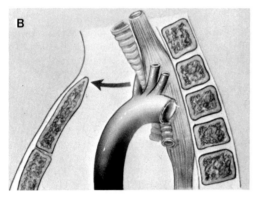

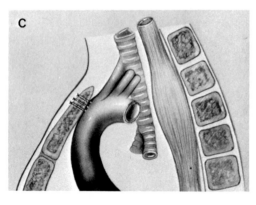

FIGURE 13.1 Mediastinal anatomy in tracheomalacia and effect of aortopexy. **A.** Sagittal view of chest showing normal relationship between aorta, trachea and esophagus. **B.** The malacic trachea can be compressed by the adjacent aorta, but when the esophagus is empty and the infant is not coughing, there is usually no appreciable airway obstruction. However, when the esophagus dilates (during swallowing or reflux), the trachea collapses between it and the aorta. Respiratory symptoms and apneic spells occur at this time. **C.** Operative procedure pulls aorta anteriorly and displaces the anterior wall of the trachea as well. The filled esophagus no longer causes critical tracheal narrowing.

bronchoscopy in children with symptomatic tracheomalacia associated with esophageal atresia[5,6] (Fig. 13.2).

Several causes have been postulated for the association between tracheomalacia and esophageal atresia. Because the trachea and esophagus are derived from primitive foregut, a faulty division that results in esophageal atresia can also be expected to affect the adjacent trachea. Evidence to support this possibility can be found in Wailoo and Emery's[4] studies, in which esophageal muscle was often present in the membranous trachea at the site of the tracheal abnormalities. Davies and Cywes[7] surmised that the dilated esophagus above the site of atresia compresses the fetal trachea and prevents its normal development. They also suggested that abnormal tracheal development could be due to the loss of intratracheal pressure in the fetus through a tracheoesophageal fistula, because the fluid that normally fills the embryonic airways may provide the mechanism of internal support for the growing trachea.

Tracheal injury and chronically elevated intrathoracic airway pressures can also produce tracheomalacia. Tracheal infection, which may occur spontaneously or in association with airway intubation, may destroy or weaken the tracheal wall. Adults with emphysema and children ventilated with high airway pressures tend to develop enlarged, thin-walled airways with widening, loss of elasticity, and flaccidity of the membranous portion of the trachea with or without histologic changes of chronic inflammation.[2]

Tracheomalacia is also seen following surgery for lesions that mechanically compress the trachea such as a vascular ring or a tumor. Although it is possible that trauma during surgery contributes to the postoperative tracheomalacia, it is more likely that long-term compression of the trachea is responsible for abnormal tracheal development. Other inflammatory lesions of cartilage, other developmental defects of cartilage, and a complete absence of tracheal cartilage are less common causes of tracheomalacia.[8,9]

The conditions associated with pure tracheomalacia which required corrective surgery at my institution in the past 10 years are shown in Table 13.1.

TABLE 13.1 Abnormalities Associated with 30 Cases of Tracheomalacia 1978–1987

Esophageal atresia	25*
Vascular ring	3*
None	3

* One patient had both esophageal atresia and vascular ring.

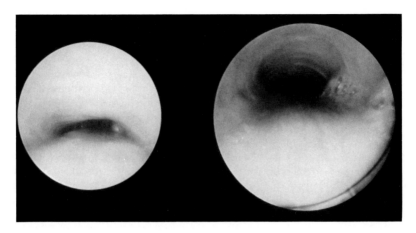

FIGURE 13.2 Tracheomalacia as seen through the bronchoscope. On the left the patient is coughing and the posterior wall of the trachea bulges anteriorly and obstructs the lumen. Following aortopexy trachea remains open during cough (right). Note the abnormal tracheal rings anteriorly and the wide membranous trachea posteriorly.

SYMPTOMS

The symptoms of tracheomalacia are largely due to airway obstruction during expiration. Most children have a typical barking cough, which is probably due to vibration of the opposing anterior and posterior tracheal walls.[6] Recurrent pneumonia is common in these patients, presumably because airway collapse during coughing prevents effective clearing of airway secretions. In some children, airway obstruction during normal ventilation is so severe that airway intubation is necessary. In others, the diagnosis of tracheomalacia is not really appreciated until the airway cannot be extubated after a surgical procedure such as repair of esophageal atresia or a vascular ring.

One of the most frequent symptoms of tracheomalacia, and perhaps the least understood, is the life-threatening "dying spell." These spells occur mostly in patients with tracheomalacia associated with esophageal atresia. Dying spells, which often do not appear until 3 months of age, are characterized by cyanosis rapidly progressing to apnea, bradycardia, and, if uninterrupted, even cardiac arrest. Characteristically, dying spells occur during feeding or within 5 to 10 minutes of a meal.

Benjamin et al[6] and Mustard et al[10] suggested that dying spells are due to a vagal reflex that arises from the tracheal wall when the trachea collapses. The experience of myself and my colleagues suggests another mechanism.[1] Transcutaneous TcPo2 monitoring during feedings in a small group of infants with spells associated with tracheomalacia showed a fall in TcPo2 during at least one feeding in four children. In these infants, bradycardia occurred as TcPo2 fell. TcPo2 and heart rate returned to normal as soon as the feeding was interrupted (Fig. 13.3). We theorize that progressive hypoxia causes the spells and that the hypoxia is due to airway obstruction caused by pressure of a dilated esophagus on the soft trachea. In patients born with esophageal atresia, esophageal dilatation is common during or just after eating because of poor esophageal peristalsis and gastroesophageal reflux.

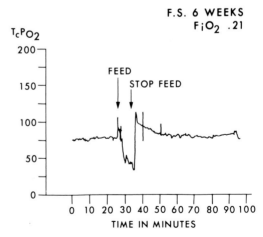

FIGURE 13.3 Transcutaneous Po2 (TcPo2) monitoring during feeding in a 6-week-old infant with tracheomalacia. TcPo2 fell during the feed and returned to resting levels when feed stopped. Bradycardia (pulse rate 60/min) noted when TcPo2 reached 25 mm Hg.

Because similar spells can be due to cardiac or neurologic disease as well as defects in swallowing, complete evaluation of the child's neurologic and cardiac status is also necessary in these cases.

DIAGNOSIS

The diagnosis of tracheomalacia should be suspected by a clinical history of apneic spells, recurrent pneumonia, or inability to extubate the airway because of expiratory obstruction, especially in children with a history of esophageal atresia, vascular ring, or a previous mass around the trachea.

Investigations to confirm the diagnosis are relatively straightforward. A narrowing of the air-filled trachea can be noted on the lateral view of a plain chest roentgenogram in almost all children with tracheomalacia whose airway is not intubated (Fig. 13.4). A better evaluation of tracheal dynamics is obtained radiographically under the image intensifier by continuous visualization of the trachea during several respiratory cycles. At the same time, the esophagus should be filled with radiocontrast material so that the relationship between the esophageal size and tracheal diameter can be appreciated. The radiocontrast study is also needed to determine if gastroesophageal reflux, esophageal stricture, recurrent tracheoesophageal fistula, and poor esophageal motility are present. Typical radiographic findings in tracheomalacia are demonstrated in Figure 13.4.

Bronchoscopy provides a definitive diagnosis in these cases (Figure 13.2). General anesthesia is usually necessary for bronchoscopy but the child must be breathing spontaneously and not paralyzed for proper evaluation of the trachea. In the symptomatic case, the tracheal lumen has an elliptical shape. Anterior vascular pulsations are usually evident and the membranous portion of the trachea is usually enlarged and bulges into the lumen, more so on the left than on the right. The cartilaginous tracheal rings may appear to be interrupted. Anterior and posterior collapse of the lumen occurs during expiration, and in severely affected cases complete airway occlusion is noted when a cough is stimulated. Because of the need for general anesthesia, bronchoscopy is usually the last test to be performed in suspected cases of tracheomalacia. In general, one should be prepared to proceed with definitive surgery at the time of bronchoscopy if it confirms the diagnosis of severe tracheomalacia.

INDICATIONS FOR SURGERY

Many children with minor degrees of airway collapse do not require specific therapy. The abnormally soft trachea tends to become more rigid with continued growth and development and symptoms can be expected to improve in the first one or two years of life.[9,11]

Symptoms that are life threatening or are likely to represent a significant chronic health hazard require surgical intervention. The major indications for surgery in our experience are noted in Table 13.2. A single dying spell due to tracheomalacia is an absolute indication for surgery. Likewise, there appears to be little justification for delaying surgical correction in the child who requires a tracheostomy or an endotracheal tube to keep his or her airway patent. Sometimes it is difficult to decide how many episodes of pneumonia are acceptable before advising surgery. Certainly more than three documented episodes in a year would be excessive, especially if a severe anatomic abnormality is seen at bronchoscopy.

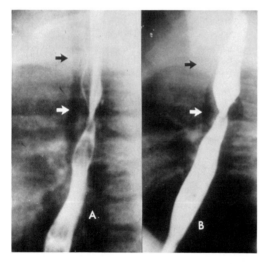

FIGURE 13.4 Lateral roentgenogram of chest focused on air-filled trachea and esophagus. **A.** During inspiration there is a slight narrowing of the tracheal lumen (between arrows) in the region of aortic arch. **B.** During expiration, collapse of trachea (between arrows) causes disappearance of air in that segment of the airway.

TABLE 13.2 Indication for Surgery in 30 Cases of Tracheomalacia 1978–1987

Dying spells	14
Recurrent pneumonia	4
Intermittent respiratory obstruction	5
Inability to extubate airway	7

Another clinical decision faced frequently is how to deal with the severely symptomatic child who is found to have both tracheomalacia and gastroesophageal reflux. When tracheomalacia has been severe by bronchoscopy, our policy has been to proceed to aortopexy and not fundoplication. In the past 10 years we treated 13 children with tracheomalacia who also had gastroesophageal reflux. All of these patients also had esophageal atresia, which is known to be associated with a high incidence of gastroesophageal reflux. Three children had had fundoplication prior to aortopexy. Only one of the remaining 10 patients required fundoplication for symptoms of gastroesophageal reflux after correction of severe tracheomalacia. Kiely et al[12] suggest that gastroesophageal reflux may be induced by upper airway obstruction and that it is advisable to correct the airway problem before fundoplication.

SURGICAL TREATMENT

Tracheomalacia can be treated by several surgical techniques. A tracheostomy will provide an internal tracheal splint and has been used by some in the hope that improvement would accompany growth.[13] Wiseman et al[14] successfully treated tracheomalacia and bronchomalacia with airway intubation and continuous positive airway pressure (CPAP) for 14 weeks. This duration of CPAP is probably not sufficient for most infants with airway collapse, because significant spontaneous improvement in tracheomalacia is unlikely before 1 or 2 years of age.[15] Johnston et al[16] used a free rib graft as a splint for the trachea in two children in whom a tracheostomy tube failed to stabilize the malacic segment. Our experience indicates that aortic suspension is an effective and safe method of treatment for most patients with tracheomalacia.[1,5,17] In a small number of cases, the abnormal airway segment is so long that aortopexy is not sufficient and the application of an airway splint is necessary.[1,18]

Aortopexy

Our original decision to use this operation for tracheomalacia was based on the favorable reports of Gross and Neuhauser[19] and of Mustard et al[10] in treating what they called the *innominate artery compression syndrome.* Many of these patients undoubtedly had what we are now calling *tracheomalacia.*[17] The rationale for the procedure assumes that the trachea will be pulled anteriorly when the aorta is suspended from the sternum if the connective tissue between the two is not disturbed. This translocation will change the configuration of the cross section of the ma-

lacic trachea from an ellipse to a circle and prevent apposition of its anterior and posterior walls. In addition, anterior displacement of the trachea will minimize its compression by the esophagus. The operation is shown in Figure 3.1.

Anesthesia for an aortopexy is planned to permit intraoperative endoscopic examination of the affected portion of the airway and immediate assessment of the adequacy of repair. For this purpose, anesthetic gases are delivered through a ventilating bronchoscope with a telescope attachment. Although the telescope takes up a portion of the lumen of the bronchoscope and resistance to airflow is increased, the anesthetist can still maintain satisfactory ventilation.

A left anterior thoracotomy through the third interspace is used to gain access to the anterior mediastinum for aortopexy. The left lobe of the thymus is excised to expose the aorta and its first branches and to create a space to translocate these vessels. The tissue plane between the aorta and trachea is not dissected because it is this attachment that pulls the trachea forward when the vessels are suspended from the sternum. Three or four 3-0 nonabsorbable sutures are placed into the adventitia and a portion of the media at the ascending aorta, the origin of the right innominate artery, and the aortic arch just beyond the origin of the innominate artery. A subcutaneous pocket is created just anterior to the upper sternum, and both ends of the vascular sutures are passed through the entire thickness of the sternum into the pocket. The sutures are pulled up simultaneously, and they are tied sequentially after bronchoscopic observation indicates a satisfactory improvement in the tracheal configuration. If the correction is not satisfactory, one or two additional sutures may be of help; otherwise a splinting procedure will be necessary.

In patients who have had a tracheostomy in place prior to surgery, we have removed it and replaced it with a nasotracheal tube one week before aortopexy. This allows the stoma to close, minimizing the possibility of bacterial contamination of the wound; this is especially important if a prosthetic splint is necessary.

Splinting Operation

Collapsing airways have been stabilized with a variety of external splints. Herzog et al[20] described the use of a free autologous rib graft to stent the adult trachea. Johnston et al[16] applied the same technique in two children, but long-term results have not been published. Rainier et al[21] first used prosthetic splinting in 23 adults with tracheomalacia due to severe and chronic obstructive lung disease. In their cases the widened membranous trachea was plicated and covered with a Dacron-reinforced Silastic prosthesis.

Since 1979 we have implanted a Silastic-reinforced Marlex mesh device, which was designed and fabricated at this institution, in eight children (Fig. 13.5).[18,22] The device has not adversely affected tracheal growth in animals or in long-term clinical follow-up.[22,23]

The indication for application of an airway splint in tracheomalacia is long segment tracheal collapse. In most of the patients splinted, aortopexy had been the primary corrective procedure. However, when bronchoscopy at the completion of the procedure indicated that aortic suspension failed to prevent tracheal collapse, the splinting procedure was undertaken under the same anesthetic. The average length of splint applied was 4.5 cm (range, 3 to 6 cm), which is about 1.5 cm greater than the length of tracheomalacia usually cured by aortopexy alone.

The exact operative technique and selection of size and shape of prosthetic splint is determined by the site and extent of airway collapse. We have a set of different size and shape splints that can be cut and modified as needed. The involved trachea can be approached either by median sternotomy or right posterior lateral thoracotomy. The splint, which is sized to encircle 75% of the circumference of the trachea, is sewn to the airway with interrupted 3-0 Dexon sutures. Application of the splint to the entire circumference of the trachea should be avoided, because this can be expected to produce tracheal stenosis.[24] As fibrous tissue grows into the interstices of the Marlex mesh, the prosthesis becomes

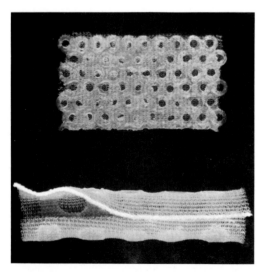

FIGURE 13.5 Marlex-Silastic airway splints. Different sizes and shapes are available at the time of aortopexy for airway splinting if necessary.

permanently fixed to the tissues. The flexible Silastic attached to the mesh is sufficiently soft and thin that erosion into the esophagus or a major artery does not occur and is very unlikely.

RESULTS OF TREATMENT
Aortopexy

The results of treating tracheomalacia by aortopexy have been the subject of several reports.[1,5,12,17] Kiely et al[12] reported on 25 aortopexies in 22 children with associated esophageal anomalies, mostly esophageal atresia and tracheal esophageal fistulas. Seventeen children had excellent results with only one long-term failure. Of interest is that symptoms worsened after aortopexy in 2 children. Both had a recurrent tracheoesophageal fistula and severe gastroesophageal reflux. Division of the fistula and fundoplication in each case proved to be curative. Over the past 10 years, we have treated 30 infants with pure tracheomalacia, and the results are given in Table 13.3. Of the 25 patients who had only aortopexy, symptoms have been relieved in 22. Of the 7 children who required surgery for inability to extubate the airway, only 1 still has a tracheostomy in place. One additional child required tracheostomy six months later. The remaining child had a vascular ring, which was unrecognized at the time of aortopexy. Dying spells recurred in the week following the operation and they ceased permanently after division of the ring. One month later, the child died unexpectedly and suddenly at home. Autopsy failed to reveal the cause of death.

Aortopexy was performed in 3 others, but when intraoperative bronchoscopy indicated that tracheomalacia persisted, an airway splint was applied at the same operation. Aortopexy has been well tolerated and operative complications have been minimal in all reports.[1,12] Evaluation of the aortic suspension by echocardiogram in a limited number of patients indicates that the aorta remains attached to the sternum for at least one year following surgery. There have been no

TABLE 13.3 Indication for Surgery in 30 Patients 1978–1987

	Number of Patients	Cessation of Symptoms
Aortopexy	25	22
Aortopexy + splint	3	3*
Splint only	2	2

* One patient required splint removal 18 months later; one patient died (see text); two patients still require tracheostomy.

reports of long-term vascular complications from aortopexy.

Splinting

Relatively few children have been treated for tracheomalacia by this method, so one must still be cautious in evaluating the results. We have applied an airway splint in 8 cases: 7 with tracheomalacia, 1 with bronchomalacia. Collapse was eliminated in all (Table 13.3). Our long-term results of airway splinting have recently been reported.[24] Five children with tracheomalacia who have been followed for more than four years were evaluated clinically and by bronchoscopy, computed tomography scan, and pulmonary function tests. Three children had had repair of esophageal atresia. The application of the splint had been preceded by aortopexy in 3. At follow-up, all children were leading normal lives. Three had mild respiratory symptoms not related to the splinting. The only long-term complication was a serous effusion that developed around the splint and compressed the trachea two years postoperatively. Removal of the splint was necessary, but the rigidity of the trachea at that time prevented recurrent airway collapse. There was no adverse effect on tracheal growth in any case.

REFERENCES

1. Blair GK, Filler RM, Cohen R: Treatment of tracheomalacia: 8 years' experience. *J Pediatr Surg* 1986;21:781–785.
2. Campbell AH, Young IF: Tracheobronchial collapse, a variant of obstructive respiratory disease. *Brit J Dis Chest* 1963;57:174–181.
3. Wittenborg MM, Gyepes MT, Crocker D: Tracheal dynamics in infants with respiratory distress, stridor and collapsing trachea. *Radiology* 1969;88:653–662.
4. Wailoo MP, Emery JL: The trachea in children with tracheoesophageal fistula. *Histopathology* 1979;3:329–338.
5. Schwartz MZ, Filler RM: Tracheal compression as a cause of apnea following repair of tracheoesophageal fistula: Treatment by aortopexy. *J Pediatr Surg* 1980;15:842–848.
6. Benjamin B, Cohen D, Glasson M: Tracheomalacia in association with congenital tracheoesophageal fistula. *Surgery* 1969;79:504–508.
7. Davies MRQ, Cywes S: The flaccid trachea and tracheoesophageal congenital anomalies. *J Pediatr Surg* 1978;13:363–367.
8. Johner CH, Szanto PA: Polychondritis in a newborn presenting as tracheomalacia. *Ann Otol Rhinol Laryngol* 1970;79:1114–1116.
9. Cox WL Jr, Shaw RR: Congenital chondromalacia of the trachea. *J Thorac Cardiovasc Surg* 1965;49:1033–1039.
10. Mustard WT, Bayliss CE, Fearon B, et al: Tracheal compression by the innominate artery in children. *Ann Thorac Surg* 1969;8:312–319.
11. Baxter JD, Dunbar JS: Tracheomalacia. *Ann Otol Rhinol Laryngol* 1963;72:1013–1023.
12. Kiely EM, Spitz L, Brereton R: Management of tracheomalacia by aortopexy. *Pediatr Surg Int* 1987;2:13–15.
13. Shapiro RS, Martin WM: Long custom-made plastic tracheostomy tube in severe tracheomalacia. *Laryngoscope* 1981;91:355–361.
14. Wiseman NE, Duncan PG, Cameron CB: Management of tracheobronchomalacia with continuous positive airway pressure. *J Pediatr Surg* 1985;20:489–493.
15. Cogbill TH, Moore FA, Accurso FJ, Lilly JR: Primary tracheomalacia. *Ann Thorac Surg* 1983;35:538–541.
16. Johnston MR, Loeber N, Hillyer P, et al: External stent for repair of secondary tracheomalacia. *Ann Thorac Surg* 1980;30:291–298.
17. Filler RM, Rossello PJ, Lebowitz RL: Life-threatening anoxic spells caused by tracheal compression after repair of esophageal atresia: Correction by surgery. *J Pediatr Surg* 1976;11:739–748.
18. Filler RM, Buck JR, Bahoric A, et al: Treatment of segmental tracheomalacia and bronchomalacia by implantation of an airway splint. *J Pediatr Surg* 1982;17:597–603.
19. Gross RE, Neuhauser EB: Compression of the trachea by an anomalous innominate artery: An operation for its relief. *AJDC* 1948;75:570–574.
20. Herzog H, Keller R, Maurer W, et al: Distribution of bronchial resistance in obstructive pulmonary diseases and in dogs with artificially induced tracheal collapse. *Respiration* 1968;25:381–394.
21. Rainier WG, Newby JP, Keble DL: Long-term results of tracheal support surgery for emphysema. *Dis Chest* 1968;53:765–772.
22. Vinograd I, Filler RM, England SJ, et al: Tracheomalacia: An experimental animal model for a new surgical approach. *J Surg Res* 1987;42:597–604.
23. Murphy P, Filler RM, Muraji T, et al: Effect of prosthetic airway splint on the growing trachea. *J Pediatr Surg* 1983;18:370–372.
24. Vinograd I, Filler RM, Bahoric A: Long-term functional results of prosthetic airway splinting in tracheomalacia and bronchomalacia. *J Pediatr Surg* 1987;22:38–41.

Tracheomalacia

Jean-Stephane Valla, MD and M. Jaubert de Beaujeu, MD

Several rare forms of tracheomalacia are life threatening because they can be complicated at any time by a rapidly fatal acute respiratory accident. The risk of sudden death prompted consultation of several children with severe tracheomalacia at our surgical unit. The medicosurgical team is faced with a difficult clinical decision in such cases: should ventilatory support be initiated with positive airway pressure, knowing that the procedure may have to be prolonged for several months and that it does not always prevent serious accidents? Should the risk be taken immediately to surgically correct the tracheal wall defect, and if so, what technique should be used?

Mention must first be made of the adverse role of tracheostomy, which should be avoided whenever possible because it both complicates treatment and aggravates tracheomalacia. At the start of the expiratory phase, the glottis is closed: this maintains a positive pressure in the trachea and prevents collapse of the tracheal walls. Although this closed glottis phase is very short (0.1 second), it counteracts the negative effects of tracheomalacia. Disappearance of this compensating mechanism after tracheostomy[1] delays decannulation. Language development in children who have had long-standing tracheostomies is also delayed.[2] We agree with Greenholz et al[3] that "direct surgical attack may replace tracheostomy in the management of selected cases of proximal and diffuse tracheomalacia."

In children, tracheomalacia usually has a congenital etiology. The one acquired case in our series[4] was secondary to accidental ingestion of hydrochloric acid, which caused esophageal and tracheal lesions. The risk of tracheomalacia in children with esophageal atresia is particularly high when there is a concomitant tracheoesophageal fistula (67% in the presence of a fistula versus 21% in the absence of a fistula), and especially when the fistula is located in the proximal trachea, above T3.[5]

Anteroposterior and lateral radiographs together with preoperative and intraoperative endoscopy are the main diagnostic techniques. Frey et al[6] recently emphasized the value of dynamic computed tomography studies (Imatron) using transverse scans, but such equipment is costly and not yet in routine use. We have had no experience with this technique.

Our experience in surgical management of tracheomalacia is limited to five cases (Table D13.1). Aortopexy, an excellent procedure that should be performed in all cases, was not used for the first two patients we treated. In our last two cases, intraoperative tracheoscopy demonstrated that aortopexy alone was insufficient and had to be complemented by tracheal splinting.

Resection of the malacic trachea with end-to-end anastomosis has been used with success by Harrison and Hendren,[7] Greenholz et al,[3] and Smith and Cavett[8] but is applicable only for cases of limited malacia. The only logical solution for extensive defects (insufficiently corrected by aortopexy) is external splinting of the trachea. If an external Silastic splint of the type developed by Filler's team is not available, the surgeon can construct a prosthesis extemporaneously. The simplest and oldest method, introduced in 1965 by Binet et al[9] consists of coating the external aspect of the trachea with an air-hardening adhesive. We have obtained excellent long-term results (20 and 18 years follow-up) using a Silastic or Histoacryl (cyano-2-acrylate-2-N-butyl) product. Surgicel mesh (case No. 4) or silastic sheets (case No. 5) can be used for reinforcement. As with other external prostheses, care must be taken not to completely encircle the trachea because this would impede growth. After a minimum follow-up period of five years, none of our patients has exhibited abnormal tracheal growth or complications due to erosion of contiguous structures. Although adhesive products appear to be well tolerated in the mediastinum, they remain

*Current Topics in General Thoracic Surgery:
An International Series*

TABLE D13.1 Experience in Surgical Management of Tracheomalacia

Case No.	Etiology	Associated Malformation	Age	Surgical Technique	Associated Procedure	Result	Follow-Up
1	Congenital	Aberrant right (retroesophageal) subclavian artery	4 mo	Pasting with Histoacryl	Section of aberrant right subclavian artery	Good	20 yr
2	Congenital	—	1 mo	Pasting with Histoacryl	—	Good	18 yr
3	Congenital	Right pulmonary hypoplasia, anomalous pulmonary venous drainage	10 mo	External splint of bone on left bronchus	Right pneumonectomy	Good	8 yr
4	Acquired	—	2 yr	External splint with Histoacryl + Surgicel	Aortopexy	Good for malacia. Post-op stenosis: resection	5 yr
5	Congenital	Esophageal atresia type III, laryngeal cleft	3 mo	External splint with Histoacryl + Silastic sheet	Esophagocoloplasty (2 mo) aortopexy, esophageal reconstruction with colon	Good	5 yr

a foreign body, like any other prosthesis, and thus cannot be considered the ideal solution.

In the future, surgical treatment of tracheomalacia will undoubtedly make increasing use of autologous grafts. One of our patients (case No. 3) was successfully managed with a rib graft, using a modification of the Herzog technique.[10] Other tissues (periosteum, cartilage) also possess the necessary biomechanical qualities; the ideal solution would be a vascularized graft, similar to the experimental model proposed by Goldstein et al.[11]

REFERENCES

1. Johnston MR, Loeber M, Hillyer P, et al: External stent for repair of secondary tracheomalacia. *Ann Thorac Surg* 1980;30:291–296.
2. Simon BM, Fowler SM, Handler SD: Communication development in young children with long-term tracheostomies: Preliminary report. *Int J Pediatr ORL* 1983;6:37–50.
3. Greenholz SK, Karrer FM, Lilly JR: Contemporary surgery of tracheomalacia. *J Pediatr Surg* 1986;21:511–514.
4. Valla JS, Jaubert de Beaujeu M: Surgical management in the treatment of infant tracheomalacia. *Chir Pediatr* 1984;4–5:265–269.
5. Bargy F, Manach Y, Wakim A: Tracheomalacia in esophageal atresia. *Chir Pediatr* 1984;4–5:261–264.
6. Frey EE, Smith WL, Grandgeorge S, et al: Chronic airway obstruction in children: Evaluation with ciné CT. *AJR* 1987;148:347–352.
7. Harrison MR, Hendren WH: Agenesis of the lung complicated by vascular compression and bronchomalacia. *J Pediatr Surg* 1975;10:813–817.
8. Smith KP, Cavett CM: Segmental bronchomalacia: Successful surgical correction in an infant. *J Pediatr Surg* 1985;20:240–241.
9. Binet JP, LaJouanine P, Guilmet T, et al: Traitement de la tracheomalacie gravissime du nourrison par application péri-trachéale du monomère Eastman 910. *Presse Médicale* 1965;74:2437–2438.
10. Herzog H: La trachéoplastie dans la sténose expiratoire de la trachée et des grosses bronches par hypotonie de la paroi membraneuse. *J Fr Med Chir Thorac* 1961;15:415–431.
11. Goldstein R, Gustafson RA, Cook L, et al: Myo-osseous intercostal pedicle flaps for tracheal reconstruction in puppies. *J Pediatr Surg* 1987;22:530–533.

Chapter 14

Aortic Arch Anomalies

*Jean Langlois, MD, Jean-Paul Binet, MD,
Jean-Louis De Brux, MD, Ulrik Hvass, MD,
and Claude Planche, MD*

In 1945, Gross[1] accomplished the first successful surgical intervention for a congenital aortic arch anomaly (AAA). By 1964, he had the largest series worldwide (129 cases). Soon after, surgical experiences increased: in 1962, 23 cases were reported by Mustard et al[2]; in 1966, 26 cases by Cooley and Halmann; in 1969, 31 cases by Lincoln et al[3]; by June 1970 we had operated on 52 children with AAA, and our present experience is 468 cases.

These vascular anomalies had nevertheless been recognized long before. Anatomical and embryologic studies had been carried out and include those by Huntington[4] in 1919, Congdon[5] in 1922, Edwards[6] in 1947, Pearson and Ronald[7] in 1968, and Corone et al[8] in 1955.

AAAs include several malformations, particularly double aortic arch, vascular rings formed by a right aortic arch and a ligamentum arteriosum, circumflex aortas, anomalous subclavian arteries, pulmonary artery sling, and tracheal compression by the innominate artery.

PATHOLOGICAL ANATOMY AND EMBRYOLOGY

For the physician or surgeon, knowledge of the embryology of the aortic arches makes it possible to understand the numerous anomalies of the aorta, great vessels, and pulmonary arteries which they may face.

Exact knowledge of the anomalies permits simple and successful operative management. One must not forget that surgery provides a lim-

ited view of the mediastinum and that the surgeon can explore only a limited part of it.

In this respect, Edwards's pathological, embryological, and clinical work[9] and classification into three groups, and Dor and Corone's[10] schematic explanations, are invaluable for the surgeon. They allow one not only to understand the malformations of the fourth and sixth pairs of branchial arches, but also to imagine the possibilities, some of which have not yet been described. In particular, they allow exact demonstration of the anomalies before surgery through interpretation of noninvasive investigations, especially the esophagogram. Aortography itself is very often useless. Consequently, we think it is important to recall some pathological and embryological data.

Comparison among different anatomical and clinical findings allowed Edwards[9] to classify AAA into three groups, taking into account the side of the mediastinum in which the descending aorta and the ligamentum arteriosum are located:

Group 1: The superior part of the descending aorta, and the ligamentum arteriosum arising from the left pulmonary artery, lie on the left of the esophagus.

Group 2: The superior part of the descending aorta, and the ligamentum arteriosum arising from the right pulmonary artery, lie on the right of the esophagus. These anomalies are exceptional.

Group 3: Multiple anomalies are included here. The descending aorta and the ligamentum arteriosum lie on opposite sides. These anomalies are relatively frequent.

The single cardiac tube of the four-week embryo is lengthened at the front as the bulbus arteriosus, which forms the ventral aorta. The ven-

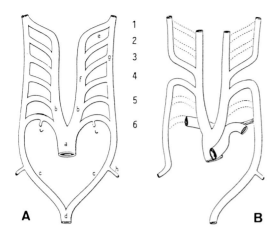

FIGURE 14.1 Aortic arch system embryology. **a.** Truncus arteriosus. **b.** Ventral aorta. **c.** Dorsal aorta. **d.** Descending aorta. **e.** Aortic arch vessels. **f.** Intermediate ventral segments. **g.** Intermediate dorsal segments. **h.** Seventh somatic artery. **i.** Pulmonary arteries.

tral aorta divides into two branches, right and left, which curve toward the back, forming the first aortic arch on each side. In the classic representation of the aortic arches (Figs. 14.1 and 14.2), the ventral aorta, arising from the truncus

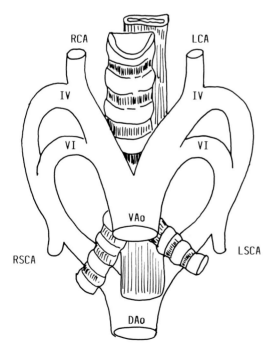

FIGURE 14.2 Ventral view of ventral and dorsal aortas, jointed on the left as on the right side by the fourth and sixth aortic arch vessels.

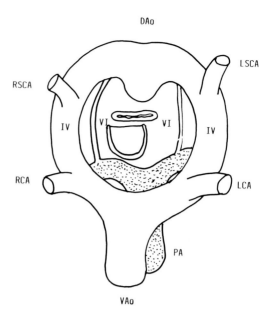

FIGURE 14.3 Cephalic view of ventral and dorsal aortas jointed by the fourth and sixth aortic arch vessels.

and running cephalad, is linked by six pairs of aortic arches to two dorsal aortas (dorsolateral with respect to the primitive bowel). The two dorsal aortas run caudad and join, forming the single dorsal aorta. The aortic segments (ventral and dorsal) connected to each aortic arch are called the *intermediate ventral* and *dorsal* segments. Each dorsal aorta gives rise to seven pairs of segmental somatic arteries. From each of the two dorsal aortas arises the future subclavian artery (seventh intersegmental artery), which migrates cephalad along the aorta. The first two pairs of arches disappear rapidly, and the fifth pair is only transitory. Hence one need consider only the third, fourth, and sixth arches.

If one imagines a bird's-eye view of the resulting system, reduced to the fourth and sixth aortic arches, the diagram would be as shown in Figure 14.3.

Study of the Fourth Arch

The fourth arch, with the two ventral and dorsal aortas, forms a ring encircling the tracheoesophageal axis. Persistence of this ring produces the *double aortic arch.* This malformation is rather frequent and can produce compression (Figs. 14.4, 14.5).

In the vast majority of cases, this vascular ring will be divided at one point. According to the location of this interruption in relation to the

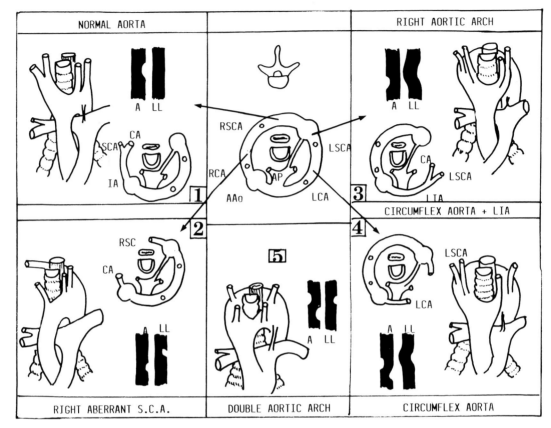

FIGURE 14.4 Classic diagram by Pierre Corone showing different anomalies formed from the primitive aortic annulus. The esophagogram is shown in both (A) anterior projection and (LL) left lateral projection.

three vessels arising from each half of the ring (third arch or common carotid artery, seventh intersegmental artery or subclavian artery, sixth arch or ductus arteriosus), a different arterial arrangement results. Four possibilities summarize almost all the cases seen:

Interruption in 1 (Fig. 14.4,1): normal disposition, with left aortic arch giving rise successively to the right innominate artery, the left common carotid artery, and the left subclavian artery.

Interruption in 2 (Fig. 14.4,2): left aortic arch with aberrant right retroesophageal subclavian artery.

Interruption in 3 (Fig. 14.4,3): circumflex aorta, with left descending aorta, right and posterior aortic arch with left innominate artery.

Interruption in 4 (Fig. 14.4,4): circumflex aorta with separated left common carotid artery (first branch of the aortic arch) and left subclavian artery, arising posteriorly.

When the descending aorta is on the right side, the first branch of the aortic arch is the left innominate artery or the common carotid artery if the left subclavian artery is in a retroesophageal position (see discussion later).

In some exceptional cases, a double interruption explains the anomaly known as *interruption of the aortic arch* (interruption in 1 and 3).

Study of the Sixth Arch

The sixth arches, left and right, arise from the dorsal aspect of the truncus arteriosus, which, on division, separates into an anterior or ventral channel, which continues as the left fourth arch and contributes to form the aortic arch; and a posterior or dorsal channel, the main pulmonary artery trunk. This is in place of the sixth right and left arches and later forms the initial part of the right and left pulmonary arteries. From these sixth arches arises a vessel that will form the extrahilar part of the definitive pulmonary artery.

Finally, the sixth arch is connected to the fourth arch in front of the position of the subclavian artery. One can thus explain the normal and abnormal dispositions of the pulmonary artery and ductus arteriosus. Normally, (1) the

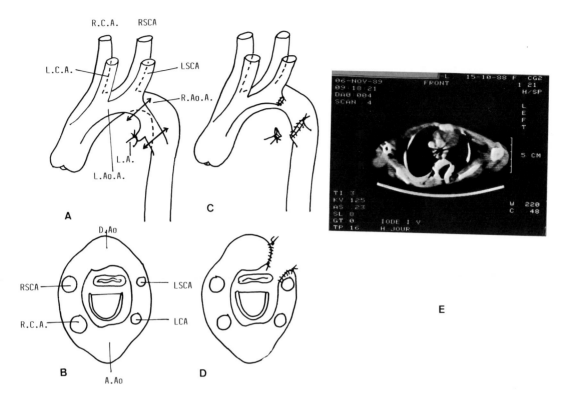

FIGURE 14.5 Double aortic arch. Clinical case with dominant right aortic arch and median descending aorta. **A.** Anatomy seen from left side. **B.** Cephalic view. **C** and **D.** After surgical cross section of the left aortic arch. **E.** Magnetic resonance imaging before surgery.

main pulmonary artery results from the division of the truncus arteriosus by the aortopulmonary septum; (2) both major branches of the pulmonary artery arise from three elements: the proximal part of the sixth arch, the primitive pulmonary artery, and the arteries of Huntington's intrapulmonary plexus; and (3) the ductus arteriosus or ligamentum arteriosum comes from the distal part of the sixth left aortic arch.

The very rare right ductus arteriosus results from the persistence of the distal part of the sixth right aortic arch.

The persistence of an anastomosis between the right and left primitive pulmonary arteries results in the possibility of an aberrant left pulmonary artery running between the trachea and esophagus.

Study of the Third Arch

Normally, the third arch gives rise to the initial part of the internal carotid artery, whether or not the segment of the dorsal aorta intermediate between the third and fourth arch disappears.

The abnormal replacement of the fourth arch by the third one, with the persisting intermediate segment, results in a rare case of *cervical aorta*, right or left.

It is necessary to point out that this description does not correspond to strict reality. The six pairs of aortic arches are indeed not present simultaneously. They develop at different periods of organogenesis. Through atresia of some segments, and persisting patency of some others, arises the normal anatomy of the aortic system as well as most of the known malformations of the aorta and its branches.

One must also point out that in some anomalies, complete or not, there may be dilated segments, such as the retroesophageal Kommerel diverticulum or a real aneurysm of the aorta or subclavian artery. Narrowed segments, even atretic ones, may also exist, leading to an abnormal isolated segment of the subclavian or innominate artery.

COMPLETE RINGS

The Double Aortic Arch

The double aortic arch is typical of the complete rings. In this type of AAA the ascending aorta is in its normal position and divides into the right and left arches, which meet again in the back to form the descending aorta.

In numerous papers, the most frequent va-

TABLE 14.1 Thoracic Vascular Rings Compressing the Esophagus and Trachea in Children: Surgical Experience

	Age over 2 years	Age under 2 years	Total
Isolated vascular rings	51	331	382
Vascular rings + associated malformations	14	72	86
Total	**65**	**403**	**468**

riety of double aortic arch (corresponding to Edwards's group[1]) is made up of the aortic isthmus and descending aorta situated to the left of the esophagus. The ligamentum arteriosum also lies on the left. In this type, the right posterior arch runs to the right of the trachea, then to the right and behind the esophagus. It gives rise successively to the right common carotid artery and to the right subclavian artery. The left arch (or anterior and left arch) lies in the normal position of the aortic arch to the left and in front of the trachea and esophagus. It gives rise successively to the left common carotid artery and to the left subclavian artery.

The double aortic arch may also belong to group 3—that is, it may result in a right-sided descending aorta. In this case, it is the left arch that runs behind the esophagus. In our surgical experience (Tables 14.1 and 14.2) this is the most frequent variety encountered.

The right and left arches are sometimes of identical diameter. Nevertheless, one of the two arches is frequently larger than the other. Classically, the right one is larger than the left. In the smaller one, the diameter is frequently irregular and some segments can be hypoplastic or atretic, being reduced to a ligament; other segments can be abnormally dilated or aneurysmal, for example a retroesophageal diverticulum. The narrowed or atretic segment can be situated proximal to the carotid artery, between the carotid and the subclavian artery, or distal to the subclavian artery. Identifying these points is important, because surgical dissection must open the ring while maintaining perfusion of the aorta distally or of the carotid and subclavian arteries.

The Right-Sided Aorta with Compression by the Ligamentum Arteriosum (Neuhauser's Anomaly)

Among the *encircling forms,* which infants usually tolerate badly, we frequently observed (60 out of 381 in our series) a particular form belonging to Edwards's group 3 (Table 14.2). In these cases, the ascending aorta lies in its normal position. The horizontal part of the aortic arch runs to the right of the trachea and esophagus, and the descending aorta runs to the right of the esophagus. The ligamentum arteriosum extends from the origin of the left pulmonary artery to the aorta at the isthmus and is situated on the right. It runs successively to the left and then behind the esophagus.

According to embryologic data, the left innominate artery, the right common carotid ar-

TABLE 14.2 Isolated Thoracic Vascular Rings Compressing the Esophagus: 382 of 468 Cases

Anomaly	Cases	>2 years	<2 years	Deaths
Double aortic arch	166	19*	147	5*
Dominant right-sided ($n = 137$)				
Dominant left-sided ($n = 28$)				
Balanced ($n = 1$)				
Retroesophageal subclavian artery	85	7	78	4
Right aortic arch ($n = 76$)				
Left aortic arch ($n = 9$)				
Right aortic branch:	60	21	39	—
Mirror branching + left ductus or ligamentum arteriosum				
Abnormally placed brachiocephalic trunk	54	2	52	—
Anomalous left pulmonary artery	8	—	8	1
Ductus sling	1	—	1	—
Circumflex aortic arch	8	3	5	—
Total	**382**	**52**	**330**	**10***

* Included one patient 47 years old.

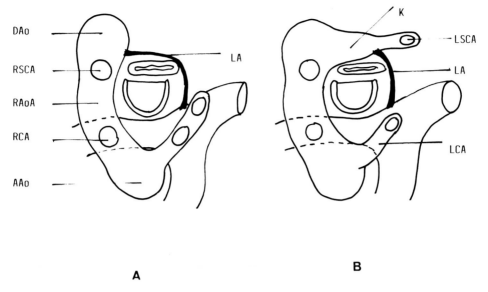

FIGURE 14.6 Two types of Neuhauser anomaly. Right aortic arch with right descending aorta and left ligamentum arteriosum. **A.** With a left brachiocephalic trunk. **B.** With a left carotid artery separated from left subclavian artery that is retroesophageal with (or without) a Kommerel diverticulum.

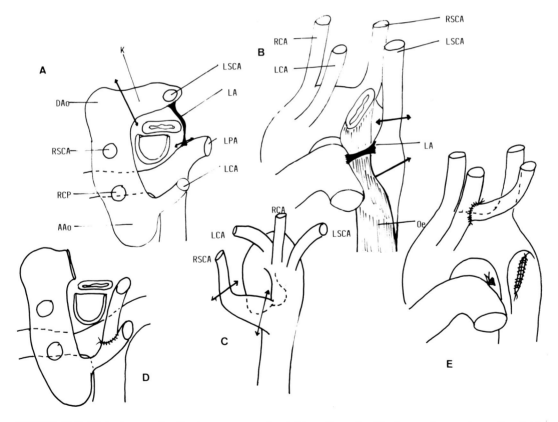

FIGURE 14.7 Clinical case of a Neuhauser anomaly: right aortic arch with descending aorta on the right side, a Kommerel aortic diverticulum, and a left subclavian artery, which are in retroesophageal position. Anatomy: **A.** Cephalic view. **B.** Left lateral view. **C.** Posterior view. **D, E.** Surgical procedure with section and anastomosis of left subclavian artery to left carotid artery.

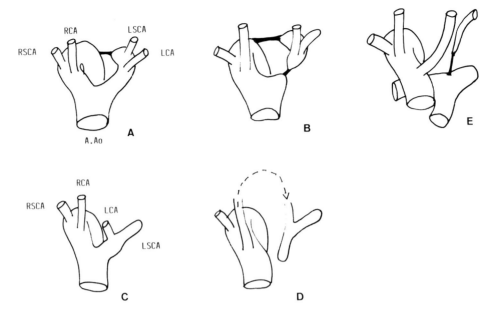

FIGURE 14.8 Isolation of left innominate artery or left subclavian artery (LSCA), with possible steal syndrome. **A.** Double aortic arch with an atretic left arch posterior segment. **B.** The same with an atretic anterior segment. **C.** Right aortic arch with a left innominate artery. **D.** The same with an isolated innominate artery. **E.** Right aortic arch with isolation of the left subclavian artery.

tery, and the right subclavian artery arise in sequence from front to back (Fig. 14.6A).

Felson and Palayew[11] demonstrated the existence of two possible types of right aortic arch (Fig. 14.6): the anterior type, which gives rise to branches as described earlier (a mirror image of the normal anatomy of a left-sided aortic arch) and the posterior type, in which there is an aberrant retroesophageal left subclavian artery. In the posterior type, according to embryologic data, the right aortic arch successively gives rise to the left common carotid artery, the right common carotid artery, the right subclavian artery, and the retroesophageal left subclavian artery, which can also develop a dilatation at its origin. If this forms a genuine aneurysm, this is Kommerel's "aortic diverticulum," which can markedly compress the esophagus and trachea.

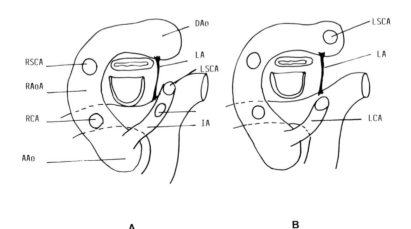

FIGURE 14.9 Cephalic view of a circumflex aorta: right and retroesophageal arch and descending aorta on the left side. There are two types: **A.** With a left innominate artery. **B.** With a carotid artery separated from left subclavian artery arising from the aortic isthmus.

Whether or not there is a Kommerel's diverticulum, the ligamentum arteriosum completes the ring. This variety is often called *Neuhauser's anomaly,* for the radiologist who first described it (Fig. 14.7).

Shuford et al[12] described in 1970 three types of AAA with a right aortic arch. They added a third anomaly to the two described by Felson and Palayew[11]: an aortic arch associated with isolation of the left subclavian artery. This is a rare anomaly, in which there is interruption of the left arch in two places: one distal to the left carotid artery, the other distal to the left subclavian artery. According to Martin et al[13] and Park,[14] isolation of the innominate artery may also occur (Fig. 14.8).

In our series, we found the situation of the descending aorta to be variable: it can be medial, behind the esophagus, or in front of the spine; it can also run to the left. In the latter case, the anomaly belongs to Edward's group 1, and is called a *circumflex aorta* (Fig. 14.9). The ligamentum arteriosum is then short, in its normal left position, and the whole anomaly is very constrictive.

THE INCOMPLETE RINGS

The Retroesophageal (or Aberrant) Right Subclavian Artery (ARSA)

The ARSA belongs to Edwards's group 1. The aortic arch runs normally in front and to the left of the trachea and mediastinum and, from front to back, gives rise to the right common carotid artery, the left common carotid artery, and the left subclavian artery; and finally the right subclavian artery arises from the deep aspect of the aortic isthmus. The ARSA runs deeply, toward the right supraclavicular space, behind the esophagus and in front of the spine.

This was the first AAA discovered. It does not always produce symptoms, is often ignored, and consequently may be the most frequent anomaly. Finally, its retroesophageal course is not obligatory. Holzapel (quoted by Mathey et al[15]) claims it can run between the trachea and esophagus, or even in front of the trachea.

The Retroesophageal (or Aberrant) Left Subclavian Artery (ALSA)

The ALSA belongs to Edwards's group 2: it originates from a right aortic arch. The ligamentum arteriosum runs toward the right pulmonary artery and is therefore different from the second type of Neuhauser's anomaly[16] previously described. It seems to be frequent (76 out of 381 cases in our series).

The aortic arch gives rise successively, from front to back, to the left common carotid artery, the right common carotid artery, the right subclavian artery, and, by its deep mediastinal aspect, the left subclavian artery, which runs behind the esophagus in front of the spine and appears high in the left hemithorax, almost at the apex of the pleura. The ALSA is sometimes dilated at its origin, and this aneurysmal aortic diverticulum can force the trachea and esophagus to the front, where compression can occur.

The Innominate Artery Compressing the Trachea

This rare anterior anomaly was described by Gross and Neuhauser[17] (Fig. 14.10). In 1971, when reviewing our first experience, we counted 22 published cases,[18] and by now we have operated on 54 cases in infants (Table 14.2).

In this anomaly, the normal aortic arch, running to the left in the anterior mediastinum, gives rise to the innominate artery, which is abnormally located to the left of the midline. It passes more or less horizontally from left to right in front of the trachea, on which it leaves an imprint. It ends by giving rise to its two branches in their normal position. Usually the tracheal wall, which is in contact with the innominate artery, is weak, and narrowing develops at this point.

This anomaly does not always cause compression: Fearon and Shortreed[19] operated on only 3, among 79 cases observed in infants.

In our series, we observed three arteries that can compress the trachea: the innominate artery, a bicarotid trunk (associated with an ARSA), or a bicarotid-subclavian trunk ("bouquet" distribution, which is a normal configuration in the horse). The latter anomaly, noted by Gross and Neuhauser,[17] caused marked compression in our series.

The Aberrant Left Pulmonary Artery or Pulmonary Artery Sling (PAS)

The PAS is an anomaly of the sixth arch. It was discovered in 1897 and was operated on for the first time in 1954 by Potts et al.[20]

In 1971, we reported our first surgical experience of 5 cases[21] and then were able to count 78 published cases, 51 of which had undergone surgery. Our present surgical experience includes 8 cases (Table 14.2). In this malformation (Figs. 14.11A, 14.12, 14.13), in infants the left pulmonary artery arises from the pulmonary arterial trunk at the level of the anterior and right edge of the tracheal bifurcation, runs successively above the right bronchus, around the right side of the trachea, between the trachea in front and

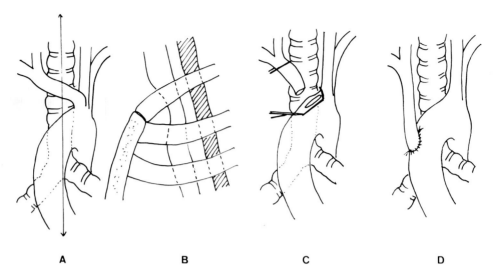

FIGURE 14.10 Right innominate artery compressing trachea arising from the aorta in the left "abnormal" position. **A.** Anatomy. **B.** Radiological findings in left lateral projection, with indentation of the anterior tracheal wall. Surgical procedure: **C.** Cutting brachycephalic trunk from aorta and **D.** Anastomosis in anatomic position.

the esophagus behind, and finally joins the left pulmonary pedicle. At its origin, the pulmonary arterial trunk lies in its normal position, and then it curves to the right and gives rise to the right pulmonary artery and to the aberrant left pulmonary artery.

Tracheal and bronchial effects are often severe, due to the compression and narrowing of the trachea by this artery. Severe structural anomalies are often associated: disappearance of the annular architecture, weakness of the tracheal wall, complete tracheal rings, extensive hypoplasia, and so on.

Many other vascular anomalies are associated with aortic malformations, such as coarctation or atresia of the aorta and ductus arteriosus.

One of us[22] successfully operated on a duc-

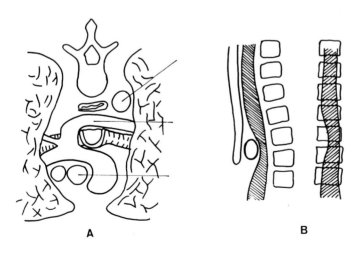

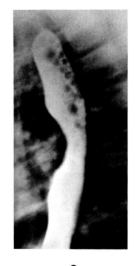

FIGURE 14.11 Left aberrant pulmonary artery (LAPA). **A.** Anatomy: cephalic view. **B.** Radiological findings in anterior and left lateral projection. **C.** Esophagogram showing the negative shadow of LAPA between trachea (clear) and esophagus (indentation of the anterior wall).

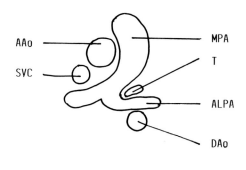

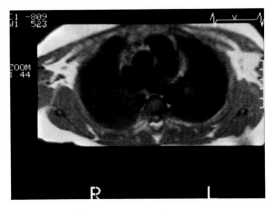

FIGURE 14.12 Left aberrant pulmonary artery: magnetic resonance imaging.

tus arteriosus sling. We also observed an exclusion of the left subclavian artery, arising from the left pulmonary artery and associated with tetralogy of Fallot.

TRACHEOBRONCHIAL ANOMALIES

Although it is impossible to prove that the vascular anomaly is responsible for the associated lesions of the trachea and bronchi, one must recognize that many tracheal and bronchial anomalies are in direct contact with the abnormal vessel and that the narrowing of the tracheobronchial lumen is generally located at that particular point.

There is, then, a limited dyskinesia at the level of the vascular anomaly, or in its proximity,

with a marked imprint of the vessel on the tracheal wall, which appears to be weak and thin and perhaps lacking any cartilage.

The severe anomalies of the architecture of the trachea and bronchi that can be associated are the following:

1. complete or partial disappearance of tracheal rings, over a variable extent, or abnormal weakness of the tracheal or tracheobronchial wall, severe dyskinesia, or tracheomalacia leading to severe respiratory troubles and postoperative complications that can require prolonged tracheal intubation and intensive respiratory care;

2. existence of a particular anomaly: lack of the membranous part of the wall with complete cartilaginous rings in the trachea and bronchi,

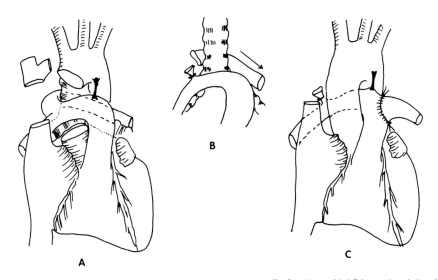

FIGURE 14.13 Left aberrant pulmonary artery. **A.** Anterior view. **B.** Section of LAPA on the right side of the trachea and translation to the left side. **C.** Anastomosis in anatomic position.

as is normally found in chickens, frequently with a narrower diameter than normal;

3. extensive hypoplasia of the trachea and bronchi, often associated with the abovementioned malformation, and which can be so severe as to preclude surgical repair of the vascular anomaly; and

4. laryngeal anomalies, which are not rare. Congenital tracheoesophageal fistula occurred twice in our series, and esophageal atresia is also frequently associated.

ASSOCIATED CARDIAC ANOMALIES

In 86 of 468 cases, we noted a congenital cardiac or aortic anomaly (Table 14.3). The most frequently associated lesions were tetralogy of Fallot, ventricular septal defect, coarctation of the aorta, and patent ductus arteriosus.

CLINICAL SYMPTOMS

The functional signs are variable and either respiratory or digestive.

Respiratory Symptoms

Stridor, which is frequently observed and of variable importance, may be permanent or intermittent. It is a hoarse or wheezing respiratory noise, audible in inspiration and expiration. In infants, it normally leads to investigation for a laryngeal

malformation, which, if discovered, does not exclude AAA. In our series, several cases have been demonstrated.

The respiratory noise can be muffled, intermittent, or even a faint purring that is heard only in decubitus or during sleep. The cough is frequent and sometimes fitful. The respiratory impairment is variable: there may be permanent dyspnea at inspiration and expiration, or it may be less severe. Feeding, crying, and anger can all trigger or worsen the dyspnea. Sometimes, in order to improve respiration, the infant pushes his or her head back by cervical hyperextension.

Sometimes, pulmonary infections with fever (bronchitis or bronchoalveolitis) reveal the anomaly. These are frequently recurrent. In our experience severe acute anoxic episodes, which may even lead to respiratory syncope or anoxic cardiac arrest, have been observed and have been triggered by eating, crying, or respiratory tract infections. Such problems require prompt resuscitation with laryngotracheal intubation, assisted ventilation, and perhaps closed chest massage.

Digestive Symptoms

The association with gastroesophageal reflux is frequent, and this diagnosis does not exclude AAA.

Feeding is often difficult and prolonged in these newborns. It can be interrupted by coughing and cyanotic attacks and can lead to acute respiratory episodes.

TABLE 14.3 Thoracic Vascular Rings in Children with Associated Malformations: 86 of 468 Cases

Anomaly	Cases	>2 years	<2 years	Deaths
Tetralogy of Fallot	14	5	9	4
Ventricular septal defect (VSD) ± patent ductus arteriosus (PDA)	17	—	17	1
Coarctation ± PDA	25	6	19	1
Coarctation + VSD + PDA	5	1	5	1
Interrupted aortic arch	4	—	3	3
PDA + HTP fixée	4	1	3	1
Aortopulmonary septal defect	1	—	1	—
Pulmonary stenosis + VSD	1	—	1	1
Pulmonary atresia + VSD	2	—	2	—
TGV + pulmonary stenosis	2	—	2	1
CCC	2	—	2	2
A-V canal + infundibular stenosis	1	—	1	—
A-V canal	1	—	1	—
Atresia tricuspid	1	—	1	—
Single ventricle + mitral atresia	1	—	1	—
Tracheoesophageal fistula	2	1	1	—
Corrected tracheoesophageal atresia	3	1	2	—
Total	**86**	**15**	**71**	**15**

HATP fixée = fixed pulmonary hypertension, TGV = transposition of great vessels, CCC = complex congenital cardiopathy.

The older child swallows slowly, seeming to fear difficulties, and thus swallowing down the "wrong way" occurs less often.

The time of onset of symptoms may vary. Some AAA may be ignored during infancy, because there are no functional troubles. Some of them are not discovered until adulthood, when severe complications[23] can arise.

The anatomical structures completely encircling the aerodigestive tract (complete double aortic arch, Neuhauser's anomaly) lead to severe and early symptoms, contrasted with incomplete structures, which compress only one face or a small portion of the trachea and cause late, modest, and intermittent symptomatology (ARSA, compressive innominate artery).

Symptoms are not always the same and depend on the type of AAA: complete rings are mainly responsible for both respiratory and digestive symptoms, compression from an abnormal innominate artery causes respiratory episodes, and aberrant subclavian arteries usually lead to digestive troubles, though they can result in respiratory symptoms as well.

Finally, a hitherto unsuspected AAA may be discovered during surgery for a congenital cardiac or other aortic anomaly, for example a coarctation or atresia of the aorta or a patent ductus arteriosus.

DIAGNOSIS

We believe there are three essential investigations for diagnosis: plain chest roentgenogram, barium contrast esophagogram, and tracheoscopy.

Chest Roentgenogram

The chest film (anteroposterior and lateral) is suggestive in 80% of cases (Backer et al[24]). Findings may include:

1. Hyperaeration of lung fields, unilateral or bilateral, especially with pulmonary artery sling (PAS).
2. Pneumonic infiltrates or atelectasis of varying degrees.
3. The location of the aortic arch and the imprint it leaves on the tracheal lumen. If the location is not clear, a double aortic arch must be suspected (Backer et al[24]); if the aortic arch runs to the right, a compressive ligamentum arteriosum must be suspected (Neuhauser's anomaly). However, a big thymus in infants frequently impedes correct interpretation of the chest roentgenogram.
4. On a lateral roentgenogram, compression of the anterior aspect of the trachea by the innominate artery is almost always visible: it is an anterior defect that narrows the tracheal lumen at the level of the sternal manubrium (Fig. 14.10B).

Barium Esophagogram

Multiple projections are necessary, especially the anteroposterior (AP) and lateral views. Cineradiography is often helpful.

In our experience, the barium esophagogram always demonstrates the existence of an AAA and very often leads to the specific diagnosis of a double aortic arch, Neuhauser's anomaly, aberrant subclavian artery, circumflex aorta, or even a pulmonary artery sling.

Even if the esophagogram is normal, one should not reject the diagnosis of AAA without ruling out an innominate artery compression.

The double aortic arch (Fig. 14.14), in its complete form, gives the following characteristic signs: (1) on the AP view, there are two indentations on the edges of the esophagus: the right one is larger and at the level of the third thoracic vertebra, and the left one is lower and smaller; (2) on the lateral view, a fixed indentation is seen on the posterior aspect of the esophagus.

For an aberrant subclavian artery, lateral views are more helpful: a semilunar or pin-shaped indentation higher than the aortic arch may be seen which forces the esophagus anteriorly. A similar image is seen in the right anterior oblique view: the indentation is obliquely pointed up and forward, due to the oblique course of the artery behind the esophagus.

A retroesophageal Kommerel's diverticulum with the aberrant left subclavian artery enlarges the posterior indentation. In addition, the ligamentum arteriosum may produce an indentation on the left side of the esophagus.

When there is a right aortic arch with compression from a ligamentum arteriosum (Neuhauser's anomaly), a double indentation is visible on the AP view: a large one on the right side corresponding to the right aortic arch, and a narrow and lower one, on the left side, corresponding to the ligamentum arteriosum.

In case of a pulmonary artery sling, an anterior indentation (Fig. 14.11), situated at the level of T4–5, corresponds to the course of the aberrant left pulmonary artery between trachea and esophagus.

Tracheobronchoscopy

This procedure follows the laryngoscopy and is intended to look for a laryngeal malformation or tracheoesophageal fistula.

We have performed tracheobronchoscopy

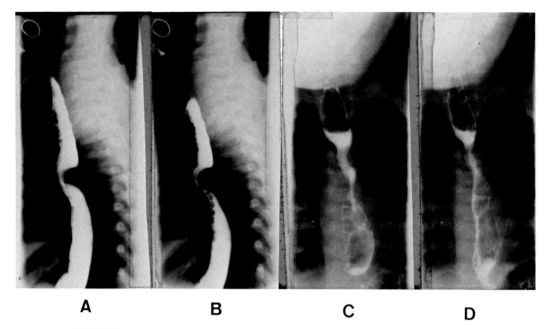

A   **B**   **C**   **D**

FIGURE 14.14 Double aortic arch: esophagogram. **A, B.** Left lateral projection. **C, D.** Anterior projection.

on almost all of our operative cases for more than 10 years. It is mandatory whenever the diagnosis is uncertain because, in every symptomatic case, a narrowing of the tracheal lumen from at least 50% to 80% can be visualized.

Endoscopy is consistently positive in our series in cases of double aortic arch, Neuhauser's anomaly, pulmonary artery sling, circumflex aorta, and innominate artery compression. For the latter diagnosis, pressing on the visible protrusion (sometimes visibly pulsatile) by the tracheoscope makes the right brachial or temporal pulse disappear.

During tracheobronchoscopy, one must also look for tracheal or bronchial anomalies: complete tracheal rings ("chicken's trachea"), varying degrees of tracheomalacia, and alteration of the tracheal bifurcation and right bronchus in case of a PAS.

Aortography, Computed Tomography (CT), Magnetic Resonance Imaging (MRI)

We seldom use aortography because in the vast majority of cases, diagnosis is made by esophagogram and tracheoscopy. CT and MRI should reduce even more the use of aortography.

Aortography can even be misleading, and in our experience, aortography failed to establish the diagnosis in two cases.

We think aortography is useful only when the diagnosis is uncertain, a specific surgical decision is to be made, and there are associated aortic arch anomalies or an AAA and a congenital cardiac anomaly. In the latter case, complete investigation with cardiac catheterization and angiography may be necessary.

We have a limited experience with CT and MRI and have not used these modalities in newborns and young infants. However, in older children CT has confirmed tracheal stenosis and the existence of a vascular anomaly in all cases (nevertheless, the exact type of vascular anomaly could not always be ascertained). Also in older children, MRI has confirmed tracheal stenosis, as well as the existence and exact type of vascular anomaly (Fig. 14.5E).

SURGICAL TREATMENT

The aim of surgical treatment is to relieve the constriction by the vascular ring by dividing and opening it, thus correcting the tracheal and esophageal compression.

Double Aortic Arch

In almost all our cases, the operative approach has been a left lateral transpleural thoracotomy through the fourth intercostal space, whatever the situation (right, left, or medial) of the de-

scending aorta and the side (left or right) of the largest arch.

As a result of good preoperative evaluation of the anomaly and a good knowledge of the different AAAs, the surgeon knows exactly which anomaly he or she is going to find.

The surgeon must successively locate the left subclavian artery, the left common carotid artery, the left aortic arch, the ligamentum arteriosum, the side (left or right) of the isthmus and descending aorta, and, if possible, the extremity of the right arch. The surgeon must also define which of the two arches is the smaller one.

Division of the smaller arch must be performed while adequate flow in the descending aorta, left common carotid artery, and left subclavian artery is maintained. Backer et al[24] recommend that the anesthesiologist monitor the radial and carotid pulses during clamping. In our experience, whenever the surgeon is in doubt, a selective clamping test of the extremity of both arches with pressure monitoring downstream (aorta, carotid artery) is carried out.

The smaller arch is divided in its distal portion, beyond where it gives rise to the subclavian artery. The ends are sutured with continuous running sutures (Figs. 14.5C and 14.5D).

The left arch is usually the smaller one, and atretic or dilated segments must be located.

Division can also be made on an atretic or narrowed segment, usually beyond the subclavian artery. If the narrowed or atretic segment lies between the left carotid and subclavian arteries, one should consider division of the subclavian artery, followed by its reimplantation into the carotid artery. In their series, Backer et al[24] stated that in 4 or 5 of 12 cases of small right aortic arch, an atretic segment existed. This fact does not seem to have had any consequence, considering that in a series of 59 patients, the approach was a left thoracotomy in 57 and a median sternotomy in 2.

The ligamentum arteriosum is always divided.

The vascular ring is opened. Finally, the trachea and esophagus must be freed from any fibrous tissue that may be potentially constrictive. The pneumogastric, recurrent, and phrenic nerves must be carefully avoided.

Right Aortic Arch with Constricting Ligamentum Arteriosum (Neuhauser's Anomaly)

We have operated on two cases through a right lateral thoracotomy. In one case, there was a large patent ductus arteriosus with severe pulmonary hypertension. The other was an adult who required cardiopulmonary bypass.[23] All other cases have been operated on via a left lateral transpleural thoracotomy through the fourth intercostal space.

The surgeon must locate the constricting ligamentum arteriosum, the left subclavian artery, and the left common carotid artery and must be aware of the existence (or absence) of a Kommerel's diverticulum behind the esophagus. One then must determine whether the left subclavian artery arises from a left innominate artery (mirror branching) or if there is an aberrant retroesophageal left subclavian artery (with or without Kommerel's diverticulum at the origin of this subclavian artery; Fig. 14.6B).

Correction of the constriction is accomplished by dividing the ligamentum arteriosum. If it exists, the Kommerel's diverticulum must be divided between two clamps. The left subclavian artery must be divided at the level of the aorta and then reimplanted into the left common carotid artery. The trachea and esophagus must also be freed from any fibrous constrictive tissue.

Aberrant (Retroesophageal) Subclavian Artery

When it is responsible for respiratory or digestive dysfunction, an aberrant subclavian artery must be divided. Whether it is a left one arising from a right aortic arch or a right one arising from a left aortic arch, the approach we have always used is a left lateral thoracotomy through the fourth intercostal space.

We have been reimplanting the subclavian artery into the corresponding carotid artery, whenever possible, for 15 years. This technique was recommended by Smith et al[25] and Jaubert de Beaujeu and Riou.[26] Its aim is to vascularize the corresponding upper limb with normal systemic pressure so as to avoid chronic ischemia or the arterial steal syndrome, as reported by Folger and Shah,[27] Midgley and Clenathan,[28] Pieroni et al,[29] and which can also be observed after the Blalock-Taussig anastomosis.

In cases of left aberrant subclavian artery, the anastomosis is easily performed in the thoracic cavity through the left thoracotomy.

In cases of right aberrant subclavian artery, reimplantation into the right common carotid artery is performed with the patient supine through a short right cervicotomy.[30] In one of our cases, we performed the entire procedure through this single cervical approach: the aberrant right subclavian artery was divided behind the esophagus and then reimplanted into the right carotid artery.

Circumflex Aorta

The circumflex aorta is a severe form of AAA and its treatment is difficult.

This form of AAA may be the consequence of the surgical treatment of a double aortic arch, of which the principal arch runs to the right, then behind the esophagus, before joining the left descending aorta. The surgical treatment, division of the small anterior left arch and the ligamentum arteriosum, may be sufficient to make the respiratory symptoms disappear. Sometimes, however, symptoms persist.

The circumflex aorta may also exist by itself: the ascending aorta runs to the right, then behind the esophagus, before joining the left descending aorta. The ligamentum arteriosum is the compressing element. When divided, symptoms may or may not disappear.

In both cases, the main aortic arch still remains in a retroesophageal position, and the opening of the vascular ring may be insufficient to relieve respiratory symptoms. The only solution is then to "shift" the aortic arch to the left after dividing it (Figure 14.15), as reported by Planché and Lacour-Gayet.[31] This technique is performed with the use of cardiopulmonary bypass (CPB) under deep hypothermia and circulatory arrest through a median sternotomy.

Innominate Artery Compression

In order to eliminate the tracheal compression, three techniques have been proposed:

Gross's Technique

Gross recommended freeing the innominate artery (through an anterolateral thoracotomy, third or fourth space) and suspending it from the periosteum of the sternum, by means of sutures placed in the adventitia of the vessel. In 1982, we counted[18] 3 failed procedures among the 18 cases reported in the literature: respiratory functional troubles had returned subsequently. Gross thought it was impossible to divide the innominate artery without producing neurological damages. It is now well known that this risk is very low.

Mustard's Technique

In two cases, Mustard et al[2] divided the innominate artery through a median sternotomy. We performed this operation in 5 cases in the beginning of our experience, and we then counted 6 further published cases. We did not observe any neurological trouble.

Nevertheless, it seems to us that in order to lessen the risk of development of atherosclerotic disease and to prevent a possible vascular steal syndrome, it is better to reestablish the vascular continuity after division of the artery.

Section Followed by Reimplantation in Anatomical Position

In our series of 53 cases, 48 had a reimplantation in the anatomical position. Through a median sternotomy, with opening of the pericardium, the innominate vein, thymus, and innominate artery are dissected free. The innominate artery is divided and then reimplanted on the anterior and right aspect of the ascending aorta, through as wide an anastomosis as possible.

One last point is worth discussing: which cases require surgical treatment? This anatomical position of the innominate artery seems to be frequent and often asymptomatic. In our series, all the infants had severe respiratory dysfunction, with narrowing of the tracheal lumen from 50% to 80%. Only these children must have surgery. In our series there has been no mortality, and the long-term results seem to be good.

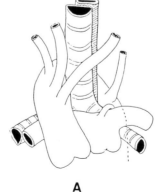
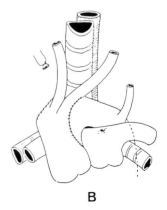

FIGURE 14.15 Surgical procedure described by Claude Planché. **A.** Circumflex aorta with the right aortic arch and left descending aorta. **B.** Under extracorporeal circulation, hypothermia, and circulatory arrest. The aorta is separated on the right side and the new aortic arch is constructed on the left side.

A   **B**

Pulmonary Artery Sling (PAS)

Potts[20] was the first to propose the three possible ways to cure this anomaly: division of the left pulmonary artery and reimplantation into its anatomical position; division of the right main bronchus and anastomosis in its anatomical position; and right pneumectomy.

Three other possibilities have also been suggested: left pneumectomy, division of the ligamentum arteriosum, and division of the left pulmonary artery.

In the choice of operative technique, one must consider several points, such as the certainty of the diagnosis (established or not before the operation), the surgical approach, and the extent of associated tracheobronchial malformations, when present.

Division of the ligamentum arteriosum or patent ductus arteriosus has been performed in 4 cases, with two survivals, by Mustard et al.[2] This procedure, although it opens the vascular ring, seems to be insufficient and is no longer used.

Right or left pneumonectomy would constitute an unnecessary mutilation, and no case seems to have been published.

During an emergency procedure without precise diagnosis, or during an exploratory right thoracotomy, the surgeon may divide the left pulmonary artery to relieve the compression of the tracheal bifurcation. This technique has been used successfully in at least 3 cases. However, we believe it is better to reestablish the vascular continuity immediately through an additional operative stage.

Division and reimplantation of the right main bronchus has been successfully accomplished in at least 1 case, with right bronchial stenosis occurring 12 years later. The left pulmonary artery then lies under the tracheal carina and under the left main bronchus.

Correction of the vascular anomaly by division, uncrossing, and reanastomosing the left pulmonary artery in its anatomical position completely frees the tracheobronchial airways from any compression. This technique is currently used. Various surgical solutions have been proposed:

Surgical approach: anterolateral thoracotomy through the fourth intercostal space, right thoracotomy, or median sternotomy.

Vascular repair: a terminoterminal anastomosis on the arterial stump or a lateroterminal anastomosis on the main pulmonary artery.

Cardiopulmonary bypass (CPB) is not indispensable. In our series, out of 8 patients, 1 was operated on without CPB. We nevertheless prefer to perform a lateroterminal anastomosis, using CPB, through a median sternotomy. It replaces respiratory function during the procedure and permits a wide anastomosis on empty and opened vessels.

Immediate results depend on the severity of the tracheobronchial dysplasia and subsequent respiratory complications. As a late result, the anastomosis can become stenosed; thrombosis of the artery and resultant nonperfusion of the left lung have been reported. Such complications have never occurred in our series.

POSTOPERATIVE COURSE AND RESULTS

Classical thoracic complications (bleeding, pleural effusion, chylothorax) are very rare. In our 15-year experience, only one adult patient (47 years old),[23] died; we have had no deaths in infancy or childhood.

Tracheal or associated tracheobronchial dysplasia ('tracheomalacia') is rather frequent and sometimes requires prolonged assisted ventilation by means of nasotracheal intubation, frequently for 4 to 5 days and up to 21 days in one case. Currently, when the tracheal wall is very weak (particularly in innominate artery compression), we try to reinforce it with biological fibrinogen sealing glue.

The operative procedure is simple and the results obtained in infants are excellent: after the first postoperative weeks or months, functional respiratory troubles disappear and respiratory function becomes normal.

In our series, we believe several children were operated on too late. They were 6, 8, and 12 years of age, and with children this old, results do not seem to be as good. Two of these children have a bad functional result: one of them had been operated on at the age of 12 years for a Neuhauser's anomaly, and the other had to be reoperated on at the age of 16, through a right thoracotomy with the use of CPB. A Dacron graft was then implanted at the aortic isthmus in order to relieve residual tracheal compression. The outcome is now satisfactory.

We observed and operated on at least two cases of complete vascular rings in adults[23]: one of these patients, after aortic valve replacement, became completely ventilator dependent and finally died.

These cases lead us to think that symptomatic AAA must be operated on during the first year of life, since the results are usually good and there is almost no mortality.

REFERENCES

1. Gross RE: Surgical relief for tracheal obstruction from a vascular ring. N Engl J Med 1945;233:586–590.
2. Mustard WT, Trimble AW, Trusler GA: Mediastinal vascular anomalies causing tracheal and esophageal compression and obstruction in childhood. Can Med Assoc J 1962;87:1301–1305.
3. Lincoln JCR, Deve Rall PB, Stark J, et al: Vascular anomalies compressing oesophagus and trachea. Thorax 1969;24:295–306.
4. Huntington W: The morphology of the pulmonary artery in the mammalia. Anat Rec 1919;17:165.
5. Congdon E. Transformation of the aortic arch system during the development of the human embryo. Contribution to Embryologie 1922;14:47–110.
6. Edwards JE. Anomalies of the derivatives of the aortic arch system. Med Clin North Am 1948;32:925–949.
7. Pearson AA, Ronald W: The Development of the Cardiovascular System. Eugene, Oregon; University of Oregon Medical School Printing Department, 1968.
8. Corone P, Nouaille J, et al: Anomalies des arcs aortiques chez le nourrisson. Arch Fr Pediatrie 1955;12:830–842.
9. Edwards JE. Malformations of the aortic arch system manifested as "vascular rings." Lab Invest 1953;2:56.
10. Dor X, Corone P: Embryologie normale et genèse des cardiopathies congénitales. Encycl Medico-Chir, Paris, Coeur-Vaisseaux 1981;3.11001 C 10, 11001 C 20, 11001 C 30.
11. Felson B, Palayew MJ: The two types of right aortic arch. Radiology 1963;81:745–759.
12. Shuford WH, Sybers RG, Edwards FK: The three types of right aortic arch. AJR 1970;109:67–74.
13. Martin EC, Mesko ZG, Griepp RB, et al: Isolation of the left innominate artery, a right arch, and a left patent ductus arteriosus. AJR 1979;132:833–835.
14. Park MK. Right aortic arch with isolation of left innominate artery. Chest 1979;76:106–108.
15. Mathey J, Binet JP, Denis B: Anomalies de développement des arcs aortiques. J Chir 1959;77:505–526.
16. Neuhauser EBD. Roentgen diagnosis of double aortic arch and other anomalies of great vessels. Am J Roentgenol Rad Therapy 1946;56:1–12.
17. Gross RE, Neuhauser EBD: Compression of the trachea or esophagus by vascular anomalies. Pediatrics 1951;7:69–83.
18. Langlois J, Binet JP, Germain M, et al: La compression de la trachée par le tronc artériel brachiocéphalique, chez le nourrisson: A propos de 4 cas. Ann Chir Thorac Cardiovasc 1971;10:171–184.
19. Fearon B, Shortreed R: Compression trachéo-bronchique par anomalies vasculaires congénitales chez l'enfant. Syndrome d'apnée. Ann Otol 1963;72:949–969.
20. Potts WJ, Holinger PH, Rosenblum AH: Anomalous left pulmonary artery causing obstruction to right main bronchus: Report of a case. JAMA 1954;155:1409–1411.
21. Langlois J, Binet JP, Planché C, et al: L'artère pulmonaire gauche aberrante: A propos de cinq cas opérés. Chirurgie 1978;104:58–73, and Arch Mal Coeur 1971;5:573–584.
22. Binet JP, Conso JF, Losay J, et al: Ductus arteriosus sling: Report of a newly recognised anomaly and its surgical correction. Thorax 1978;33:72–75.
23. Georges JL, Brux JL de, Langlois J, et al: Aortic arch anomalies in adults: A rare cause of tracheooesophageal compression: Report of two cases [in French]. Ann Chir: Chir Thorac Cardiovasc 1989;43:99–104.
24. Backer CL, Ilbawi MN, Idriss FS, DeLeon SY: Vascular anomalies causing tracheoesophageal compression: Review of experience in children. J Thorac Cardiovasc Surg 1989;97:725–731.
25. Smith JM, Reul GJ, Wuragh DC, Cooley DA: Retro-oesophageal subclavian arteries: Surgical management and symptomatic children. Card Vascul Disease, Texas Heart Institute 1979;6:333–334.
26. Jaubert de Beaujeu M, Riou RJ: Réimplantation aortique de l'artère sous-clavière droite anormale: A propos de trois cas chez le nourrisson. Chir Pédiatr 1978;19:197–200.
27. Folger GM, Shah KD: Subclavian steal in patients with Blalock-Taussing anastomosis. Circulation 1965;31:241.
28. Midgley FM, Clenathan JE: Subclavian steal syndrome in pediatric age group. Ann Thoracic Surg 1977;24:252–267.
29. Pieroni DR, Brodsky ST, Row RD: Congenital subclavian steal: Report of a case occurring in a neonate and a review of the literature.
30. Langlois J, Binet JP, Hafez A, et al: Artère sous-clavière rétro-oesophagienne: Section et réimplantation dans la carotide primitive par cervicotomie. Nouv Press Méd 1982;11:47–49.
31. Planché C, Lacour-Gayet F: Aortic uncrossing for compressive circumflex aorta: Three cases [in French.] Presse Méd 1984;13:1331–1332.

Aortic Arch Anomalies

Phillip G. Ashmore, MD, FRCS(C)

The material in this chapter is drawn from the combined experience of the authors over more than 20 years. They have treated a large number of patients with this important abnormality with excellent results.

The embryological background that results in abnormal development of the aortic arch is thoroughly described. Although some of the embryological events are not completely understood, the authors present a clear and logical explanation of the various abnormalities, and any surgeon undertaking treatment of these conditions should read (and reread) these embryological considerations.

A few points could be stressed which have led to inaccurate diagnosis in my own experience. It is important to recognize that in some instances localized dilatation of the vascular ring can occur (eg, the diverticulum of Kommerel). These diverticula may compress the mediastinal structures in such a way that treatment is required. It is also necessary to recognize that stenotic or atretic areas that occur in the aortic arch development may not always be in the usual location, or may be multiple, and must be identified before appropriate and successful surgical treatment can be employed. The authors have pointed out that the Kommerel diverticulum is particularly likely to be seen where there is a right-sided aorta and a compressive ligamentum arteriosum. They refer to the potential problem of compression of the trachea with an abnormal innominate artery. There is considerable difference of opinion about the management of this condition, which will be mentioned later.

The tracheobronchial abnormalities associated with aortic arch lesions are an important problem that the surgeon must always keep in mind. The trachea that has been compressed throughout embryological development and early life does not always immediately return to normal size and function, but it usually will over time. It is important to recognize the anatomical situation when normal growth and development of the trachea is not likely to occur.

Early diagnosis of the clinical syndromes associated with aortic arch anomalies is enhanced if the primary physician or pediatrician has a high index of suspicion of the existence of this abnormality in any child with otherwise unexplained stridor or dysphagia. One cannot bring this to the attention of colleagues too often, because delay in the diagnosis of one of these lesions, particularly when the airway is obstructed, can lead to disastrous consequences. The authors review the signs and symptoms thoroughly. One small diagnostic point that I have found commonly present is that the cough that is so common in these children usually has a harsh bark-like quality similar to that noted in the child following correction of esophageal atresia with tracheoesophageal fistula. This has been likened to a seal bark, though not all physicians have an opportunity to become familiar with this sound in their everyday experience. It is also important to point out that dysphagia may be absent or minimal initially but that it may become more obvious when solids are added to the child's diet. Usually the aberrant retroesophageal subclavian artery produces swallowing difficulties, but as the authors point out, there are patients with retroesophageal subclavian artery in whom respiratory symptoms are prominent.

I entirely agree with the authors that plain AP and lateral films of the chest and a barium study of the esophagus are most important diagnostic tools in identifying both the presence and the nature of the aortic arch abnormality. In their practice they almost routinely use tracheoscopy, and the need for this investigative procedure is more controversial, especially when the outline of the air-filled column of the trachea can be assessed by plain films or other means. The hazards of tracheoscopy must be stressed, especially in inexperienced hands or when one does not expect to encounter an aortic arch le-

655 Avenue of the Americas, New York, NY 10010
Current Topics in General Thoracic Surgery:
An International Series

sion creating tracheal deformity. Even in experienced hands, tracheoscopy can precipitate severe or complete respiratory obstruction. I believe it is probably not necessary to carry out tracheoscopy in the majority of cases, but certainly when one suspects a condition such as a pulmonary artery sling, tracheoscopy may be essential in assessing the intrinsic problems of the trachea. Once again, however, the need for special care must be stressed. It is very difficult to be certain of the anatomical structure of the trachea and of the likelihood of its relief by simple division of the vascular ring. Attempts to pass the bronchoscope beyond the stenotic area to assess its distensibility may produce edema and subsequent total respiratory obstruction. In my hospital if my colleagues or I carry out tracheoscopy, particularly in patients suspected of having a pulmonary artery sling, it is done in the operating room just before starting the surgical procedure. It can then be repeated after the vascular anomaly is corrected to assess the postoperative appearance of the trachea.

The authors believe aortography does not have much to offer in terms of definitive diagnosis. This has not been my experience. Especially in difficult cases and when an expert radiologist is present to plan the procedure and interpret the results, aortography has been useful frequently in my preoperative assessment.

Some mention should be made of the place of echocardiography. The authors apparently have not made use of this modality; however, my colleagues and I have found it useful as a screening method, and with increasing use and experience we are finding it possible to diagnose the presence and type of aortic arch lesions with increasing frequency.

There are practical problems of using CT or MRI scanning in infants and small children because they must either be anesthetized or heavily sedated to prevent movement. Our early experience with MRI is most promising, and excellent images have been obtained of both double aortic arch and pulmonary artery sling abnormalities. I must stress the necessity of interpretation by one experienced in interpreting images of this nature. Presently we can obtain superb images of anomalies of the aortic isthmus and its descending portion (eg, coarctation and recurrent coarctation) and it is the opinion of our radiologists that MRI will become the method of choice in identifying the presence and nature of aortic arch abnormalities (J.A.G. Culham, written communication, 1990).

The authors have extensive experience with the surgical treatment of these lesions and have come to a number of logical conclusions. I agree

that a left thoracotomy through the fourth intercostal space is the ideal approach for most cases. During the operation the anatomy must be reassessed as completely as possible and the most prominent arch identified. Unusual areas of complete or severe obstruction must be anticipated, and if doubt exists, selective clamping of the arch and monitoring of downstream pressure is essential. Obviously the tools to carry out these pressure studies must be immediately available in the operating room.

We had an unfortunate experience many years ago when the presence of a diverticulum of Kommerel in association with a constricting ligamentum arteriosum was not recognized. Division of the ligamentum gave some relief of symptoms, but this was not complete, and studies much later identified the presence of a diverticulum producing continued tracheal distortion. It will be necessary for this to be dealt with at a second operation.

I can only reiterate the importance of dividing the ligamentum arteriosum in every case.

In the management of aberrant right subclavian artery it has not been our practice to reimplant the vessel into the right carotid artery. We have not observed either chronic ischemia of the affected limb or the arterial steal syndrome in any of our cases observed over many years. Incidentally, neither have we noted this after the "native" Blalock-Taussig anastomosis. If, however, reimplantation can be done easily and without complications, as seems to be the case in the authors' series, it may be an appropriate addition to the operative procedure.

The management of patients with respiratory symptoms apparently due to tracheal compression by the innominate artery deserves comment. The authors appropriately point out that abnormal origin of the innominate artery seems frequent in the absence of any functional problems. It seems that there is great variability in the frequency of surgery for innominate artery compression among centers experienced in the management of airway problems in children. It is also true that a skilled bronchoscopist can often eliminate the right radial or temporal pulse by manipulating the bronchoscope even when no tracheal compression is present. Suffice it to say that a period of conservative management before undertaking surgery is desirable, and in many cases, over time, the obstructive symptoms will disappear. Only when the child's condition is deteriorating and when severe tracheal obstruction can be clearly demonstrated should innominate decompression or reimplantation be carried out.

There is still no consensus as to the best surgical approach in the management of pulmonary artery sling. To begin with, it is not agreed that surgery with cardiopulmonary bypass is necessary in every case. Although the authors recommend this method and have used it with success in most of their cases, other recent reports from large institutions[1] still recommend division and reimplantation of the left pulmonary artery through a left thoracotomy without bypass. The rather high incidence of late pulmonary artery obstruction has been noted by some, and there is no doubt that intrinsic tracheal obstruction occurs in some patients and is not adequately relieved by section and reanastomosis of the left pulmonary artery.

We have operated upon a number of patients without cardiopulmonary bypass with successful results and have encountered no known cases of late left pulmonary artery obstruction (based on postoperative echocardiographic assessment). We have had two cases who were almost moribund when presented for surgery on the basis of severe tracheal obstruction triggered by tracheoscopy. One of these suffered further tracheal obobstruction and cardiac arrest when we attempted to dissect the left pulmonary artery from the trachea without cardiopulmonary bypass, and this patient subsequently died.

In addition, early reports in the French literature[2] and, more recently, from the group at Boston Children's Hospital[3] describe division and resuture of the right main bronchus or of the stenotic trachea as a means of repositioning the pulmonary artery without dividing it, thereby avoiding the possible late development of pulmonary artery thrombosis. The patients reported by Jonas et al[3] have done well after their tracheal resection and resuture using polydioxanone absorbable suture material. They suggest that division and resection of the stenotic area of the trachea (under cardiopulmonary bypass) allowing replacement of the pulmonary artery without the necessity of dividing it may be the preferred way to manage this lesion.

As a result of our experience we have developed the following surgical protocol as an effective and safe method of managing the pulmonary artery sling.

1. After the diagnosis has been established, the patient is prepared for surgery under cardiopulmonary bypass.
2. Under anesthesia careful tracheoscopy is carried out through the endotracheal tube using a small flexible bronchoscope.
3. Cardiopulmonary bypass is established and the chest opened through a midline sternotomy.
4. The pulmonary artery is freed, divided, and placed anterior to the trachea and then reanastomosed to the left of the trachea.
5. After cardiac function has been reestablished and cardiopulmonary bypass discontinued, we again examine the trachea using the flexible bronchoscope. If serious distortion remains, cardiopulmonary bypass is reinstituted and tracheal resection can be accomplished easily with minimal risk.

REFERENCES

1. Backer CL, Ilbawi M, Idriss F, DeLeon SY: Vascular anomalies causing tracheoesophageal compression. *J Thorac Cardiovasc Surg* 1989;97:725–731.
2. Lochard J, Vert P, Chalnot P: Trajet aberrant de l'artère pulmonaire gauche comprimant l'origine de la bronche souche droite. *Ann Chir Thorac Cardiovasc* 1963;2:458–461.
3. Jonas RA, Spevak PJ, McGill T, Castaneda AR: Pulmonary artery sling: Primary repair by tracheal resection in infancy. *J Thorac Cardiovasc Surg* 1989;97:548–550.

Chapter 15

Aerodigestive Tract Foreign Bodies

Gerald B. Healy, MD

INTRODUCTION

The aspiration of foreign bodies into the aerodigestive tract is an important cause of morbidity and mortality. This problem is responsible for more than 3000 deaths per year in the United States, with children under 2 years of age most commonly affected. At this age children become quite oral and frequently place objects into their mouths, increasing the chance of aspiration.

Those patients who survive the acute stage may present even the most experienced endoscopist with a challenge in diagnosis and treatment. Fortunately, advances in radiology, anesthesia, and endoscopic instrumentation have led to improved patient care in this area. These advances have also pointed to the need to develop a qualified team consisting of the radiologist, the anesthesiologist, and the endoscopist.

Certain objects are more commonly aspirated into one anatomic location versus another. Bones usually lodge in the pharynx, whereas coins are more common in the upper third of the esophagus. Meat and other soft objects may lodge superior to a stricture or may become impacted in patients who have motility disorders of the esophagus. Aspiration into or through the larynx occurs more frequently in children than in adults, with the most common foreign body being a peanut. Other objects, such as parts of toys and organic material, may also be aspirated into the airway by children.

Diagnosis

The diagnosis of acute aspiration is usually straightforward. Initially, there may be a dramatic

episode of choking, coughing, gagging, or wheezing. Frequently there may also be an associated hoarseness, aphonia, or dysphonia. Objects impacted in the larynx or trachea may also cause audible stridor (usually biphasic or expiratory).

An accurate history is mandatory, and parents should be questioned carefully regarding the possibility of foreign body aspiration in any patient with respiratory symptomatology or swallowing disorders. Unfortunately, historical facts given by parents and/or the patient may be overlooked or underappreciated by the primary care physician, and thus it is not uncommon for patients to be treated for other disorders such as asthma or recurrent pneumonia for a long period of time. Many aspirations also occur in the same age group that has a high incidence of these disorders. Unexplained recurrent pneumonia, respiratory illness, or other conditions that do not respond to appropriate medical management should always raise the suspicion of an aspirated foreign body.

A careful physical examination is extremely useful in establishing the presence or absence of foreign body. This is especially true in those cases where objects may be lodged in the respiratory system. Differences in examination findings between the right and left side of the chest should always raise one's suspicion, and thus foreign body must rank high in the differential diagnosis of such patients.

Objects lodged in the pharynx typically impale themselves in lymphoid tissue or in the vallecula. Small fishbones, for example, frequently protrude from the medial surface of the tonsil or from the posterior aspect of the lingual tonsil into the pharyngeal area.

Objects inhaled into the respiratory tract rarely become impacted in the larynx and usually pass directly into the trachea or bronchi. There appears to be a predilection for the right main-stem bronchus because of its direct continuity with the trachea.

Esophageal impaction will frequently demonstrate signs and symptoms of swallowing difficulty. This may include pain, regurgitation of undigested food, or increased salivation. However, the absence of these signs or symptoms does not rule out the possibility of an esophageal foreign body.

Radiologic Evaluation

Plain roentgenograms of the neck and chest are basic to the evaluation of any patient suspected of having aspirated a foreign object, but in and of themselves they do not constitute a complete examination.

The cross-sectional area of the airway increases during inspiration, and thus foreign objects tend to move peripherally during this phase of respiration. If the object is positioned to allow air flow during inspiration with occlusion during expiration, it will act as a check valve. This results in overinflation of the lung distal to the object in question and depression of the ipsilateral hemidiaphragm, with shift of mediastinal structures to the opposite side. If the object completely obstructs the airway as it progresses distally, complete endobronchial obstruction ensues with resulting atelectasis (Fig. 15.1).

Fluoroscopy is quite helpful in detecting the presence of a foreign body in the airway. Mediastinal shift and diaphragmatic movement is compared on both sides of the chest; obvious changes are helpful in determining the presence and location of a foreign object.

In cases of aspirated esophageal foreign bodies, contrast material should be used with caution. Unsuspected complete obstruction by a nonradiopaque object may force aspiration of the contrast material into the respiratory tract. If the history and physical examination is clearly pointing to the possibility of an object in the esophagus and plain roentgenograms do not reveal evidence, endoscopic evaluation should be undertaken without the use of contrast. Overall, it must always be remembered that a normal roentgenographic study does not rule out the presence of a foreign body either in the airway or the esophagus. It should also be remembered that objects that have become impacted high in the esophagus may produce symptoms of laryngeal irritation or respiratory distress because of the highly compliant partition between the trachea and the esophagus in the pediatric age group (Fig. 15.2). Dysphagia may be a later finding in these patients, but its absence should not lead to a low level of suspicion. Thus any patient suspected of having an airway foreign body who undergoes a negative airway endoscopy should also have a complete examination of the esophagus at the same time to rule out this possibility.

Equipment

It is imperative that the endoscopist have a complete selection of appropriate endoscopes before attempting any foreign body extraction. This includes a full range of rigid and flexible laryngoscopes, bronchoscopes, and esophagoscopes in sizes appropriate for both neonates and older children. The use of flexible endoscopes for foreign body removal, however, is somewhat limited in children due to the unavailability of appro-

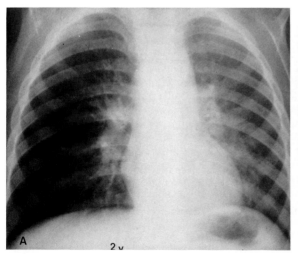 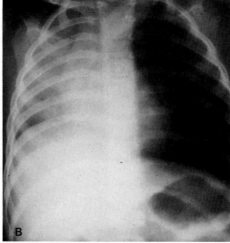

FIGURE 15.1 A. Obstructive emphysema of right lung caused by foreign body in right main bronchus. B. Obstructive emphysema of left lung with mediastinal shift.

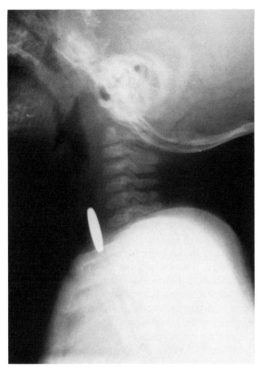

FIGURE 15.2 Coin in cervical esophagus causing respiratory symptoms by compression of posterior tracheal wall.

priate forceps. In addition, a wide selection of extraction forceps must also be available. It is beneficial to have appropriate telescopes for magnification to allow for better definition of the foreign body position and configuration.

MANAGEMENT
General Principles

Once the diagnosis of foreign body aspiration is suspected, the burden of proof of its presence or absence is on the endoscopist. A complete examination of the aerodigestive tract should be undertaken, preferably with the patient under general anesthesia. Extraction with rigid instrumentation with control of the airway is still the method of choice.

Care must be taken not to distress the patient who presents with adequate pulmonary ventilation. A favorable situation must not be converted to a nonfavorable one by shortcuts or aggressive invasive tests. Heroic manipulation, such as the Heimlich maneuver, should be reserved for those patients in immediate danger of asphyxiation.

Before any procedure is undertaken the en-doscopist and anesthesiologist should carefully evaluate all pertinent radiographs as well as the characteristics of the suspected foreign body. This will allow a plan of action to be developed in order to avoid a crisis situation. The endoscopist must then survey all equipment that will be necessary for the procedure. If possible, an exact replica of the foreign body in question should be obtained, so that appropriate extraction forceps can be selected.

Procedure

After a careful assessment and plan has been developed by the endoscopist and the anesthesiologist, the induction of general anesthesia begins. Manipulation is minimized and a slow, careful mask induction is undertaken until the patient reaches a satisfactory depth of anesthesia while still maintaining spontaneous respirations. An intravenous line is then placed, and the pharynx and larynx are topically anesthesized with 0.5% Xylocaine solution. An oximeter is utilized to monitor adequate ventilation. If the foreign body resides in the esophagus, the airway is secured before esophagoscopy is undertaken. Otherwise, endoscopic evaluation will proceed as described in the appropriate sections to follow.

Positioning is extremely important in ensuring both an adequate examination and the comfort of the endoscopist. The patient should be placed in the reverse Trendelenburg position to allow direct, straight-line eye contact between the endoscopist and the endoscope being utilized. A roll is placed under the shoulders and the head hyperextended. Care should be taken to protect the gingiva or teeth as the endoscopy proceeds. Eye protection is also provided.

Larynx

The extraction of laryngeal foreign bodies is the most difficult to achieve safely. Because this is the narrowest point of the airway, the chance for complete obstruction is greatly enhanced. The patient should be taken to a deep level of anesthesia while maintaining spontaneous respirations. At this point a small catheter may be placed through the nose into the hypopharynx so that anesthetic and O_2 insufflation can be utilized to maintain the desired level. Topical anesthesia is then applied to the larynx (0.5% aerosolized Xylocaine). The endolarynx is carefully visualized and the foreign body inspected. Forceps are utilized to carefully extract the object. The patient is immediately ventilated by mask to maintain oxygenation. Bronchoscopy is then performed to ensure that no further objects or parts of objects reside within the airway.

Tracheobronchial Tree

Foreign bodies in this location should always be removed with rigid instruments. An introducing laryngoscope is used to inspect for the presence of a foreign object in the larynx, as well as for the purpose of inserting a ventilating broncho-scope. The bronchoscope with telescopic attachment is utilized to inspect the trachea, bronchi, and all divisions. After the foreign body has been located, the endoscopist must be careful not to dislodge it so that it may move more peripherally (Fig. 15.3). Careful examination of the object and its relationship to surrounding structures should be undertaken. At this point a decision is made as to whether the object may be extracted through the bronchoscope or is too large. In this case it must be brought to the tip of the bronchoscope, and then both the bronchoscope and the foreign body are extracted as a unit. The anesthesiologist must be alerted before the actual extraction takes place so that the patient's level of anesthesia is of sufficient depth to avoid laryngospasm as removal occurs and continuous ventilation is facilitated. Once the object has been removed from the airway, a complete reinspection is undertaken to rule out the presence of a second foreign body. At this point many endoscopists will inspect the esophagus to be certain that no object is present in that location as well.

Esophagus

The extraction of esophageal foreign bodies has generated considerable discussion as to what may be the most appropriate methodology. Traditionally these objects have been removed with the use of a rigid esophagoscope under general anesthesia with complete control of the airway. This is probably the safest and most reliable method. The use of flexible instrumentation for this purpose is somewhat restricted due to limitation in the variety of extraction forceps. However, flexible instruments are quite useful in patients with meat impactions in the distal third of the esophagus or when a stricture is present.

In the past few years the use of a Foley catheter has been advocated for the extraction of coins in the upper third of the esophagus. In this technique, radiologic control is utilized and general anesthesia is not employed. The patient is placed in the Trendelenburg position and the coin is extracted into the pharynx where it is hoped that it will be expectorated by the patient. Obviously, the shortcomings of this procedure are that more than one object may be present and that the airway is not controlled. Food may also be present proximal to the coin, and this would not be radiopaque. In this case, extraction with the Foley catheter may fill the pharynx with undigested food, thus risking aspiration. Advocates maintain that this is indeed a safe technique, and in fact saves the patient from general anesthesia. Opponents maintain that the procedure is usually carried out by radiologists who are not trained endoscopists, and should a crisis occur in the radiology suite there may not be sufficient equipment or experienced personnel present to reverse a life-threatening situation.

If rigid instrumentation is used, the patient should be carefully induced by the anesthesiologist, usually using a rapid sequence induction. Once the airway is secured, the oropharynx and esophagus are inspected and the foreign body visualized. Appropriate forceps are then used to extract the object. Following extraction the esophagus is completely examined to rule out the presence of a second foreign body.

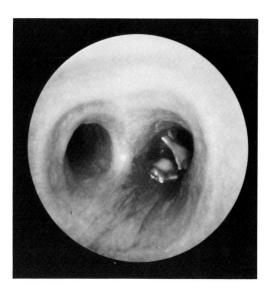

FIGURE 15.3 Peanut shell visualized in right main bronchus.

CONCLUSION

Sophistication in radiology, anesthesia, endoscopy equipment, and endoscopic techniques should make the removal of foreign bodies from the aerodigestive system safe and reliable for patients. These procedures should not be undertaken by the unskilled or occasional endoscopist. It takes only seconds for total airway occlusion to occur followed by asphyxiation. There are no shortcuts to the solution of these challenging clinical problems.

SUGGESTED READINGS

1. Holinger PH: Foreign bodies in the air and food passages. *Trans Am Acad Ophthalmol Otolaryngol* 1962;66:193.

2. Jackson C: *Bronchoscopy and Esophagoscopy,* Philadelphia, Penn: WB Saunders Co, 1950.

3. McGill, TJ: Foreign bodies in the aerodigestive tract. In: Cummings CW, ed. *Otolaryngology—Head and Neck Surgery.* St. Louis, MO: CV Mosby, 1986; chap 132.

Aerodigestive Tract Foreign Bodies

Guy J. Dutau, MD, François C. Bremont, MD, and Annie C. Sengelin, MD

INTRODUCTION

The number of cases of aspiration of foreign bodies in France has been estimated at 700 per year, which corresponds to an annual incidence of 4 per 10,000 children under the age of 4 years. In 1981, 65 children in France aged from 1 to 14 years died as a result of aspiration of a foreign body, according to the estimate of the Institut National de la Santé et de la Recherche Médicale (INSERM). In fact, these statistics are inexact because sudden infant death syndrome is included in the same category as foreign body aspiration, whereas the former usually involves inhaled vomit. In our unit, the annual number of respiratory foreign bodies (RFB) has increased since 1978–1979; since 1980 the yearly average has been 18 to 20 cases (Fig. D15.1). These figures correspond to an incidence of 1.09 per 1,000 children up to the age of 15 years admitted to our hospital in Toulouse.

DIAGNOSIS

The procedures for diagnosis of RFB are the same in Western European countries as in the United States. The easy diagnosis of foreign bodies in the larynx or trachea (10% of RFB) is distinguished from that of bronchial foreign bodies (BFB), which are sometimes more problematic and which make up 90% of our figures. In our experience, the penetration syndrome is either unknown or overlooked in 25% of cases. On average, the time elapsed since aspiration of the RFB is 17 days, and in 10% of our observations it is longer than 30 days. The possibility of RFB should therefore be borne in mind in the presence of any unexplained acute or subacute respiratory illness, in particular lung disorders that

are chronic or which recur in the same area and recurrent attacks of asthma, in spite of appropriate treatment with bronchodilators. Though roentgenograms are not specific they may be of help: in 58% of our cases, there was obstructive emphysema, whereas pulmonary atelectasis was present in only 6% of cases. In 25% of children,

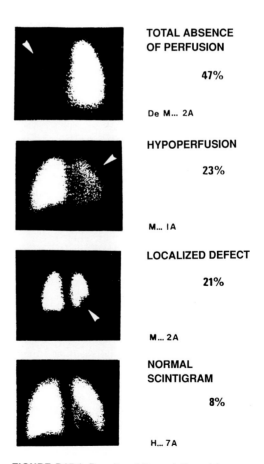

TOTAL ABSENCE OF PERFUSION

47%

De M... 2A

HYPOPERFUSION

23%

M... IA

LOCALIZED DEFECT

21%

M... 2A

NORMAL SCINTIGRAM

8%

H... 7A

FIGURE D15.1 Results of the scintigraphic examination (technetium 99 by intravenous infusion).

197

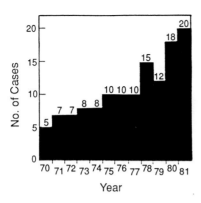

FIGURE D15.2 A graph showing foreign bodies of the tracheobronchial tree (pediatric age group, 1970–1981).

Meticulous preparation and premedication
   Valium   (0.1 mg/kg IM up to age 10 yr)
   Atropine (0.01 mg/kg)
Local anesthesia using 1% lidocaine
General anesthesia (GA)
   Atropine   (0.015 mg/kg)
   Pentobarbital sodium (5 mg/kg)
   Suxamethonium   (1 mg/kg)
   Maintenance of GA with oxygen and 0.5% halothane
Rigid tube bronchoscopy under direct laryngoscopy
Continuous ECG surveillance
Extraction of the respiratory foreign body through the
   tube, more rarely as a unit (tube plus foreign body)
Complete inspection of both bronchial systems
GA again deepened and intubation after suxamethon-
   ium (1 mg/kg)
Awakening "on the catheter," expulsion by the patient

however, the lung roentgenogram may apparently be normal.

Complementary investigations may thus be useful. In our experience, lung tomography and computed tomography are of no value (five of six scans were false negatives). However, scanning with technetium 99m is revealing: the scintigrams are abnormal in 90% of RFB, with the exclusion of laryngotracheal foreign bodies. Total absence of perfusion of a pulmonary area is observed in nearly half the cases (Fig. D15.2). In addition, the scintigram has more value in court proceedings than a roentgenogram, whose interpretation may be open to question.

TREATMENT PROCEDURES

The general principles of foreign body extraction put forward by Gerald B. Healey are in complete accordance with ours. In our opinion, general anesthesia is essential for endoscopy of a child with a suspected BFB, and a rigid endoscope must be used. The main elements of the protocol we have developed are shown in Table D15.1. Our protocol has the following advantages:

the patient can be ventilated, and if necessary O_2 insufflation can be used during the procedure;

ideal conditions for extraction are obtained, generally through the tube of the bronchoscope;

both bronchial systems can be easily and thoroughly inspected to ensure that extraction is complete;

anesthesia can be deepened before removal of the rigid tube, immediately followed by reintubation with a catheter; and

awakening "on the catheter" which is then spontaneously expelled, avoids laryngospasm after removal of the tube. Endobronchial aspiration can be carried out as necessary and

the inhalation of mucous matter or gastric fluids can be avoided in these patients, who are often nauseated.

Apart from these laryngotracheal foreign bodies, we do not consider extraction to be of extreme urgency. For long-standing RFB, adequate preparation with antibiotics and intravenous corticosteroids, ultrasonic aerosols, and physical therapy result in better conditions for extraction.

Some RFB may prove impossible to remove at the first attempt or even during a second intervention one week later after increased medical treatment. These are long-standing foreign bodies, lodged at some distance or out of reach below an established bronchial stricture, or they may be impossible to remove for technical reasons. They are removed surgically by bronchotomy or lobectomy as necessary, but such procedures were required in less than 3% of our cases.

Finally, although transpulmonary migration is extremely rare, it is a possibility with RFB of vegetable origin causing a pneumocutaneous fistula. We have observed one such case (caused by *Hordeum murinum,* or wall barley).

ETIOLOGY AND PREVENTION

Vegetable RFB (Figs. D15.3, D15.4) are by far the most frequent (79%) and half of these are peanuts. Among nonvegetable RFB (Figs. D15.5, D15.6) are a large number of small objects (often parts of toys), bones, projectiles from peashooters, pebbles, screws, and so on. Table D15.2 provides a more detailed list.

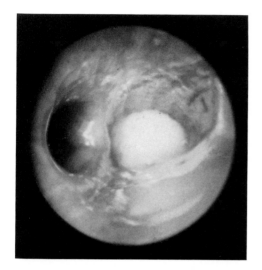

FIGURE D15.3 Peanut in the left inferior bronchus.

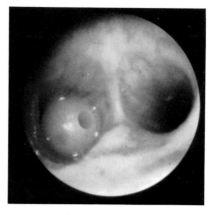

FIGURE D15.6 Pearl of necklace in the left main bronchus.

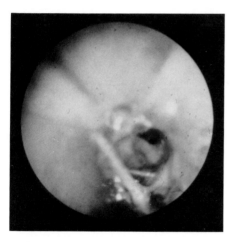

FIGURE D15.4 Buffalo grass in the right inferior bronchus.

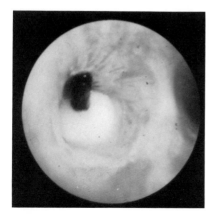

FIGURE D15.5 Toy bear's eye in the right main bronchus.

TABLE D15.2 Nature of Respiratory Foreign Bodies (RFBs)

Vegetable RFB: 81 cases (79%)	
peanuts	47
hazelnuts, almonds, pistachios	10
apple peel	3
Treets	3
chestnuts	2
sweetcorn	2
lime flowerheads	2
hordeum murinum (wall barley)	2
beans	1
watermelon seeds	1
lentils	1
olives	1
beetroot	1
unspecified	5
Nonvegetable RFB: 22 cases (21%)	
bones	3
small toys	2
plastic objects	2
screws	2
metal ball	1
toy bear's eye	1
reed of whistle	1
biro pen	1
lead shot	1
pin (of hand-grenade)	1
ring	1
Q-tip	1
sugared almond	1
eggshell	1
pebble	1
meat	1
toasted bread	1

Personal statistics, 1981.

Preventive measures are simple: observe safety guidelines for toys of children younger than 3 years; chicken and especially rabbit should not be fed to small children; chewable tablets should not be given before the age of 3 years; and above all, no peanuts or similar foods should be given before the age of 7 years. It is estimated that if peanuts were no longer given to young children, three-quarters of RFB could be avoided.

Awareness of respiratory sequelae due to RFB is recent. The insult takes place at a critical age—from one to three years—which corresponds to the phase of rapid multiplication and maturation of pulmonary structures. It is therefore not surprising that various sequelae have been described, including bronchiectasis, bronchial strictures, and hypoplasia of a pulmonary area. In 1981, we were the first to study these sequelae using the perfusion test with xenon 133, which demonstrates regional pulmonary perfusion and ventilation of perfused areas. We have observed deficiencies affecting perfusion and especially ventilation of the areas adjoining the extracted foreign body. Mean reduction in perfusion varies between 6.5% (short term) and 4.5% (long term), whereas ventilatory deficiency is more marked: 22% initially, 17% after 6 months, and 14% after 18 months to 2 years after extraction. These sequelae are explained not only by intraluminal obstruction but also by the under-lying bronchial infection, the presence or absence of a constricting endobronchial granuloma, and the duration of postoperative antibiotherapy. Statistical study of two groups of RFB defined according to the time elapsed since aspiration showed that ventilation was reduced to a significantly greater extent in long-standing aspirations (more than 15 days) as compared with more recent foreign bodies (less than 15 days). Prevention of these sequelae thus requires diagnosis as early as possible, rapid extraction before the crucial limit of 10 to 15 days, and treatment with antibiotics and, above all, corticosteroids for at least 15 days after extraction.

SUGGESTED READINGS

1. National Safety Council: *Accident Facts*. Chicago, Ill: National Safety Council, 1981;7.
2. Dutau G, Sablayrolles B, Petrus M, et al: Séquelles respiratoires à court et moyen termes des corps étrangers bronchiques. *Revue Française des Maladies Respiratoires* 1981;9:358.
3. Institut National de la Santé et de la Recherche Médicale: Causes médicales de décès, année 1981: Résultats définitifs. France. Le Vésinet: INSERM.
4. Law D, Kosloske AM: Management of tracheobronchial foreign bodies in children: A reevaluation of postural drainage and bronchoscopy. *Pediatrics* 1976;58:362–367.
5. Piquet JJ, Desaulty A. Incidence et gravité des corps étrangers bronchiques: Résultats et perspectives. *Journal Français d'ORL* 1981;30:503–508.

PART V

Diaphragmatic Defects

Chapter 16

Congenital Diaphragmatic Hernia

Jan C. Molenaar, MD, PhD, FAAP, Frans W. J. Hazebroek, MD, PhD,

Dick Tibboel, MD, PhD, and Albert P. Bos, MD

INTRODUCTION

From the days when congenital diaphragmatic hernia (CDH) was first described and treated surgically, it has been interpreted as a purely anatomical defect of the diaphragm. Nowadays there is growing awareness that CDH is primarily an anatomical and functional disorder of the fetal lungs with a high mortality (40% to 80%) despite optimal postnatal care and therapy.[1,2]

Prenatal diagnosis of CDH has drastically influenced the conventional statistics of its incidence and mortality. In 1953, Gross reported survival of 55 out of 63 patients operated for CDH.[3] These good results, however, must be attributed to the selection of his patients: the youngest patient operated upon was 22 hours old.

Adzick and coworkers recently reported a series of 38 consecutive cases of CDH diagnosed in utero: there were only 9 survivors despite optimal postnatal therapy, including extracorporeal membrane oxygenation (ECMO).[1] Their results showed that prenatal diagnosis of CDH before 25 weeks of gestation in 14 fetuses turned out to be lethal for all. Polyhydramnios proved to be associated with a poor prognosis: only 2 out of 22 patients survived. The authors recommend consideration of surgical intervention before birth and neonatal lung transplantation using ECMO as a "bridge to transplant."

Prenatal sonography has made it possible to accurately diagnose CDH and to understand the natural history of this malformation, because many of the afflicted fetuses have lethal associated nonpulmonary anomalies (hidden mortal-

ity). The incidence of CDH has been calculated as one in 4000 live births.[4] This figure, however, has also become less important as prenatal diagnosis has become more relevant for the prognosis.

EMBRYOLOGY

In the development of the diaphragm, two phases can be identified: (1) development of the septum transversum and (2) closure of the pleuroperitoneal canals. The primary body cavity, or intraembryonic coelom, is formed as early as the fourth week of gestation as an inverted U-shaped tube from which the pericardial, pleural, and peritoneal cavities subsequently develop. At the cranial border of the embryo the position of the septum transversum is changing markedly from somite C-1 to L-1 between 2 mm crown-rump length (CRL) and 28 mm CRL (ca. 8 weeks) due to active growth of the developing heart and lungs. According to O'Rahilly and Boyden,[5] the pulmonary primordium appears at the caudal end of the laryngotracheal sulcus as early as 2.0 to 3.5 mm CRL (Streeter's horizon 10; ca. 3 weeks).

The septum transversum is a mesodermal structure. The lumbar part of the future diaphragm is formed from mesodermal cells around the aorta and more laterally from mesoderm of the posterior body wall behind the suprarenal, the mesonephric ridge, and the gonad.[6] There are no arguments that point to a primary defective development of the septum transversum as the cause of diaphragmatic hernia.

The pleuroperitoneal canals close at approximately 52 days of gestation,[6] at which stage the intestines have not yet returned from the umbilical herniation. The processes involved in closure of the pleuroperitoneal canals are not yet fully understood.[7] Until recently the original theory of Broman was widely accepted,[8] in which nonclosure of the pleuroperitoneal canals was thought to result in a dorsolateral diaphragmatic defect permitting subsequent protrusion of bowel into the thoracic cavity. The resulting compression of the lung(s) was believed to give rise to pulmonary hypoplasia (mechanical theory).

The publications of Iritani,[9] on an experimental mouse model, and Bohn and coworkers,[10] on humans, point to pulmonary hypoplasia as the primary defect in congenital diaphragmatic hernia. The literature on the pathogenesis of posterolateral diaphragmatic defects has been reviewed by Kluth et al; they also described the process of closure of the pleuroperitoneal canals in the normal Sprague-Dawley rat.[7]

Recently our group, in collaboration with Kluth, studied the embryogenesis of diaphragmatic hernia following induction with 2,4-dichlorophenyl-p-nitrophenyl ether as described by Kimbrough et al[11] and by Costlow and Manson.[12] A marked difference was observed between lung growth in normal controls and that in animals with diaphragmatic hernia. At the site of the still-open pleuroperitoneal canal a part of the liver was found both in left-sided and right-sided defects. The bowel loops were found only in the physiological umbilical hernia and returned to the abdominal cavity in later stages of development. These observations support the theory that pulmonary hypoplasia is the primary event in cases of diaphragmatic hernia.

ANATOMY

Congenital diaphragmatic hernia occurs on the left side in the majority of cases (85% to 90%). In large defects it is often difficult to identify a posterior rim of muscle. However, by opening the peritoneum covering the posterior wall just superior to the kidney and adrenal gland, a posterior rim can nearly always be found which can be used for surgical repair. Usually the anterior rim of the defect is reasonably well developed and recognizable. The larger the defect the poorer the prognosis.

The contents of the chest vary; nearly any abdominal organ can be positioned in the thoracic cavity. A thoracic position of the stomach has a considerably adverse effect on the prognosis.[13] Malrotation of the intestine is always present. Both lungs are hypoplastic with a lung weight/body weight index and radial alveolar count lower than normal.[14] The luminal area is reduced due to muscularization and increased medial thickness.[15] Cardiac anomalies are frequent. The high frequency of chromosomal abnormalities necessitates karyotyping as soon as the prenatal diagnosis has been made.

SYMPTOMS

The classic symptom triad of left-sided CDH consists of cyanosis, dyspnea, and dextrocardia. The abdomen is usually flat and remains scaphoid. In right-sided CDH there is respiratory distress with the apical heartbeat in the normal or extreme left position. Most patients present with these symptoms immediately or soon after birth. A late onset of symptoms indicates a better chance of survival, with almost 100% survival when symptoms remain absent for 24 to 48 hours or longer after birth. It is very likely that pulmonary hypoplasia is absent in these cases and that the anomaly is limited to the definition of its name, congenital diaphragmatic hernia. A chest roentgenogram shows air-filled intestinal loops. Congenital cystic adenomatoid malformation of the lung often shows the same picture but usually with a normal abdominal gas pattern and a low but normal diaphragm.

TREATMENT

Continuous nasogastric tube suction and a Gastrografin enema are indicated to decompress the stomach and the bowel and to limit further compression of the hypoplastic lungs due to bowel loop distension. Endotracheal intubation is mandatory and mask ventilation should be avoided because this will fill the intestines with air.

In most centers emergency surgery is performed, and only a short time ago it was advocated that surgery be performed even in the delivery room.

The operative technique has been described in many textbooks.[16] In our hospital we never use sophisticated reconstructive surgical procedures to close large defects. A liberal use of prosthetic material—Lyodura or Goretex—is advocated for these cases.[17]

The strategy of early operation has been changing since 1986, when Cartlidge and coworkers first reported delayed surgical repair after a period of stabilization.[18] Further experiences with delayed surgical repair have been published by the group from the Hospital for Sick Children, Toronto,[19] and by our group.[20,21]

Implementation of a delayed surgical repair protocol means admittance of all patients to a pediatric surgical intensive care unit for preoperative stabilization. The stomach and bowel are decompressed by continuous suction using a nasogastric tube with a double lumen. The infants are paralyzed, sedated, and mechanically ventilated using a time-cycled, volume-controlled ventilator with frequencies of 60 to 80 breaths per minute. Ventilatory support is aimed at arterial pH values of 7.45, or even at alkalotic levels (7.50 to 7.55), at $Paco_2$ between 25 and 30 mm Hg, and at Pao_2 between 100 and 150 mm Hg. Blood pressure and arterial blood gas values are monitored using preductal and postductal indwelling catheters or with transcutaneous Po_2 monitors if indwelling catheters cannot be inserted. Metabolic acidosis is treated vigorously with sodium bicarbonate or TRIS buffer. Circulatory failure is treated with plasma, dopamine, and dobutamine.

Cardiac evaluation is carried out in all patients, using ultrasound to exclude structural cardiac anomalies, to assess myocardial contractility, and to evaluate right-to-left shunting through the ductus arteriosus or the foramen ovale. In case of right-to-left shunting due to persistent pulmonary hypertension, several drugs have been advocated to lower pulmonary vascular resistance: tolazoline, nitroglycerine, sodium nitroprusside, and prostacyclin.[22] However, these drugs are not specifically aimed at the pulmonary vasculature and have deleterious side effects, especially systemic hypotension.

Adequate oxygenation of the high-risk CDH patient, however, is entirely dependent on the degree of pulmonary hypoplasia and of persistent pulmonary hypertension.

Surgical correction follows when the patient's condition is considered optimal, the pulmonary vascular system has become stable, and there is no evidence of persistent pulmonary hypertension. Recent research by our group showed an activation of the arachidic acid cascade leading to a rise in levels of thromboxane (a compound with vasoconstrictive properties) in CDH patients in the immediate postoperative period.[23] In other words, the surgical procedure may provoke persistent pulmonary hypertension in a susceptible pulmonary vascular bed.

Ventilatory parameters have proved their use in prediction of survival in CDH patients.[24–27] Hazebroek and coworkers found that (1) satisfactory ventilatory parameters on admission will remain good during the preoperative stabilization phase and will not be affected by its duration or by subsequent surgery, forecasting survival; (2) unsatisfactory ventilatory parameters on admission may improve with preoperative stabilization, giving these patients a chance of survival; and (3) poor ventilation parameters on admission that fail to improve with preoperative stabilization will not improve with surgery or postoperatively, forecasting death.[20] Although this de-

layed surgical approach did not lead to a significant decrease of the mortality, which was as high as 50%, it does enable selection of patients.

In patients who do not improve, alternative treatment may be considered, such as ECMO, which has proved to be a viable therapeutic option for some infants who otherwise would not have survived.[28–30] Adzick and coworkers added ECMO to their delayed surgical repair protocol but could not show any improvement in survival.[1]

Further improvement in the treatment of the pathophysiology of CDH can be achieved only when its etiology and pathogenesis have become better understood. Many questions concerning pulmonary vascular abnormalities, the extent of lung hypoplasia, and its reaction pattern to artificial ventilation need to be answered. But these factors are hard to evaluate in the clinical situation. A number of researchers have used experimental animals, inducing diaphragmatic hernia in a relatively late stage of fetal development.[31–37] Only Adzick and coworkers interfered with pulmonary development early in gestation.[30] All these experiments involve rather small numbers, high costs, and the need for surgical intervention to obtain a CDH model.

In 1984, Iritani reported successful generation of neonatal CDH in mice after oral administration of 2,4-dichlorophenyl-p-nitrophenylethen (Nitrofen) for prolonged periods during gestation.[9] His report, however, does not include details about pulmonary development or morphometrical analysis of the lungs. Tenbrinck and coworkers recently reported experimental attempts to induce CDH in rats by administering a single dose of Nitrofen on the 10th day of gestation.[38] This rat model was used to evaluate lung development and the presence of lung hypoplasia by morphometrical analysis. They found that a single dose of Nitrofen given five days before the normal closure of the diaphragm in the rat leads to a high incidence of diaphragmatic hernia, mainly on the right side, however, but with pulmonary hypoplasia comparable to the human situation. The lung weight/body weight index and the radial-alveolar counts were significantly lower in animals with CDH. This animal model offers a good opportunity to study abnormal lung development early in gestation in relation to ventilatory capacity and postnatal pulmonary vascular reactivity. In these studies no statistical correlation could be found between the size of the defect and the ipsilateral lung weight, whereas a significant decrease of lung weight could be observed on both the contralateral side and the ipsilateral side.

Among researchers in this field there is growing awareness that pulmonary hypoplasia is the primary anomaly in CDH, developing early in gestation independently of the position of the developing bowel. Compression of the hypoplastic lungs by air-filled distending intrathoracic bowel loops most likely has a late, and strictly postnatal, secondary deteriorating effect.

Prenatal correction of the fetus with CDH, as advocated and initiated by Longaker et al,[39] should therefore be considered highly experimental; besides, it is probably aimed at the wrong target: the defective diaphragm. Postnatal lung transplantation or prenatal acceleration of pulmonary growth, as described by Crombleholme et al,[40] should be the targets for further experimental research.

REFERENCES

1. Adzick NS, Vacanti JP, Lillehei CW, et al: Fetal diaphragmatic hernia: Ultrasound diagnosis and clinical outcome in 38 cases. *J Pediatr Surg* 1989;24:654–658.
2. Nguyen L, Guttman FM, de Chadarevian JP, et al: The mortality of congenital diaphragmatic hernia: Is total pulmonary mass inadequate, no matter what? *Ann Surg* 1983;198:766–769.
3. Gross RE: Surgery of infancy and childhood. Philadelphia, Penn: WB Saunders, 1953;428.
4. Stauffer UG, Rickham PP: Congenital diaphragmatic hernia and eventration of the diaphragm. In: Rickham PP, Lister J, Irvings JM, eds. *Neonatal surgery.* London: Butterworths, 1978;163–178.
5. O'Rahilly R, Boyden EA: The timing and sequence of events in the development of the human respiratory system during the embryonic period proper. *Z Anat Entwickl Gesch* 1973;141:237–250.
6. Wells LJ: Development of the human diaphragm and pleural sacs. *Contr Embryol Carneg Instn* 1954;35:107–137.
7. Kluth D, Petersen C, Zimmerman HJ: The developmental anatomy of congenital diaphragmatic hernia. *Pediatr Surg Int* 1987;2:322–326.
8. Broman I: Ueber die Entwicklung des Zwerchfells beim Menschen. *Verh Anat Gesellschaft* 1902;16:9–17.
9. Iritani I: Experimental study on embryogenesis of congenital diaphragmatic hernia. *Anat Embryol* 1984;169:133–139.
10. Bohn D, Tamura M, Perrin D, et al: Ventilatory predictors of pulmonary hypoplasia in congenital diaphragmatic hernia, confirmed by morphologic assessment. *J Pediatr* 1987;11:423–431.
11. Kimbrough RD, Gaines TB, Linder RE: 2,4-Di-chlorophenyl-p-nitrophenyl ether (TOK), effects on the lung maturation of rat fetus. *Arch Environ Health* 1974;28:316–320.
12. Costlow RD, Manson JM: The heart and diaphragm: Target organs in neonatal death induced by nitrofen (2,4-dichloro-phenyl-p-nitrophenyl ether). *Toxicology* 1981;20:209–227.
13. Burge DM, Atwell JD, Freeman NV: Could the stomach site help predict outcome in babies with left sided congenital diaphragmatic hernia diagnosed antenatally? *J Pediatr Surg* 1989;24:567–569.
14. Askenazi SS, Perlman M: Pulmonary hypoplasia: Lung weight and radial alveolar count as criteria of diagnosis. *Arch Dis Child* 1979;54:614–618.
15. Geggel RL, Murphy JD, Langleben D, et al: Congenital diaphragmatic hernia: Arterial structural changes and persistent pulmonary hypertension after surgical repair. *J Pediatr* 1985;107:457–464.
16. Anderson KD: Congenital diaphragmatic hernia. In: Welch K, Randolph J, Ravitch M, et al, eds. *Pediatric Surgery.* Chicago, Ill: Year Book Medical Publishers, 1986;589–601.
17. Bax N, Collins D: The advantage of reconstruction of the dome of the diaphragm in congenital posterolateral diaphragmatic defects. *J Pediatr Surg* 1984;19:484–487.
18. Cartlidge PHT, Mann NP, Kapila L: Preoperative stabilization in congenital diaphragmatic hernia. *Arch Dis Child* 1986;61:1226–1228.
19. Langer JC, Filler RM, Bohn DJ, et al: Timing of surgery for congenital diaphragmatic hernia: Is emergency operation necessary? *J Pediatr Surg* 1988; 23:731–734.
20. Hazebroek FWJ, Tibboel D, Bos AP, et al: Congenital diaphragmatic hernia: Impact of preoperative stabilization: A prospective pilot study in 13 patients. *J Pediatr Surg* 1988;23:1139–1146.
21. Tibboel D, Bos AP, Pattenier JW, et al: Preoperative stabilization with delayed repair in congenital diaphragmatic hernia. *Z Kinderchir* 1989;44:139–143.
22. Drummond WH, Lock JE: Neonatal "pulmonary vasodilator" drugs: Current status. *Dev Pharmacol Ther* 1984;7:1–20.
23. Bos AP, Tibboel D, Hazebroek FWY, et al: Congenital diaphragmatic hernia; impact of prostanoids in the perioperative period. *Arch Dis Child* 1990;65:994–995.
24. Bartlett RH, Roloff DW, Cornell RG, et al: Extracorporeal circulation in neonatal respiratory failure: A prospective randomized study. *Pediatrics* 1985;76:479–487.
25. Bohn D, James I, Filler R, et al: The relationship between $Paco_2$ and ventilation parameters in congenital diaphragmatic hernia. *J Pediatr Surg* 1984; 19:666–671.
26. Prince R, Ballantine T: Formula for calculating mean airway pressure. *J Pediatr* 1983;102:164–165 (correspondence).
27. Raphaely RC, Downes JJ: Congenital diaphragmatic hernia: Prediction of survival. *J Pediatr Surg* 1973; 8:815–823.
28. Beck R, Anderson KD, Pearson GD, et al: Criteria for extracorporeal membrane oxygenation in a population of infants with persistent pulmonary hypertension of the newborn. *J Pediatr Surg* 1986;21:297–302.
29. Heaton J, Redmond CR, Graves ED, et al: Congenital diaphragmatic hernia: Improving survival with ECMO. *Pediatr Surg Int* 1988;3:6–10.
30. Langham MR Jr, Krummel TM, Bartlett RH, et al: Mortality with extracorporeal membrane oxygenation following repair of congenital diaphragmatic hernia in 93 infants. *J Pediatr Surg* 1987;22:1150–1154.
31. Adzick NS, Outwater KM, Harrison MR, et al: Correction of congenital diaphragmatic hernia in utero: IV. An early gestational fetal lamb model for pulmonary vascular morphometric analysis. *J Pediatr Surg* 1985;20:673–680.
32. DeLuca U, Cloutier R, Laberge JM, et al: Pulmonary

barotrauma in congenital diaphragmatic hernia: Experimental study in lambs. *J Pediatr Surg* 1987; 22:311–316.

33. Haller JA, Signer RD, Golloday ES, et al: Pulmonary and ductal hemodynamics in studies of simulated diaphragmatic hernia of fetal and new born lambs. *J Pediatr Surg* 1976;11:675–680.

34. Harrison MR, Jester JA, Ross NA: Correction of congenital diaphragmatic hernia in utero: I. Intrathoracic balloon produces fetal pulmonary hypoplasia. *Surgery* 1980;88:174–182.

35. Harrison MR, Bressack MA, Churg AM, et al: Correction of congenital diaphragmatic hernia in utero: II. Simulated correction permits fetal lung growth with survival at birth. *Surgery* 1980;88:260–268.

36. Harrison MR, Ross NA, de Lorimier AA: Correction of congenital diaphragmatic hernia in utero: III. Development of a successful surgical technique using abdominoplasty to avoid compromise of umbilical blood flow. *J Pediatr Surg* 1981;16:934–942.

37. Pringle KC, Turner JW, Schofield JC, et al: Creation and repair of diaphragmatic hernia in the fetal lamb: Lung development and morphology. *J Pediatr Surg* 1984;18:131–140.

38. Tenbrinck R, Tibboel D, Gaillard JLJ, et al: Experimentally induced congenital diaphragmatic hernia in rats. *J Pediatr Surg* 1990;25:426–429.

39. Longaker MY, Golbus MS, Filly RA, et al: Maternal outcome after open fetal surgery: A review of the first 17 human cases. *JAMA* 1991;265:737–741.

40. Crombleholme TM, Adzick NS, Hardy K, et al: Pulmonary lobar transplantation in neonatal swine: A model for treatment of congenital diaphragmatic hernia. *J Pediatr Surg* 1990;25:11–18.

Congenital Diaphragmatic Hernia

Desmond Bohn, MB, BCh, FRCP(C)

Despite all the advances in pediatric surgery, anesthesia, and intensive care in the past 30 years, little or no impact has been made on the survival rate in congenital diaphragmatic hernia. Over that period, the emphasis in treatment has gradually shifted away from the concept that diaphragmatic hernia is a neonatal surgical emergency requiring urgent surgical intervention, to the extent that some centers are now strongly advocating deferred surgical repair.

When Gross[1] described the first attempts at operative treatment of CDH in 1946 and again in 1953, the problem seemed to be of a surgical nature and have a surgical solution. At that time the cause of the hypoxia, acidosis, and hypercarbia was considered to be compression of the ipsilateral lung by abdominal contents. Logic dictated that the removal of intestine and viscera from the thoracic cavity would relieve the lung compression and the lung would then expand and oxygenation would improve. Unfortunately, despite urgent surgical intervention, the numbers of infants who died after repair of their hernias remained frustratingly high at a time when neonatal mortality in general was falling.

In the 1960s and 1970s great emphasis was placed on neonatal resuscitation and transport in the hope that these infants would arrive in better condition with fewer iatrogenic complications, resulting in greater numbers of survivors. There was, however, still no change in mortality. In the late 1970s abnormalities of the pulmonary vascular bed in association with CDH were first described, which resulted in a plethora of pulmonary vasodilators being used in an attempt to reduce shunting at both a ductal and preductal level. As the Rotterdam group have correctly observed in Chapter 16, the drugs that are used are not selective pulmonary vasodilators and have pronounced effect on the systemic circulation as well. In most instances, this results in a drop in systemic vascular resistance, which has to be corrected by use of either intravenous fluids or inotropes. Although the pulmonary vascular bed is definitely abnormal in CDH, the morphometric abnormalities are not nearly as severe as those seen in ideopathic persistent pulmonary hypertension of the newborn (PPHN). The morphometric analysis published by myself and my colleagues has shown that the major abnormality is the deficiency of alveolar number along with the accompanying pulmonary vessels, so there is in reality a pulmonary hypoplasia, not only in terms of alveoli, but also a severe reduction or hypoplasia of the pulmonary vascular bed.[2]

These false dawns in the treatment of CDH have led us to question our fundamental understanding of what is the primary anomaly in this disease. The group from Rotterdam have reexamined one of the basic assumptions in CDH, which is that pulmonary hypoplasia is caused by inhibition of lung growth due to compression by abdominal viscera. This explanation has always seemed to be somewhat oversimplistic as it fails to explain why pulmonary hypoplasia exists in the contralateral as well as the ipsilateral lung. They have reexamined the whole embryological development of the diaphragm and lung bud, based on previous published work by Iritani, who has shown that the drug nitrofen results in the development of diaphragmatic hernia and pulmonary hypoplasia in experimental animals. The Rotterdam group have extended these observations and undertaken a detailed morphometric analysis of the lungs in these animals and shown that the lungs are severely hypoplastic, confirming that this is a primary failure of lung development.

In the past few years, several new therapies have been introduced for the treatment of these severe forms of CDH. These include ECMO, high frequency oscillatory ventilation (HFOV) and intrauterine repair.[3–6] The results from the animal model produced by the Rotterdam group would suggest that intrauterine repair of CDH is highly unlikely to be successful in influencing mortality. Those who advocate intrauterine repair assume

655 Avenue of the Americas, New York, NY 10010
Current Topics in General Thoracic Surgery:
An International Series

that lung compression is a major factor in the failure of lung development, but these embryological studies suggest that this is not in fact the case and, therefore, prenatal surgery is unlikely to result in normal lung growth and development.

The other fundamental assumption that has recently been called into question is that blood gases and lung function improve after surgery. Studies from this center in fact suggest the converse is true. Following repair of CDH, both respiratory system compliance and CO_2 elimination in fact deteriorate and in some instances this precipitates the onset of acidosis and hypoxia and results in premature death. Because lung compression is not part of the gas exchange problem, there is no rationale for performing emergency surgical repair.

In an attempt to improve ventilation and blood gas exchange, ECMO and HFOV have been used more frequently over the past few years. There is no doubt that both these therapies improve oxygenation, normalize CO_2, and correct acidosis in CDH. In the case of HFOV, this improvement is usually only temporary, but it has enabled adoption of a delayed approach to surgical repair. In the case of ECMO, it still remains to be proved whether the widespread introduction of this technique will result in increased survival. If these infants are truly dying of severe pulmonary hypoplasia, it's unlikely that 7 to 10 days of ECMO therapy would allow sufficient time for lung growth and development to occur. It has certainly been some centers' experience that a significant proportion of infants with CDH failed to be weaned from bypass or died from severe bronchopulmonary dysplasia. The national ECMO registry figures show that with the more widespread use of the technique, the number of nonsurvivors treated with ECMO is actually rising. There is an obvious need for a proper randomized, controlled trial of the use of ECMO in CDH. If it indeed has a place, only severely affected infants should be placed on ECMO prior to surgery and probably have their surgical repair performed on bypass. This approach has already been successfully employed in several centers in North America.

REFERENCES

1. Gross RE: Congenital hernia of the diaphragm. Am J Dis Child 1966;71:579.
2. Bohn D, Tamura M, Perrin D, et al: Ventilatory predictors of pulmonary hypoplasia in congenital diaphragmatic hernia, confirmed by morphologic assessment. J Pediatr 1987;111:423–431.
3. Heiss K, Manning P, Oldham K, et al: Reversal of mortality for congenital diaphragmatic hernia with ECMO. Ann Surg 1989;209:225–230.
4. Tamura M, Tsuchida Y, Kawano T, et al: Piston-pump-type high frequency oscillatory ventilation for neonates with congenital diaphragmatic hernia: A new protocol. J Pediatr Surg 1988;23:478–482.
5. Bohn D, James I, Filler R, et al: The relationship between Paco2 and ventilation parameters in predicting survival in congenital diaphragmatic hernia. J Pediatr Surg 1984;19:666–671.
6. Harrison MR, Langer JC, Adzick NS, et al: Correction of congenital diaphragmatic hernia in utero: V. Initial clinical experience. J Pediatr Surg 1990;25:47–57.

Chapter 17

Phrenic Nerve Palsy

Jacob C. Langer, MD, FRCS(C)

Elevation of a hemidiaphragm in childhood was first described in 1947 by Bisgard,[1] who reported an infant with congenital eventration of the diaphragm. Plication of the diaphragm to treat phrenic nerve palsy was popularized by Bingham in the 1950's.[2] Early reports described the condition in newborns subjected to birth trauma, in association with tumors or infections of the mediastinum, or occasionally without any clear cause. In the latter group of patients bilateral involvement was relatively common,[3] and associated anomalies such as cardiac defects, tracheomalacia, neurologic abnormalities, and chromosomal anomalies[4] were often present. Other causes of paralysis such as spinal muscular atrophy[5] and Werdnig Hoffman disease[6] have also been described.

The advent of sophisticated cardiac surgical techniques in recent years has resulted in an additional group of patients with iatrogenic injury to the phrenic nerve. Although this complication is relatively rare (occurring in approximately 1% to 2% of cardiac procedures[7–9]), operative injury has become the most frequent cause of diaphragmatic paralysis.

Phrenic nerve palsy results in paralysis and elevation of the diaphragm, with attenuation of the diaphragmatic musculature. Children with this condition may be asymptomatic or may develop varying degrees of respiratory embarrassment, including recurrent pneumonia, respiratory distress, or chronic ventilator dependence. This chapter will review the spectrum of disease, the pathophysiology of the resultant respiratory failure, and the current approaches to treatment.

PATHOPHYSIOLOGY

Respiratory distress in phrenic nerve palsy is caused by ipsilateral alveolar hypoventilation and by paradoxical movement of the contralateral hemidiaphragm.[10] The problem is particularly severe in newborns and infants because of their reliance on diaphragmatic excursion for ventilation[11] and their relatively weak intercostal musculature, as well as a mobile mediastinum and compliant rib cage, which tends to accentuate the paradoxical movement of the contralateral hemidiaphragm.[12,13] The ventilatory muscles of newborns are more susceptible to fatigue than those of older infants,[14] and their small bronchi become easily obstructed by retained secretions, particularly in the supine position.[15] The effectiveness of continuous positive airway pressure (CPAP) in improving ventilation in many of these children suggests that splinting of the airways, either at a mechanical or at an alveolar level, plays an important role in the reversal of the pathophysiology.[16]

DIAGNOSIS AND PREOPERATIVE MANAGEMENT

Chest roentgenograms often show an elevated hemidiaphragm (Fig. 17.1). In an infant on positive pressure ventilation, however, the affected hemidiaphragm may be pushed down to a normal level.[17] The diagnosis may be confirmed by fluoroscopy or real-time sonography[17] during spontaneous respiration or with electrical stimulation of the phrenic nerve.[18,19] The right side is affected more frequently. Bilateral involvement, though rare, is more commonly seen in congenital cases and usually involves the anterior portion of the diaphragm.[4] Some patients present with recurring episodes of atelectasis and pneumonia. The episodes often respond to antibiotics, and no fur-

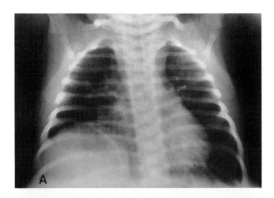

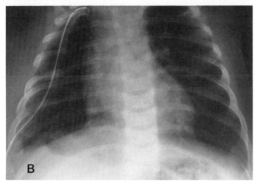

FIGURE 17.1 A. Chest roentgenogram of a 2-week-old child with phrenic nerve palsy on the right side. **B.** The same patient after operative plication of the right diaphragm.

ther treatment is necessary. Although surgical plication of the diaphragm is extremely effective in this situation, it is advised only for patients who are not adequately controlled by more conservative means.

For patients presenting with respiratory distress, initial management is supportive. Occa-sionally oxygen therapy is sufficient, though in-tubation and positive pressure ventilation are often required to maintain adequate gas ex-change. Phrenic nerve injury during an intra-thoracic procedure usually presents postopera-tively because of difficulty in weaning from the ventilator. Once a patient with irreversible phrenic nerve palsy is ventilator dependent, the most effective treatment is surgical plication.

Congestive heart failure from associated car-diac anomalies,[7] hyaline membrane disease from prematurity,[4] or pneumonia may complicate the respiratory embarrassment caused by paralysis of the diaphragm. Treatment of these conditions is necessary to optimize the patient's condition before surgical intervention is considered.

OPERATIVE PLICATION OF THE DIAPHRAGM

The indications for operative management of phrenic nerve palsy are somewhat controversial. The excellent results from plication have led some authors to recommend that this procedure be performed as soon as the diagnosis is made.[20] Because of the significant incidence of sponta-neous recovery in cases of traumatic phrenic nerve injury, others have suggested a two- to three-week period of observation on CPAP before plication.[21] It seems clear that infants who cannot be stabilized on CPAP will not benefit from pli-cation, whereas those who are stable on CPAP but cannot be weaned from the ventilator may do very well with this technique.[22–24] Infants with true congenital eventration and no history or as-sociated stigmata of birth trauma will probably not improve spontaneously and should undergo plication early.[4] Similarly, if the phrenic nerve is knowingly and irreparably damaged during re-

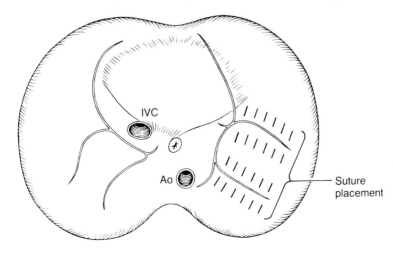

FIGURE 17.2 Operative plica-tion of the diaphragm (transab-dominal approach). Several rows of sutures are placed using a heavy, nonabsorbable material. Care is taken to avoid branches of the phrenic nerve.

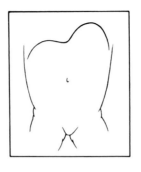

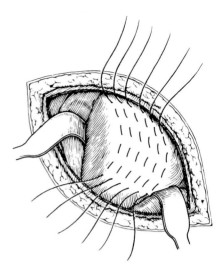

FIGURE 17.3 Operative plication of the diaphragm (transabdominal approach). All sutures are placed before tying. Sutures should incorporate enough tissue to prevent cutting through and technical failure.

section of a mediastinal tumor, early or concomitant plication is indicated.

Plication of the diaphragm increases both tidal volume and maximal breathing capacity in animal models[25] and has been empirically successful in many clinical series.[4,12,20,24,26–29] The operation can be performed through either a laparotomy or a thoracotomy. The transthoracic route is preferred in cases requiring a concomitant cardiac surgical procedure.[24] The technique is illustrated in Figures 17.2 to 17.4. Several rows of sutures are placed, taking care to avoid phrenic nerve branches. It is important to use heavy, nonabsorbable sutures and to include enough tissue to adequately flatten the involved hemidiaphragm and to prevent technical failure. In cases of bilateral eventration, both sides can

be approached through an upper transverse abdominal incision.

RESULTS OF PLICATION

In general, plication of the diaphragm is extremely effective in improving respiratory function. Patients presenting with either respiratory distress or recurrent pneumonia are usually cured, with no recurrence of symptoms. Postoperative ventilator dependence due to paralysis of the hemidiaphragm responds dramatically to plication, with almost all patients being weaned within a week of the procedure.[24] A typical example is shown in Figure 17.5. It is important to realize, however, that primary pulmonary pathology, residual cardiac failure, or abnormalities

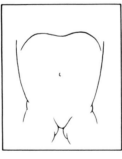

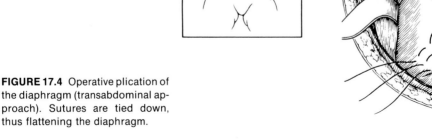

FIGURE 17.4 Operative plication of the diaphragm (transabdominal approach). Sutures are tied down, thus flattening the diaphragm.

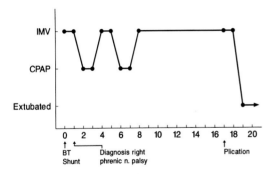

FIGURE 17.5 Typical pattern of ventilatory support in a patient with postoperative phrenic nerve palsy. *(Reproduced from Langer et al,[24] with permission.)*

of the upper airway such as tracheal stenosis or bronchomalacia may compromise the effectiveness of the operation.

Postoperative morbidity and mortality are largely related to associated or preexisting pneumonia, congestive heart failure, and congenital anomalies, as well as complications of prolonged intubation.[4,24] Recurrent eventration has been described and may be due to inadequate plication, breakdown of the suture line, or stretching of the attenuated diaphragmatic musculature by chronic respiratory distress or airway obstruction.[4,24,27]

Little information exists regarding long-term function after plication of the diaphragm. Most authors report normal function at follow-up, with the majority of patients remaining free of respiratory symptomatology.[12,20,24] More sophisticated assessment using pulmonary function or exercise tolerance testing has yet to be reported.

FUTURE DIRECTIONS

Several authors have reported successful reinnervation of the diaphragm with phrenic nerve repair done two weeks[30] to four months[31] after transection of the nerve. Although this technique holds promise, especially for cases where a transected nerve is recognized immediately, return of function takes approximately six months.[30,31] The long period of persistent paralysis limits the usefulness of this approach in most situations.

Pacing of the diaphragm using electrical stimulation of the phrenic nerve has been used extensively for patients with central apnea syndromes and quadriplegia.[32] Pacing is technically possible—and generally effective—even in infants and children.[33,34] However, pacing of the diaphragm requires an intact phrenic nerve and is therefore unsuitable for most infants with paralysis of the diaphragm.

REFERENCES

1. Bisgard JD: Congenital eventration of the diaphragm. *J Thorac Surg* 1947;16:484–491.
2. Bingham JAW: Two cases of unilateral paralysis of the diaphragm in the newborn treated surgically. *Thorax* 1954;9:248–252.
3. Aldrich TK, Herman JH, Rochester DF: Bilateral diaphragmatic paralysis in the newborn infant. *J Pediatr* 1980;97:988–991.
4. Smith CD, Sade RM, Crawford FA, et al: Diaphragmatic paralysis and eventration in infants. *J Thorac Cardiovasc Surg* 1986;91:490–497.
5. McWilliam RC, Gardner-Medwin D, Doyle D, et al: Diaphragmatic paralysis due to spinal muscular atrophy. *Arch Dis Child* 1985;60:145–149.
6. Mellins RB, Hays AP, Gold AP, et al: Respiratory distress as the initial manifestation of Werdnig Hoffman disease. *Pediatrics* 1974;53:33–40.
7. Hong-Xu Z, D'Agostino RS, Pitlick PT, et al: Phrenic nerve injury complicating closed cardiovascular surgical procedures for congenital heart disease. *Ann Thorac Surg* 1985;39:445–449.
8. Watanabe T, Trusler GA, Williams WG, et al: Phrenic nerve paralysis after pediatric cardiac surgery. *J Thorac Cardiovasc Surg* 1987;94:383–388.
9. Markland ON, Moorthy SS, Mahomed Y, et al: Postoperative phrenic nerve palsy in patients with open-heart surgery. *Ann Thorac Surg* 1985;39:68–73.
10. Mickell JJ, Oh KS, Siewers RD, et al: Clinical implications of postoperative unilateral phrenic nerve paralysis. *J Thorac Cardiovasc Surg* 1978;76:297–304.
11. Laing IA, Teele RL, Stark AR: Diaphragmatic movement in newborn infants. *J Pediatr* 1988;112:638–643.
12. Greene W, L'Heureux P, Hunt CE: Paralysis of the diaphragm. *Am J Dis Child* 1975;129:1402–1405.
13. Hagan R, Bryan AC, Bryan MH, et al: Neonatal chest wall afferents and regulation of respiration. *J Appl Physiol* 1977;42:362–367.
14. Keens TG, Bryan AC, Levison H, et al: Developmental pattern of muscle fiber types in human ventilatory muscles. *J Appl Physiol* 1978;44:909–913.
15. Clague HW, Hall DR: Effect of posture on lung volume: Airway closure and gas exchange in hemidiaphragmatic paralysis. *Thorax* 1979;34:523–526.
16. Robotham JL: A physiological approach to hemidiaphragmatic paralysis. *Crit Care Med* 1979;7:563–566.
17. Oh KS, Newman B, Bender TM, et al: Radiologic evaluation of the diaphragm. *Radiol Clin North Am* 1988;26:355–364.
18. McCauley RGK, Labib KB: Diaphragmatic paralysis evaluated by phrenic nerve stimulation during fluoroscopy or real-time ultrasound. *Radiology* 1984;153:33–36.
19. Laroche CM, Mier AK, Moxham J, et al: Diaphragm strength in patients with recent hemidiaphragm paralysis. *Thorax* 1988;43:170–174.
20. Shoemaker R, Palmer G, Brown JW, et al: Aggressive treatment of acquired phrenic nerve paralysis in infants and small children. *Ann Thorac Surg* 1981;32:251–259.
21. Lynn AM, Jenkins JG, Edmonds JF, et al: Diaphragmatic paralysis after pediatric cardiac surgery: A retrospective analysis of 34 cases. *Crit Care Med* 1983;11:280–282.

22. Haller JA, Pickard LR, Tepas JJ, et al: Management of diaphragmatic paralysis in infants with special emphasis on selection of patients for operative plication. *J Pediatr Surg* 1979;14:779–785.

23. Robotham JL, Chipps BE, Shermeta DW: Continuous positive airway pressure in hemidiaphragmatic paralysis. *Anesthesiol* 1980;52:167–170.

24. Langer JC, Filler RM, Coles J, et al: Plication of the diaphragm for infants and young children with phrenic nerve palsy. *J Pediatr Surg* 1988;23:749–751.

25. Marcos JJ, Grover FL, Trinkle JK: Paralyzed diaphragm-effect of plication on respiratory mechanics. *J Surg Res* 1974;16:523–526.

26. Schwartz MZ, Filler RM: Plication of the diaphragm for symptomatic phrenic nerve paralysis. *J Pediatr Surg* 1978;13:259–263.

27. Wayne ER, Campbell JB, Burrington JD, et al: Eventration of the diaphragm. *J Pediatr Surg* 1974;9:643–651.

28. Otte JB, Mignon T, Kartheuser A, et al: Eventrations et paralysies diaphragmatiques chez l'enfant. *Acta Chir Belg* 1982;82:559–568.

29. Jaubert de Beaujeu M, Valla JS, Berard J: Eventrations et paralysies diaphragmatiques chez l'enfant. *Ann Chir: Chir Thorac Cardio-vasc* 1981;35:241–245.

30. Merav AD, Attai LA, Condit DD: Successful repair of a transected phrenic nerve with restoration of diaphragmatic function. *Chest* 1983;84:642–644.

31. Brouillette RT, Hahn YS, Noah ZL, et al: Successful reinnervation of the diaphragm after phrenic nerve transection. *J Pediatr Surg* 1986;21:63–65.

32. Baer GA, Talonen PP: International symposium on implanted phrenic nerve stimulators for respiratory insufficiency. *Ann Clin Res* 1987;19:399–402.

33. Glenn WWL: Pacing the diaphragm in infants. *Ann Thorac Surg* 1985;40:319–320.

34. Hunt CE, Brouillette RT, Weese-Mayer DE, et al: Diaphragm pacing in infants and children. *PACE* 1988;11:2135–2141.

Phrenic Nerve Palsy

Jean Paul Binet, MD and Alain Serraf, MD

Phrenic nerve palsy, as a result of cardiac surgical procedures, has been extensively reviewed. It seems to occur after 1% to 2% of all kinds of cardiac operations. Rarely symptomatic in adults, because accessory muscles of respiration can compensate for the loss of diaphragmatic function, it may, however, be life threatening in infants and small children. Weak intercostal musculature, horizontal orientation of the rib cage, mobile mediastinum, and recumbent position aggravate the paradoxical motion of the paralyzed diaphragm. Phrenic nerve paralysis (PNP) has been attributed to insults such as nerve transection, nerve stretch, electrocautery injury, or cryoinjury from iced slush pericardial lavage. Controversy still exists as to whether long-term ventilatory support or early surgical diaphragmatic plication provides better management of these patients. This retrospective review of 109 patients evaluates factors predisposing to PNP, the magnitude of the complications of such injury, and patient management.

PATIENTS AND METHODS

From January 1, 1978, to December 31, 1988, a total of 9149 cardiac operations were performed in patients younger than 15 years at the Marie Lannelongue Hospital (3509 closed, 5640 open). Phrenic nerve palsy was suspected when weaning from ventilatory support was unsuccessful or when postoperative chest roentgenograms showed elevation of either side of the diaphragm. This was then confirmed by fluoroscopic demonstration of immobility or paradoxical motion of the affected hemidiaphragm. None of these patients had abnormal elevation of the diaphragm on preoperative chest roentgenograms.

Using these criteria, 109 patients were iden-

tified as having PNP. There were 60 males and 49 females. The mean age was 37 months (range, 1 day to 15 years) and their mean weight was 11.3 ± 8.7 kg. Basic cardiac anomalies are listed in Table D17.1.

All operative notes were reviewed, and a definite cause of injury was assigned only when specific reference to the phrenic nerve was made. All respiratory complications were recorded, and sepsis was considered as a complication only when pulmonary source was proved. Comparisons were performed by standard statistical methods, and ratios are expressed with ±70% confidence limits.

RESULTS

Phrenic nerve palsy occurred in 1.2% ($n = 43$) of closed procedures and in 1.2% ($n = 66$) of open heart operations, and its frequency was 1.2% in a total of 9149 operations performed in our institution between January 1978 and Decem-

TABLE D17.1 Basic Cardiac Pathology

Pathology	n
Tetralogy of Fallot	30
Transposition of great arteries	18
Pulmonary atresia	
Intact septum	2
Open septum	4
Atrioventricular Canal	7
Double outlet right ventricle	4
VSD	13
ASD	4
Single ventricle	3
TAPVR	5
Valve	6
Truncus Arteriosus	1
Coarctation	8
PDA	4

TABLE D17.2 Open Heart Procedures Leading to PNP

Procedure	PNP (n)	PTS (n)	%
Senning	11	179	6.1
Repair of TAPVR	5	111	4.5
Repair of Fallot	22	745	2.9
Arterial switch repair of TGA	4	309	1.3
Valves	6	420	1.4
AVC	5	431	1.1
VSD	9	1007	0.9
ASD	4	750	0.5

ber 1988. Procedures leading to PNP are listed in Tables D17.2 and D17.3.

There were 49 right PNPs after 13 right thoracotomies and 36 median sternotomies. Left PNP was diagnosed in 60 patients after 24 left thoracotomies and 34 median sternotomies. In two other patients, one underwent a bilateral thoracotomy and the other a right thoracotomy leading to left PNP. Twelve injuries to the phrenic nerve were sustained during reoperation; five of these procedures were performed through the previous thoracotomy and seven through the previous sternotomy.

TABLE D17.3 Closed Procedures Leading to PNP

Procedure	PNP (n)	PTS (n)	%
Blalock-Taussig shunt			
Right	14	320	4.4*
Left	8	374	2.1
Isolated repair of coarctation	8	397	2.0*
Banding	7	352	1.9
PDA	4	253	1.6
Mediastinal tumor	2	42	4.7

* $p < .02$.

Open-heart operations that predisposed to PNP were, in order of decreasing incidence (see Table D17.2), Senning repair of TGA (6.1%), repair of TAPVR (4.5%), and repair of tetralogy of Fallot (2.9%). In the group of closed procedures, the right Blalock-Taussig shunt had the higher incidence of PNP ($p < .02$). Furthermore, operations that needed autologous pericardial harvesting resulted in a significantly higher rate of PNP ($p < .0001$).

Four patients (3.7%), with PNP died during the same hospital stay. No death was related to the PNP or to associated complications. All were due to the basic cardiac anomaly.

Ventilatory support longer than 21 days was required in 21 patients (1 to 3 weeks in 18 patients and shorter than 1 week in 70 cases). Duration of ventilatory support was correlated with age ($r = 0.36$, $p < .0005$).

Thirty patients experienced 39 complications related to PNP (Table D17.4). All of these complications occurred in younger patients ($p = .001$) and were part of the indications for diaphragmatic plication in 11. Seventeen children underwent a diaphragmatic plication in this series (15.6%). The mean elapsed time between primary operation and plication was 37.5 ± 25 days. Subsequent extubation was possible in 15 patients 3.3 ± 2.5 days after plication. Two other patients needed a new plication because of inefficacy of the first procedure, but both of them were then successfully extubated. The mean age of patients undergoing diaphragmatic plication was 3.9 ± 3.3 months versus 42 months for the nonplicated group of patients ($p = .0004$).

TABLE D17.4 Respiratory PNP-Related Complication

Complication	n	%
Atelectasis	22	20.2
Pneumonia	7	6.4
Chylothorax	5	4.6
Pleural effusion	4	3.6
Sepsis	1	0.9

PART VI

Chest Wall Deformities

Chapter 18

Pectus Excavatum, Pectus Carinatum, and Isolated Defects of the Rib Cage

Juro Wada, MD, FACS and Wolfgang R. Ade, MD

INTRODUCTION

Under the supervision of the senior author (JW) more than 2500 operations for anterior chest wall deformities have been performed since 1957. From the cosmetic and functional standpoints, for pectus excavatum, as well as for the two predominating forms of pectus carinatum (keeled type and pouter pigeon type), operative correction is advisable before puberty, as after this period scoliosis becomes prominent in pectus excavatum and lordosis of the thoracic spine in pectus carinatum. Correction also benefits the patient's personality development and prevents long-term complications of these disorders, such as impairment of respiratory function. It can thus increase life expectancy.

In patients up to 14 years of age, the method of choice for pectus excavatum correction is sternocostal elevation (SCE) similar to the methods of Brown and Ravitch; in patients 15 years or more sternal turnover (STO)[1] is suggested. The latter was pioneered by the senior author and used clinically for the first time in July 1959 in Sapporo. In pectus carinatum, sternal turnover or a suitably modified version of sternocostal elevation may be indicated, depending on the anatomical character of the deformity.

The senior author carried out his first operation on pectus excavatum at the beginning of 1955 and first reported his findings in 1958.[2] In 35 years under his supervision nearly 2500 operations for chest wall deformities have been performed. In the period from 1957 to 1977 at a time when surgical therapy for pectus excavatum was not practiced at most hospitals and conservative treatment was still advocated by certain authors,[3] 455 operations were carried out at Sapporo Medical College, followed by 2000 operations from 1977 to 1987 at Tokyo Women's Medical College Hospital. To understand these figures, the reader should realize that Sapporo is in Hokkaido, the northernmost of the main islands of Japan, with a population of less than 6 million, compared with the Kanto area (Greater Tokyo), which has approximately 20 million people. In Tokyo, the Japanese Funnel Chest Center, founded by the senior author at Tokyo Women's Medical College, saw patients from all over Japan and from Hawaii, Italy, Peru, Taiwan, and other countries.

More than 100 reports on clinical findings and various studies in the field of chest wall deformities have been published, mainly in Japanese surgical journals. These data have been collected in a comprehensive volume, *Thorax Deformity* (*Kyokaku Henkei*), published in 1987.[1] The clinical findings in this chapter are based on the work of the senior author published in the work cited, unless another source is given. The evolution of the idea for the sternal turnover operation is depicted in a Japanese paper on the resection of aneurysms of the ascending aorta.[4] The first publication in an American journal appeared in 1961,[5] and other publications have followed. For the interested reader three articles published abroad that report on the surgical experience in Sapporo are cited.[6–8] In the United States, Haller's vast experiences with the management of pectus excavatum receives extensive interest.[29]

Current Topics in General Thoracic Surgery: An International Series

PECTUS EXCAVATUM

Pathology of Pectus Excavatum

Morphology of Pectus Excavatum

Since the historical description of pectus exca-vatum by Brauhinus in 1594,[9] various designa-tions for the condition, including chondroster-non, foveated chest, funnel breast, funnel chest, koilosternia, schusterbrust, thorax en embudo, thorax en entonnoir, and trichterbrust, have been used. In this deformity the sternum and the costal cartilages curve backward toward the spine. The deformity may involve the ribs.

The depression usually starts in the region of the symphysis manubriosternalis and is man-ifested as a funnel with sloping walls; the deepest point is usually seen cephalad to the processus xyphoideus, the free end of which frequently pro-trudes forward. In general, the deformity mani-fests itself gradually from birth, becoming more and more pronounced during the first 1 or 2 years of life. As the bony chest is still soft in infants less than 6 months to 1 year, some infants have excessive retraction of the sternum during ex-piration. This "pseudopectus excavatum," which disappears gradually by age 2 or 3, should be con-sidered in the differential diagnosis of pectus ex-cavatum.

Before school age, frequently the depression in pectus excavatum is symmetrical; after the second period of accelerated growth, that is, from 13 to 16 years, markedly assymetrical deformities are increasingly seen. At the same time scoliosis with right convexity of the lower thoracic spine and left convexity of the upper thoracic spine to-gether with a left rib hump are observed.

After puberty, in girls, right anterior chest wall depression is frequently accompanied by hy-poplasia of the right mammary gland (Fig. 18.1). From the beginning of scoliosis formation, pul-mocardial symptoms worsen, and surgery should be considered before scoliosis develops, that is, at the latest around the age of 15.

Depending on the depression, the sterno-vertebral distance shortens, the mediastinal or-gans are displaced, the pulmonary arteries be-come compressed, the heart moves markedly to the left, or in severe cases the cardiac apex even reaches the axillary line.

Patients who have funnel chest are generally tall and asthenic. They have a flat chest with a central depression. With increasing degree of se-verity, the circumference of the chest decreases, and the abdomen, in comparison with the flat chest, appears belly-shaped and protruding. In Marfan's syndrome, these findings become pro-nounced during puberty. The ribs and the costal

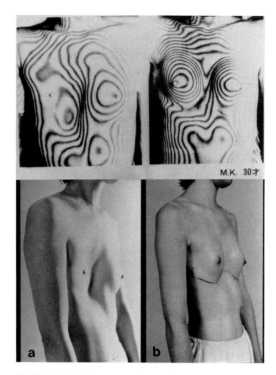

FIGURE 18.1 A. Preoperative and **B** postoperative chest configuration (sternocostal elevation and mammaplasty) in a 30-year-old woman.

cartilages that form the chest cage bend poste-riorly toward the sternum with acute anterior an-gulation. Phrenoptosis is frequently seen. This morphological arrangement is responsible for the characteristic pattern of impaired respiratory movement associated with this deformity caused by the compression of major intrathoracic organs with impediment of air exchange, thus favoring frequent respiratory tract infections during child-hood.

Pulmonary and Cardiac Symptoms

The symptoms of pectus excavatum can be di-vided into those caused by compression of the thoracic organs and those caused by the dis-torted shape of the breast.

Although frequently the objective and sub-jective symptoms are mild, as soon as pulmonary function improves after surgery, in many cases for the first time physical fitness and ability to practice sports increase and normalization of the personality features is seen. Furthermore, in pre-school children not infrequently the disposition to respiratory tract infections seen before surgery disappears. In general, in these patients the res-piratory tract symptoms are predominant. More than 50% complain of recurrent bronchitis, bronchial asthma, severe adenoids, and so on.

Younger children infrequently have cardiac symptoms. With increasing age, most exhibit some, such as dyspnea on effort, tachycardia, increased fatigability, and cardiac pain. Objective findings include systolic murmurs, pronounced changes of the heart rate on postural changes, rapid changes of blood pressure, or both. After puberty in our patients, tachycardic attacks occurred in 27% and cardiac murmurs in 15.7%. These symptoms were accompanied by dyspnea on effort in 31.4% and increased fatigability in 22.9%.

Symptoms overlooked before the operation are frequently noted in retrospect, through increased activity, a more positive attitude, and a more cheerful personality.

Wada's Marfan Index (Fig. 18.2) enables the physician to be vigilant not to miss seemingly latent cases of this syndrome. Coincidence of various congenital anomalies is not rare (Table 18.1).

Personality Features

An introverted disposition develops after entry into kindergarten when there is increasing exposure of the deformity to others. This is seen in about 20% of patients, and frequency increases with age. At the end of puberty, the number of patients with an introverted disposition in our series reached 35.7%.

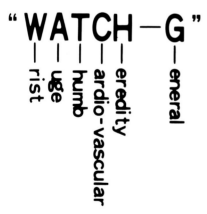

FIGURE 18.2 Wada's acronym for memorizing what to look for when Marfan's syndrome is suspected (wrist: wrist sign; *Auge* [German]: eye symptoms; thumb: thumb sign; cardiovascular: cardiovascular symptoms). In the case of cardiac pathology, funnel chest correction and intracardiac surgery can be carried out at one stage.

TABLE 18.1 Disorders Associated with Pectus Excavatum[a]

Disorder		
Scoliosis	(>15 years of age)	50%
Cardiac murmurs		30%
Marfan syndrome	20	3%
Cardiac pathology	18	
AHD	5	
CHD	3	
Malposition	4	
Arrhythmia	3	
Pericardial defect	2	
Congenital anomalies	16	2.6%
Multiple anomalies	4	
Poland syndrome	3	
Cockayne syndrome	Bone cyst	
Prune belly syndrome	Myopathy	
Short sternum	Enteropia	
Thick sternum		
Diaphragmatic relaxation	Morbus	
Severe mental	Recklinghausen	
depression	6	
Total	60	9%

[a] In certain patients there are multiple associated disorders.

Assessment and Documentation of the Deformity

Funnel index The Wada Funnel Index allows simple and fast evaluation of the deformity. Its calculation is explained in Fig. 18.3.

Moiré topography As another method for objectively estimating the extent of a chest wall deformity, moiré topography[10] has been introduced. Recently a computer-based method for scanning the moiré lines and calculating the dimension of the deformity has come into use (Figs. 18.4 and 18.5). This enables the physician to follow the development of the deformity over time and facilitates objective assessment of surgical results.

Chest roentgenogram In chest roentgenograms, the heart silhouette is displaced to the left, the aortic arch and the truncus pulmonalis cannot be distinguished, and overall a right-angled triangle with the spine as the hypotenuse is seen. The right lower lung field shows apparent increased transradiancy, with the bronchial artery silhouettes taking an oblique course. The right cardiac outline is usually identical with the right sternal edge. Also typical of this disorder is the course of the anterior parts of the ribs, which form an acute angle with the lateral and anterior facies of the sternum. In the second oblique view, cases with a diminished Holzknecht's space and

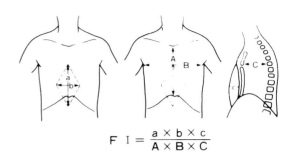

$$F \ I = \frac{a \times b \times c}{A \times B \times C}$$

a   horizontal / depression

b   transverse / depression

c   depth

___

A   length of sternum

B   horizontal / thorax

C   Louis angle to shortest distance
                        ant vertebra

FIGURE 18.3 Wada Funnel Index (FI).

aortic window are seen. These are both signs of displacement of the heart and great vessels through compression by the deformed chest wall. In the lateral view, inward arching of the sternum is seen and in the most severe cases the dorsal surface of the sternum appears almost to touch the ventral surface of the spine. The diaphragm frequently is lower than normal, and for this reason the longitudinal diameter of the chest is increased. This means that the freedom of movement of thorax excursions during respiration is restricted.

Computerized axial tomography and magnetic resonance imaging Two other pictorial modalities, computerized axial tomography

(CAT) and magnetic resonance imaging (MRI), are available. These methods have made it possible to demonstrate compression of the heart effectively (Fig. 18.6).

Cardiac angiography In cardiac angiography, cases of compression of the right atrium and the right ventricle against the left surface of the spine are also seen and a pressure difference in the inferior vena cava, which ascends at the right side of the spine, is observed in some cases. Compression phenomena are sometimes also seen in the course of the right coronary artery (Fig. 18.7), which may be displaced. Such findings may be explained as the expression of right ventricular hypertrophy but, as in pectus excavatum,

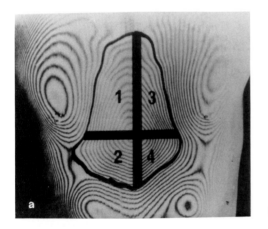

24-YEAR-OLD MALE 62kg, 179.5cm
BODY SURFACE AREA 1.73m^2

Funnel Volume			
205.0ml			
Right		Left	
124.3ml		80.7ml	
1	2	3	4
73.9ml	50.4ml	51.7ml	29.0ml

FIGURE 18.4 Calculation of the volume of the concavity based on moiré topography. The concavity can be divided into four segments, and their volumes in the inspiratory and expiratory phases can be calculated accurately. Left: Moiré topogram. Right: Calculated funnel volume.

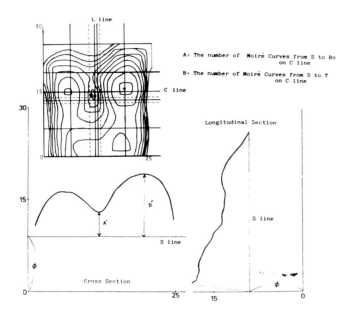

FIGURE 18.5 Computer analysis of moiré topogram (left upper graph), cross section (left lower graph), and longitudinal section (right).

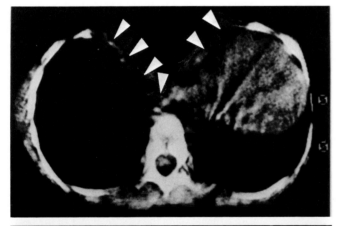

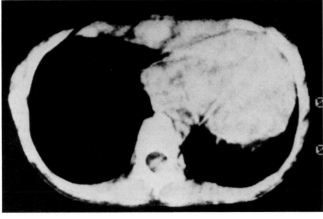

FIGURE 18.6 Computer tomograms before and after sternal turnover operation.

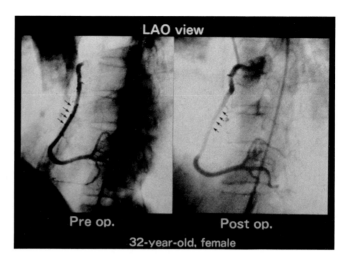

FIGURE 18.7 Preoperative coronary angiography (left anterior oblique [LAO] view) in a 32-year-old woman shows deviation of the right coronary artery due to compression by the sternum (left) that disappeared after sternal turnover operation.

compression and displacement of the heart, flat chest, and bathycardia are not infrequently observed, and it does not necessarily follow that a hypertrophy exists.

Coronary arteriography in a series of severe funnel chest patients revealed displacement of the right coronary artery in 18 of 33 consecutive cases. This finding may explain cardiac arrhythmias and palpitations seen in these patients.

Echocardiography A high incidence of cases with concomitant mitral valve prolapse and/or annuloectasia of the aortic valve is noted in severe cases of pectus excavatum.

Cardiac Function

In some asymptomatic cases a weak systolic murmur between the second and fourth intercostal spaces at the border of the sternum is the principal auscultatory finding, and during heart catheterization in some instances elevated left ventricular end-diastolic pressure can be measured.

Two main pathomechanisms explain the impairment of cardiac function: (1) impairment based on the chest wall deformity, compression, or displacement of intrathoracic organs, or all three abnormalities; (2) Secondary cor pulmonale. In the first case, in advanced age, symptoms resembling those of constrictive pericarditis may be present. It cannot be said, however, that the degree of the chest wall deformity always matches that of cardiac impairment. Further, in certain cases correction of compression of the heart fails to improve cardiac function. It is difficult, therefore, to explain all the symptoms by compression alone.

Development of secondary cor pulmonale may be explained by (1) the anterior chest wall deformity and (2) changes in the physiological curvature of the spine (kyphoscoliosis), as these changes may not allow full expansion of the lungs and thus cause compensatory emphysema. In addition, changes in the course of the pulmonary arteries may occasionally contribute to an increase in the afterload of the right ventricle leading to right ventricular hypertrophy and cor pulmonale as old age is approached. This may be the cause of limited longevity in individuals with severe deformity, as is frequently seen in Marfan's syndrome.

Electrocardiography

Distinct P inversion in lead V_1 (Fig. 18.8), which, in contrast to mitral stenosis, does not change after exercise, and negative T waves are frequently observed in otherwise healthy children and adults with chest wall deformities. These electrocardiographical (ECG) findings sometimes disappear after surgery, but may also persist.

Some patients exhibit incomplete right bundle-branch block, which is frequently associated with a deviation of the electrical axis of the heart to the right.

Pulmonary Findings

Pulmonary function In general, pulmonary function is somewhat impaired. In severe cases the vital capacity at about 50 years of age is reduced to 70% to 80% of the normal values. Further, in the fourth decade of life the maximal expiratory flow at 75% and 25% of the vital capacity may exhibit values lower than normal for healthy persons without thoracic deformity. In pectus excavatum patients, also, even if total lung capacity is normal, the residual volume is increased, but decrease in vital capacity of 25% to 30% of the normal values is rarely seen. This may be attrib-

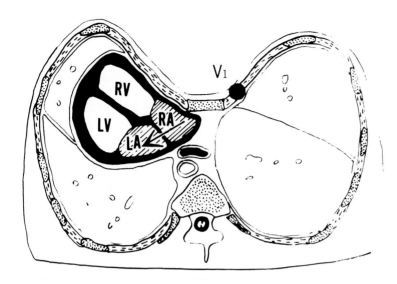

FIGURE 18.8 Cross section at the level of V_1 shows negative terminal force as seen from the arrow that represents the vector of the P wave.

uted to the wide margins of the normal values. Nevertheless, according to the experience of the authors, an increase in vital capacity amounting to roughly 30% of the preoperative values is usual. For this reason the authors believe that pectus excavatum causes a mean decrease in vital capacity of 30% when compared to that of healthy persons.

Fiberoptic bronchoscopy Bronchial narrowing (most frequently of the left main bronchus) is observed in certain patients.

Epidemiology of Pectus Excavatum

Prevalence

The senior author's mass survey of schoolchildren in northern Japan (Hokkaido) in the late 1950s, before family planning became popular, indicated an overall prevalence of pectus excavatum of about 0.2%, with a male predominance of approximately four to one. These data were collected before the liberalization of abortion in Japan and are, therefore, not distorted by the reduced birth rates that make judgments of the somatic manifestation rate of hereditary defects unreliable. For reference only, realizing the limitations of data based on hospital populations, two European studies are mentioned. Hümmer's German patients show a sex distribution of 1.86 men to 1 woman[11] and Lacquet's Dutch patients, of 3 men to 1 woman.[12] Among 1236 unselected consecutive patients operated on at the Department of Thoracic Surgery of Tokyo Women's Medical College, 77% were men and 23% were women, and among 354 patients seen at Sapporo Medical College, 80% were men and 20% women, making the ratio four to one.

Family History and Genetic Background

The hereditary element in the causes of pectus excavatum is strong. In a study comprising 581 patients, 20 revealed the deformity in siblings of the same parents or in one parent and one sibling. In about 20% of family histories, a prior example of the deformity was found. This finding corresponds fairly well with the 25% indicated by Lacquet.[12] The tendency toward dominant inheritance is strong. On the basis of various factors the degree of somatic manifestation varies, however, and multifactorial propagation is most probable.

However, careful investigators must not limit themselves to history taking and examination of the patient. They should also see the parents in order to exclude the presence of a familial chest wall deformity. In the case of children it may be necessary to take the family history in the absence of the child, as the parents may not wish to allude to their own deformity in front of the child. Nevertheless, even the most diligent investigator may not be able to establish the chest wall configuration of the grandparents.

Surgical Treatment of Pectus Excavatum

When Is Surgery Indicated?

Morphological considerations The funnel index mentioned previously (Figure 18.4) yields a measure of the degree of severity of the deformity on the basis of morphological criteria. This index has proved useful for assessing whether or not surgery is indicated. The funnel index allows a measurement of the ratio of the

TABLE 18.2 Severity Grading of Pectus
Excavatum Based on the Wada
Funnel Index

FI	Grade	Severity of Deformity	Indication for Surgery
FI < 0.2	1	Mild	No
0.3 > FI > 0.2	2	Moderate	Yes
FI ≥ 0.3	3	Severe	Yes

depth of the funnel and the dimensions of the chest. For a normal chest configuration it is zero. Physical build and age do not affect it appreciably. The author's assessment based on the grading is given in Table 18.2.

The degree of the deformity can also be evaluated by filling the funnel with a liquid and measuring its volume. Among the imaging methods mentioned, moiré topography yields the clearest results.

Proper age for operation. Bearing in mind the occurrence of pseudo pectus excavatum in small infants and the risk of development of introverted personality traits after school entry, as well as the increased occurrence of scoliotic deformation of the spine with approaching adolescence, the ideal age for surgery is during the fourth to seventh year of age. Correction at this time provides space for the intrathoracic organs and thereby allows their normal development. This prevents the frequent cardiac and pulmonary complications that occur when severe deformities are not corrected during childhood.[13] An early operation is also supported by the fact that, in adults and especially in elderly patients, the operation becomes technically more demanding. Nevertheless in adults after successful surgery improvement in outlook is also obvious.

Contraindications. Apart from considerations valid for all major surgical procedures, no special contraindications are observed. Some authors consider Marfan's syndrome, an entity in which pectus excavatum frequently occurs, a contraindication, but in the series reported here, good cosmetic and functional results have been noted in these patients.

Operative Methods

Sternal turnover procedure (STO). In the summer of 1959, a middle-aged man with an apple-sized pulsating aneurysm of the ascending aorta consulted the senior author. The aneurysm had eroded the chest wall, and thoracotomy seemed to be out of the question. At that time temporary removal of parts of the skull during

surgery and use of bone paste for filling bone defects were the techniques applied in orthopedic surgery. After careful consideration Wada excised the anterior chest wall en bloc together with the aneurysm and replaced the chest wall in situ. This operation, performed on April 13, 1959, was the first excision of an aneurysm of the ascending aorta in Japan.[4] Wada then considered turning over the sternum as a method for treating pectus excavatum. After confirmative animal studies, on July 23, 1959, a boy of 11 years had the first sternal turnover procedure.[14]

A midline or submammary skin incision is followed by osteotomy/chondrotomy of the ribs and myotomy of the intercostal muscles on both sides, but slightly medial to the edges of the deformity, starting caudal at the costal arch. For chondrotomy the costal cartilages are grasped on either side of the planed transection with towel clips, lifted upward, and transected subperichondrially. The cartilage stumps attached to the sternum are stripped from the perichondrium and resected. A transverse osteotomy is placed one intercostal space cephalad of the cranial end of the deformity, and the entire deformed portion of the sternum is removed (Fig. 18.9A). The intercostal muscles and the transverse muscles of the thorax are trimmed off as far as possible, and multiple incisions are made into the deformed part to elongate the sternum and restore its normal curvature. At the same time, the costal cartilages attached bilaterally to the sternum are cut down to a suitable length. Then the free fragment is turned over on its longitudinal axis and fixed with a metal wire to the sternal stump. Techniques for preserving the rectus muscles, as well as the internal mammary vessels, intact have also been reported, but more than 25 years of clinical experience indicate that they do not necessarily produce good results.

Sternal turnover with overlapping (STO-O). In cases in which the deformity extends into the manubrium the simple sternal turnover procedure is not sufficient to provide complete correction. In these patients the sternum is turned over and fixed in a position overlapping the superior sternal stump (Fig. 18.9B). Through this step the costal stumps of the sternum are placed about one intercostal space cephalad of their original site, thereby increasing the anteroposterior diameter of the thorax (Fig. 18.9C).

Sternal turnover with overlapping and costal elevation. In cases of pectus excavatum with marked asymmetry of the deformity, the free fragment is reshaped through multiple incisions and turned over, and the sternum is overlapped

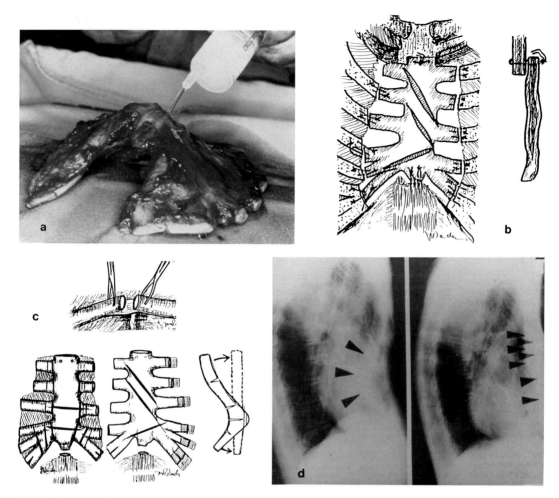

FIGURE 18.9 A. The removed bone fragment is being irrigated by antibiotic solution. **B.** Towel clips are useful in dividing cartilages or ribs subperichondrially or subperiosteally. Left: Sternum is severed from the xyphoid process. Multiple incisions are made into the sternum. Right: Muscles are trimmed off. The inner surface is also given liberal cuts until the fragment maintains flatness by itself. **C.** The fragment is trimmed into shape to fit into the defect of the anterior bony chest wall as illustrated. In many instances, placing it anterior to the manubrium yields good cosmetic results in cases in which correction would not be possible otherwise. Wire sutures are used for the sternum. Cartilages and ribs are sutured with heavy (Tevdec) material. The xyphoid is sutured to the corpus sterni. After placing fine suction tubes anterior to and posterior to the sternum, the pectoralis muscles are approximated and the skin is closed. The suction tubes are connected to a vacuum suction pump overnight. The patient is ambulatory within a few days. **D.** Left: Concavity is marked by three arrows. Right: Overlapping of the sternum is marked by the anterior four arrows.

as described. Costal elevation is performed to relieve compression of the intrathoracic organs and achieve good cosmetic results. It is not necessary for the sternum to lie accurately in the midline after the operation if a sufficient anteroposterior diameter is achieved.

Elevation of the deformed chest wall.
Sternocostal elevation (SCE) has been widely adopted in patients up to the age of 15. It is sim-ilar to the methods described by Brown[15] and Ravitch.[16] In young patients, the sternum frequently moves forward into its normal position after the costal cartilages and intercostal muscles have been detached from it. If the overgrown costal cartilages are trimmed to appropriate lengths bilaterally and their anterior ends are elevated and then reconnected with the sternum, the sternum is kept stable in the elevated position and increased anteroposterior diameter of the chest cage is achieved.

Costal elevation, also called costoplasty, is used in highly asymmetrical deformities. The deformed costal cartilages, the ribs of the deformed hemithorax that descend in the anterior-inferior direction, or both are freed from their posterior perichondrium/periosteum, the overgrowth of the cartilages is resected, and the lateral anterior ends are elevated. If necessary, partial osteotomies are performed to increase the anteroposterior diameter of the thorax. The cartilages are then reattached to the anterior surface of the sternum.

Sternal elevation was used frequently until some years ago. The deformed cartilages are subperichondrially resected, then wedge osteotomy of the sternum at the level of Louis' angle is performed. The sternum is aligned in the correct position. To keep it there, a wire is positioned to support the sternum. After stabilization has been reached some months postoperatively, the metal is removed in a second operation. For this reason, the technique is not used in current practice.

Combined procedures at one stage. Eleven open heart procedures, three pulmonary resections, nine pacemaker implantations, seven mammaplasties, five removals of thoracic subcutaneous implants that had been inserted at other hospitals for cosmetic correction of the chest contour, and 11 other minor surgical procedures have been carried out together with pectus operations (Table 18.3). In all cases the results were very gratifying.

In cases of Marfan's syndrome combined with a severe pectus excavatum deformity, surgical treatment becomes difficult and complex. In adult patients radical correction is the only way to achieve good results; therefore, STO or STO-O is the method of choice. Patients with Marfan's syndrome who require intracardiac operations for annuloaortic ectasia, valve replacement,

TABLE 18.3 Simultaneous Funnel Chest and Cardiac Surgery Procedures

Patient No.	Age/Sex		
1	5F	PC + VSD	STO + Clos
2	26M	FC + AVF	STO-O + Ligat
3	9F	FC + VSD	STO + Clos
4	20F	FC + VSD	CP + Clos
5	23F	FC + VSD	CP + Clos
6	34M	FC + AR	STO-O + AVR
7	25M	FC + MS	STO + OMC
8	17M	FC + MR	STO + MVR
9	19M	FC + MR + TR	STO + MVR
10	31F	FC + MR + TR	STO + MVR + T-TAC
11	20M	FC + AAE + AR	STO + Bentall

F: female, M: male, FC: funnel chest, PC: pigeon chest, AAE: annuloaortic ectasia, AR: aortic regurgitation, AVF: coronary arteriovenous fistula, MR: mitral regurgitation, MS: mitral stenosis, TR: tricuspidal regurgitation, VSD: ventricular septal defect, STO: sternal turnover, CP: costoplasty, AVR: aortic valve replacement, Bentall: Bentall operation, Clos: closure, MVR: mitral valve replacement, OMC: open mitral commisurotomy, T-Tac: tricuspidal annular constriction (according to the method of J. Wada).

or myocardial revascularization are the most challenging. In this situation STO is the method of choice in order to have a broad operating field for the cardiovascular repair. A wide-blade retractor, shown in Fig. 18.10, is recommended. During the cardiac procedure the bone fragment can be preserved in sterile ice slush containing cardioplegic and antibiotic solutions. Meticulous surgical repair guarantees the same good results we have experienced.

Postoperative Course and Long-Term Results

In the majority of cases the patient can be extubated immediately after awakening from anesthesia. In the presence of hypertrophy of the tonsils or adenoids, extubation is delayed. After that,

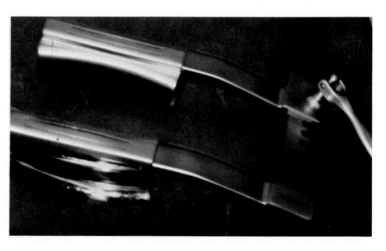

FIGURE 18.10 Sternal spreader for one-stage sternal turnover and intracardiac operations.

TABLE 18.4 Reoperations After Pectus Excavatum Correction (up to August 1986)

CP → STO-O	1
SCE → SCE	1
STO-O → Bil. mammoplasty	1
STO → SCE	2
STO → STO-O	6
Total	11

Bil.: bilateral, CP: costoplasty, SCE: sternocostal elevation, STO: sternal turnover, STO-O: sternal turnover with overlapping.

with coughing encouraged at regular intervals, sufficient expectoration of bronchial secretions is achieved. Small negative-pressure suction tubes are placed anterior and posterior to the sternum for decompression of surgically created dead space and for removal of blood. Patients walk within a few days and are usually discharged within 1 week. For about 3 months active physical exercise is to be avoided. Full activity is allowed after 6 months.

The safety of the sternal turnover procedure and its excellent long-term results have been demonstrated in a large number of patients with more than 10 years of follow-up study. The objections to this technique that have been raised, for example, extent of surgery and risk of avascular necrosis of the sternal fragment, have proved groundless, and the sternal turnover procedure has become the method of choice for the treatment of chest deformities in older patients; in young patients, whose skeleton and the costal cartilages are still soft, the authors give preference to sternocostal elevation.

In our surgical series of 2500 cases, mortality was zero. Complications and recurrences were no problem, although few cases required reoperation because of poor long-term results. These patients were again operated on, as shown in Table 18.4, with gratifying results. These cases confirmed our opinion that there need be no concern about necrosis of the sternal fragment. Bone marrow histological study of the sternum showed slight degenerative changes consistent with the technectium 99m (^{99m}Tc) scintigraphic findings.

The patients' personality features became more cheerful and extroverted. Thus it can be said that the long-term results were really gratifying.

Conclusions

Pectus excavatum is a depression of the anterior chest wall that can affect the intrathoracic organs markedly and causes ECG changes through compression and displacement of the heart. Further, in severe cases and in elderly patients, the respiratory function is severely impaired, making operative correction during the early years of life highly desirable. Early surgical treatment also has a positive effect on psychological development and prevents the complications that accompany long-standing chest wall deformities. Until the 15th year of age sternocostal elevation should be given preference; in older patients sternal turnover is advised.

PECTUS CARINATUM

Pathology of Pectus Carinatum

The term *pectus carinatum* is used synonymously with chicken breast, pigeon breast, pyramidal chest, sternal kyphosis, thorax cuneiforme, thorax en carene, and other terms. Robicsek provides an excellent description of this condition.[17]

Various classifications have been published. However, concerning the operation for the repair of lateral or asymmetrical pectus carinatum, Robicsek writes, "The operation . . . has to be tailored to the extent and location of the deformity and it may be very simple or quite extensive." Since this applies to all carinatum deformities, the authors use a broad classification of keeled-type deformities (pyramidal chest[18]*, chondroglandilar prominence, typical caudal keel chest, Ravitch's "truly keeled chest,"[19]), pouter-pigeon-type deformities (pectus arcuatum,[20] Ravitch's pouter pigeon chest,[19] chondromanubrial type), and other deformities. Fig. 18.11 shows typical lateral chest roentgenograms of a keeled-type and a pouter-pigeon-type deformity.

In the keeled-type deformities, the chief complaints of many patients are sternal prominence and pseudo-Harrison's grooves. These bilateral depressions at the level of the fifth and sixth ribs may be attributed to overgrowth of the third and fourth ribs, including their cartilages; nearly normal length of the fifth ribs; and overgrowth of the sixth and seventh ribs.

The pouter-pigeon-type deformities are described by some authors as variants of pectus excavatum since the sternum in sagittal view follows a Z-shaped form with the manubrium and the upper cartilages tilting forward.

Surgical Treatment of Pectus Carinatum

For the operation in general the same principles can be applied as for pectus excavatum. Improvement of respiratory and cardiac function, with

* Ravitch uses the term *pyramidal chest* for the variant in which the sternum is relatively straight and rises significantly anterior to the level of the manubrium.

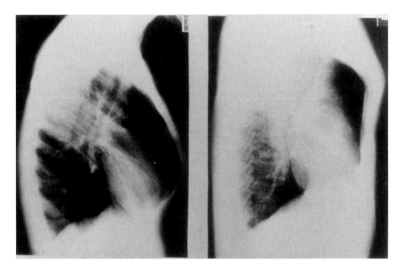

FIGURE 18.11 Pigeon chest. Left: Keeled type. Right: Pouter pigeon type.

cosmetic correction of the anterior chest wall are the goals. The senior author[1] has reported a series of 31 cases in which sternal turnover was used in 9 cases, shortening of the cartilages of ribs T-2 or T-3 to T-7 in 14 cases, and combined procedures in 7 cases (shortening of the cartilages with sternal osteotomy, 4 cases; STO with left costoplasty, 1 case; STO with bilateral costoplasty, 1 case; shortening of the cartilages with interposition of cartilage and repeat surgery, 1 case). In 1 case only mitral valve replacement for mitral regurgitation was carried out, without correction of the chest deformity.

Before the operation, the retrosternal space

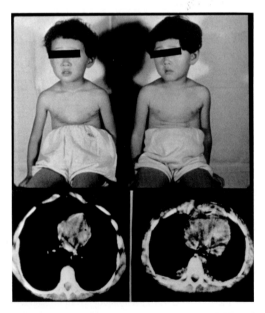

FIGURE 18.12 Pigeon chest in twins. Pre-SCE and post-SCE CAT chest scan of the girl on the left.

has to be assessed carefully by CAT or MRI to determine the extent of the operation. If this is neglected, compression of the heart after the operation may occur. In one of the cases reported by the senior author the chest cage actually had to be reopened after the operation because of impairment of diastolic dilatation of the heart.

Sternal Turnover Procedure

In general, the operation is the same as for pectus excavatum. According to the marked length differences of the ribs in carinatum disorders, it is advisable to trim the cartilages when the sternal fragment is reattached.

SCE-Type Procedure

As described for costal elevation, the deformed cartilages are resected and the sternum is replaced. Preoperative and postoperative CT findings are shown in Figure 18.12.

Combined Procedures

On the basis of the extent and anatomical nature of the deformity, combinations of various methods are used, as mentioned previously.

ISOLATED DEFORMITIES OF THE CHEST CAGE

Sternal Fissures

True ectopia cordis with the pulsating heart protruding anteriorly far beyond the chest wall has been a challenging condition for the surgeon. There is a bad prognosis in most cases because of associated multiple anomalies.[21] True ectopia cordis is rare, however, and in the three principal types of split sternum (superior sternal cleft, clefts of the entire sternum, distal sternal cleft) according to the classification of Ravitch,[22] "the heart is generally unusually prominent and only appears to be ectopic." Shao-tsu[23] published a classification of ectopia cordis and gave the following relative frequencies for the various forms of the condition:

Thoracic ectopia cordis:	58%
Thoracoabdominal ectopia cordis:	17%
Abdomial ectopia cordis:	13%
Cervical ectopia cordis:	2%
Others:	10%

The senior author has reported a foraminiform defect of the sternum at the level of the fifth rib, which was seen as an incidental finding in a pectus excavatum patient and can be interpreted as an abortive form of a distal sternal cleft.

Ravitch[22] gives detailed advice concerning the treatment of this disorder.

Poland's Syndrome

Poland's syndrome[24] is characterized by absence of the pectoralis major or its costosternal portion, hypoplasia of the breast and pectoral subcutaneous tissue, and, in the more severely affected, absence or hypoplasia of the pectoralis minor, absence of costal cartilages, and syndactyly, brachydactyly, ectromelia, or all three.[25] The senior author has reported on 12 patients (8 males, 4 females), of whom 3 had hand anomalies. In 9 patients the right thorax side was affected. In 2 patients, Wada successfully used latissimus dorsi muscle flaps to ameliorate the defect.

Other Disorders

Costochondral incurvation,[19] asymmetrical congenital deformity of the ribs,[26] complex anomalies of ribs and vertebrae (absent, deformed, fused, supernumerary ribs; fused bony paravertebral bars),[22,27] and Jeune's syndrome[28] are rare conditions that the pediatric surgeon should keep in mind. Imaginative surgical procedures have been described that, when successfully applied to these conditions, benefit the patient.

REFERENCES

1. Wada J: *Thorax Deformity* [Kyokaku Henkei], Bunkodo, Tokyo: Bunkodo, 1987.
2. Wada J, Matsufuji K: Surgical treatment of the funnel chest (Rodokyono Gekachiryo). *Nihon Iji Shimpo* 1958;1783:37–40.
3. Vidal J, Perdriolle P, Brakin B, et al: Conservative treatment for deformities of the anterior chest wall. *Rev Chir Orthop* 1977;63:595–608.
4. Wada J, Tashiro T, Nakase E, et al: Two cases of successful resection of aneurisms of the ascending aorta. *Surgery* [Shujutsu] 1960;14:75.
5. Wada J: Surgical correction of the funnel chest "sternoturnover." *West J Surg Obstet Gynecol* 1961;69:358–361.
6. Wada J, Ikeda T, Iwa T, Ikeda K: Sternoturnover, an advanced new surgical method to correct funnel chest deformity. *J Int College Surg* 1965;44:69–76.
7. Wada J, Ikeda K, Ishida T, Hasegawa T: Results of 271 funnel chest operations. *Ann Thorac Surg* 1970;10:526–532.
8. Wada J, Ikeda K: Clinical experience with 372 funnel chest operations. *Int Surg* 1972;57:707.
9. Brauhinus Schenck von Grafenberg J: De partibus vitalibus, thorace contentis. In: *Observationum Medicarum, Rararum, Novarum, Admirabilium, et Monstrosarum, Liber Secondus.* Freiburg, 1594.
10. Wada J, Todo K, Inao M: Moiré topography in funnel chest deformity. *Thorac Surg* [Kyobugeka] 1974;10:1.
11. Hümmer HP: *Die Trichterbrust—Stadien- und Formgerechte Korrektur,* Munich, Bern, Vienna: W. Zuckschwerdt Verlag, 1985.
12. Lacquet LK: Surgical correction of congenital deformities of the anterior chest wall. *Verh K Acad Geneeskd Belg* 1985;47(2):27–47.
13. Schmitt W: Zur Brustwandstabilisierung nach Trichterbrustoperationen. *Chirurg* 1962;33:440.
14. Wada J: "Sternal turnover," editorial. *Ann Thorac Surg* 1974;17:296.
15. Brown AL: Pectus excavatum (funnel chest): Anatomic basis, Surgical treatment of the incipient stage in infancy, and correction of the deformity in the fully developed stage. *J Thorac Surg* 1939;9:164–184.
16. Ravitch MM: The operative treatment of pectus excavatum. *Ann Surg* 1949;129:429–439.
17. Robicsek F: Pectus carinatum. In: Wada J, ed. *Thorax Deformity* [Kyokaku Henkei], Tokyo, Japan: Bunkodo, 1987.
18. Peters JT: Erklärung für das Zustandekommen des pyramidenförmigen Thorax. *Klin Wochschr* 1924;3:1535–1537.
19. Ravitch MM: *Deformities of the Chest Wall and Their Operative Correction.* Philadelphia, Penn: WB Saunders Co, 1977.
20. Lester CW: Pigeon breast (pectus carinatum) and other protrusion deformities of the chest of developmental origin. *Ann Surg* 1953;137:482–489.
21. Breschet G: Mémoire sur l'ectopie de l'appareil de la circulation et particulièrment sur celle du coeur. *Répertoire Gén d'Anat et de Physiol Pathologiques et de Clinique Chirurg* Paris 1826;1–59.
22. Ravitch MM: Disorders of the sternum and the thoracic wall. In: Sabiston DC Jr, Spencer FC, eds. *Gibbon's Surgery of the Chest,* 4th ed. Philadelphia, Penn: WB Saunders Co, 1983;318–360.
23. Shao-tsu L: Ectopia cordis congenita. *Thoraxchirurgie* 1957;5:197–212.
24. McDowell F: On the propagation, perpetuation, and parroting of erroneous eponyms such as Poland's syndrome. *Plast Reconstr Surg* 1977;59(4):561–563.
25. Giachero E, Casale A, Bogetti P, Garavoglia M: *Ann Chir Plast Esthet* 1984;29(2):141–144.
26. Ravitch MM: Asymmetric congenital deformity of the ribs, collapse of the right side of the chest. *Ann Surg* 1980;191:534.
27. McEwen GD, Conway JJ, Miller WT: Congenital scoliosis with a unilateral bar. *Radiology* 1968;90:711.
28. Kaufmann HJ, Kirkpatrick JA, Jr: Jeune thoracic dysplasia—a spectrum of disorders? *Birth Defects* 1974;10(9):101–116.
29. Haller JA, Jr: Evolving management of pectus excavatum based on a single institutional experience of 664 patients. *Ann Surg* 1989;209(5):578–582.

DISCUSSION

Pectus Excavatum, Pectus Carinatum, and Isolated Defects of the Rib Cage

J. Alex Haller, Jr, MD

It is both an honor and a formidable undertaking to comment on the world's largest series of operations for correction of chest wall deformities, presented by Professor Wada of Tokyo. It is a particularly intimidating assignment because I have been a longtime personal friend and student of the late Dr. Mark Ravitch, whom many consider the American father of chest wall reconstructions.[1] Not the least impressive aspect of Professor Wada's enormous accumulated experience is the fact that his chest surgery is now embodied in its own institute, the Juro Wada Commemorative Heart and Lung Institute of the Yuden Clinic & Akasaka Hospital Medical Center, Tokyo, Japan!

Basically, Professor Wada believes the indications for correction of congenital chest wall deformities are *structural abnormality,* which frequently leads to *functional and physiological derangements* in later childhood and young adulthood, and the important correction of the *cosmetic concerns* of the patient. With these indications, I wholeheartedly agree.

In patients less than 14 years of age, he prefers an operation that he calls "sternal costal elevation," which is based on the Ravitch procedure, but in teenagers and adults, he has developed a unique and, to me, radical sternal turnover operation, which removes the sternum, trims its muscles, turns it over, and then reimplants it in the anterior chest wall. For the less common pectus carinatum abnormalities he prefers this turnover operation or a suitably modified version of sternal costal elevation.

Professor Wada believes, "The deformity manifests itself gradually from the point of birth"; with this I disagree because I think that the pectus

excavatum deformities are *established in utero,* are present at birth, and then progress at varying velocities until the pubertal growth spurt, when even moderate deformities may become quite marked.[2,3] He comments on the gradual change of a symmetrical to an asymmetrical pectus excavatum in teen age but gives no explanation. I believe this asymmetry results from a shift of the heart into the left chest that, during the pubertal growth spurt, becomes more marked and lifts up on the left side of the sternum, rotating it toward the right, and thus gives the appearance of an ectopic position in the teenager. Professor Wada does not discuss the dynamic factors of the chest wall, which I believe are important. The overgrowth of the length of the costal cartilages holds the sternum in its posterior fetal position and does not allow it to move forward as the chest organs grow. This is best illustrated by asking the child to inhale and noting that the lungs expand laterally and the sternum hardly moves forward at all. This abnormal dynamic feature of chest wall function is thus a reflection of the overgrowth of the costal cartilages and accounts both for the continuing increase in severity and for the functional abnormality. I agree strongly with Dr Wada's feeling that both pulmonary and cardiac dysfunction result from this marked depression of the sternum. I suspect that most of the pulmonary functional abnormality is due to this complex restrictive force on the chest wall and that the cardiac dysfunction is due to displacement and anterior compression of the heart.[4,5]

Professor Wada has developed the simple and useful Wada Funnel Index, which is quite helpful in defining the severity of the deformity. Others have used different approaches, including the moiré measurements and the pectus index of Welch and others in Boston. I have preferred an even simpler index, which is determined from the CAT scan. This pectus index is derived from mea-

Current Topics in General Thoracic Surgery:
An International Series

suring the anteroposterior (AP) diameter of the sunken chest to the vetebral body, divided into the transverse diameter of the chest.[6] If this figure is greater than $2\frac{1}{2}$, then the pectus deformity is significant and will probably require operative intervention. If the index is greater than 4–5, even at 5 or 6 years of age, this clearly predicts a progressive lesion that will require ultimate operative correction.

Professor Wada's discussion of the pathophysiology of cardiac and pulmonary dysfunction is excellent and is both logical and understandable. His implication in the discussion of the epidemiology of pectus excavatum that it is genetically determined and sex-linked (it occurs in boys in a ratio somewhere between 4:1 and 3:1) is interesting, but, except in Marfan's syndrome,[7] no genetic defect has yet been documented. Professor Wada concludes, "A multifactorial propagation is most probable," which is to say that we remain ignorant of a specific genetic defect. Wada has chosen the ideal age for repair, between 4 and 7 years of age, and I would agree with this if the evaluating surgeon can be certain of the severity and the progression of the defect. Earlier operative correction makes no sense in terms of stress to the child; the results are excellent anytime up to the pubertal growth spurt.

I certainly agree with Professor Wada that Marfan's syndrome,[7] the connective tissue abnormality, is not a contraindication to correction, but I believe strongly that such patients need to have substernal stainless steel bar support in addition to the basic Ravitch operation because recurrence can be expected in 20% to 30% of such patients if they do not have the additional bar support. I cannot comment on the incidence of recurrence after the Wada turnover operation since it has not been used by me nor have such series been reported in the world literature except that from Tokyo.

The sternal turnover operation certainly deserves comment because it was originated by Professor Wada and has not gained worldwide acceptance. The major concern has been the devascularization of such a large, free bone graft, but, remarkably enough, in Professor Wada's hands, ischemic necrosis and infection have not been frequent complications. Most of us have not been brave (or foolish?) enough to adopt his proposal since we have had excellent results with less radical procedures. As he points out, there is a real appeal to this procedure if it is to be combined with open heart surgery for Marfan's syndrome, for example; but even then the threat of massive bleeding and infection, while using cardiopulmonary bypass, has deterred most North American surgeons from adapting this combined approach. Indeed, I have recom-

mended a staged management of Marfan's patients with heart disease and pectus excavatum. We carry out the pectus excavatum repair a few months to a few years before the open heart surgery. This more conservative (timid?) approach has yielded good results in a small number of such complicated patients, and there have been no complications. We now have had experience in managing 12 Marfan's syndrome patients in this staged fashion, and Professor Wada mentions 11 open heart procedures that he has performed, using the Wada turnover operation combined with the intracardiac repair. The bottom line is the remarkable figure that in his 2500 cases there has been no mortality and complications have been minimal.

Remarkably enough, the same radical turnover procedure is proposed for pectus carinatum, which has no demonstrable associated physiological problems and can be very nicely corrected with a modified Ravitch procedure. The cosmetic results are excellent, and we prefer a more conservative approach. He mentions Poland's syndrome and his experience with 12 cases, but these are not referred to in the references.[8] We have had a similar experience, but I am not certain how this compares with the operative correction in Wada's hands.

I would like to add my admiring salute to a master thoracic surgeon who has had remarkable experience and who has generously shared that experience with many colleagues over the years. His institute is a fitting living memorial to him and to his colleagues.

REFERENCES

1. Haller JA: Operative management of chest wall deformities in children: Unique contributions of southern thoracic surgeons. *Ann Thorac Surg* 1988;46:4.
2. Haller JA, Scherer LR, Turner CS, Colombani PM: Evolving management of pectus excavatum based on a single institutional experience of 664 patients. *Ann Surg* 1989;209:578.
3. Haller JA, Peters GN, Mazur D, White JJ: Pectus excavatum—a twenty year experience. *J Thorac Cardiovasc Surg* 1970;60:375.
4. Haller JA, Turner CS: Diagnosis and operative management of chest wall deformities in children. *Surg Clin North Am* 1981;61:1199.
5. Haller JA, et al: Operative correction of pectus excavatum. *Ann Surg* 1976;184:554.
6. Haller JA, Kramer SS, Lietman S: Use of CT scans in selection of patients for pectus excavatum surgery: A preliminary report. *J Pediatr Surg* 1987;22:904.
7. Scherer LR, Arn PH, Dressel DA, et al: Surgical management of children and young adults with Marfan syndrome and pectus excavatum. *J Pediatr Surg* 1988;23:1169.
8. Haller JA, Colombani PM, Miller D, Manson P: Early reconstruction of Poland's syndrome using autologous rib grafts combined with a latissimus muscle flap. *J Pediatr Surg* 1984;19:423.

PART VII

Thoracic Tumors

Chapter 19

Primary Chest Wall Tumors in Infancy and Childhood

Georges Lemoine, MD and Michel Deneuville, MD

Primary chest wall tumors (PCWTs) are uncommon in childhood and infancy and most are likely to be malignant. Malignant chest wall neoplasms represent 1.8% of all pediatric malignant tumors.[1] They consist of a variety of extrapleural neoplasms originating from skeletal chest wall or surrounding soft tissues. Primary tumors of the bony chest wall have been reported to comprise 5% of all intrinsic bone tumors.[2] PCWTs are defined as neoplasms located in the region bordered at the highest level by the clavicles, inferiorly by the rib margin, and medially by the medial border of the scapula.[3] This definition excludes tumors arising in the scapula as well as spinal or paraspinal neoplasms. Mediastinal or pulmonary tumors involving the chest wall or skeletal metastases to the rib are also excluded.

A large majority of PCWTs have traditionally been called Ewing's sarcoma, which was first described in 1921 by Ewing as a "diffuse endothelioma of the bone."[4] In 1979 Askin[5] described a distinct clinicopathological entity characterized as a "malignant small cell tumor of the thoracopulmonary region in children."

Surgical resection plays a role both in diagnosis and in therapeutic management. For benign neoplasms, a resectional biopsy provides a radical resection; for malignant tumors identification of histological type is mandatory for the choice of adequate chemotherapy. For the last decade, a combination of preoperative chemotherapy, wide radical chest wall resection of a residual tumor, and aggressive chemotherapy, irradiation, or both has been the key to successful management and reasonable likelihood of cure.

PATHOLOGY
Benign Primary Chest Wall Tumors

Benign PCWTs are exceedingly rare. Most involve only one rib and remain small. Various histological types are encountered, including osteochondroma, osteoblastoma, and tumor-related disorders such as aneurysmal bone cyst, eosinophilic granuloma, and fibrous dysplasia.[6,7]

Resectional biopsy ensures diagnosis and provides curative resection; the prognosis is invariably excellent after excision, except for osteochondroma, which tends to recur. On occasion, benign PCWT, mostly hourglass lipoma or mesenchymal hamartoma, may enlarge enough to compress vital intrathoracic structures.[8–10] Vascular dysplasia involving the chest wall is often massive, leading to the problems common to all dysplasias wherever located. Surgical resection is seldom indicated. Complications can be successfully managed by transcatheter embolization.[11]

Malignant Primary Chest Wall Tumors

Most of the PCWTs encountered in childhood and infancy are malignant. The vast majority of these lesions have traditionally been called either Askin's tumors, Ewing's sarcomas, or neuroectodermal tumors. However, they have recently been considered as a single entity known as "malignant round small cell tumors."[12,13] Other soft tissue sarcomas involving the chest wall (osteosarcoma, synovial cell sarcoma, and so on) are rare.[2,5,13,14] Preoperative chemotherapy has been found beneficial in these massive neoplasms as it provides effective tumor reduction and facilitates complete resection of the gross residual tumor.

TUMOR ASSESSMENT

The majority of PCWTs lack clinical features indicating that a tumor is benign or malignant. Pain or the asymptomatic presence of a chest wall mass is the most common complaint of patients. Computerized axial tomography (CAT) scan and magnetic resonance imaging (MRI) have clarified dramatically the extent of the tumor in the chest wall and the invasion of intrathoracic structures. MRI requires no contrast medium and gives no radiation exposure. Its ability to display the lesion in coronal and sagittal planes is helpful in precisely defining encroachment on versus violation of essential neurovascular and bony structures.

Histological confirmation requires needle biopsy or excisional biopsy. The latter is carried out, in our experience, after failure of needle biopsy. Large tumor samples are readily obtained without pleural violation. Frozen section examinations are helpful to ensure that samples are adequate to provide definite diagnosis.

SURGICAL PROCEDURES

The technical rules of chest wall resection remain the same whatever the nature of the neoplasm.

The majority of PCWTs are approached through a posterolateral thoracotomy, as most neoplasms commonly involve the posterior or middle arch of the ribs. In anterior lesions, an anterolateral approach can be used and facilitates sternal resection, if required.

Operative Resection

The level of thoracic incision is guided by the location of the neoplasm. Posterolateral thoracotomy is advisable for a majority of lesions. It allows a large exposition of the entire rib cage and complete rib resection from costosternal to spinal articulation with easy ligation of intercostal vessels.

Latissimus dorsi muscle must be transected as low as possible to preserve a potential muscular flap. All other muscles must be spared unless they are involved by the neoplasm. In such cases, en bloc resection of full-thickness chest wall must be performed.

The pleural space is penetrated one space below or deep to the known rib involvement so that full assessment of the intrathoracic extent and resectability can be made from inside the pleural cavity.

Massive neoplasms usually require a second thoracotomy approach through the same skin incision to delimit the bulky skeletal tumor clearly. It permits complete assessment of fixation to intrathoracic structures and facilitates en bloc resection.

Anterior transection of the chondrosternal joint is first performed with ligation of the intercostal vascular bundle. Complete transection of intercostal muscles using electrocautery is then carried out to the spine. En bloc resection is achieved posteriorly with disarticulation of the involved rib from the transverse process of the vertebra. The intercostal arteries must be carefully ligated.

All attached intrathoracic structures (lung or diaphragm) must be resected "en bloc" with the neoplasm. Combined lung resection proceeding with wedge resection or regular lobectomy must provide a tumor-free margin.

Frozen section examinations are mandatory to ensure that all resection margins are free of tumor.

Reconstruction of the Chest Wall

A small skeletal defect like that after a single rib resection does not need to be repaired unless for cosmetic reasons.

A posterior defect under the scapula does not require prosthetic reconstruction because the scapula covers the bony defect if no more than two ribs are removed. The trapezium and rhomboid muscles provide adequate tissue to fill the defect so that no physical abnormality is detectable and no flail chest results.

Surgical defects of the lower or the anterior chest wall or occurring after full-thickness resection require reconstruction using muscle flaps, prosthesis, or both.

In children, primary chest wall tumors require in most cases removal of one to three ribs. In young patients, the defect must be closed to prevent lung herniation and flail chest in all locations not under the scapula.

Many methods and materials have been reported in reconstruction of the rib cage.[15] The most commonly used are synthetic meshes (Marlex mesh and the Goretex patch). Both are well tolerated, and fibrous ingrowth of tissue is excellent.[13,15,16]

However, for a few years, we have favored a resorbable mesh of polyglactin 910 (Vicryl) to repair chest wall defects in children. This surgical mesh has demonstrated several desirable characteristics. It provides elasticity in both directions and is less likely to fracture when flexed than the more rigid mesh. The placement of the mesh under appreciable tension is easy and provides adequate structural stability. When used in four layers cut to fit the side and shape of the defect (Fig. 19.1) and securely sutured to

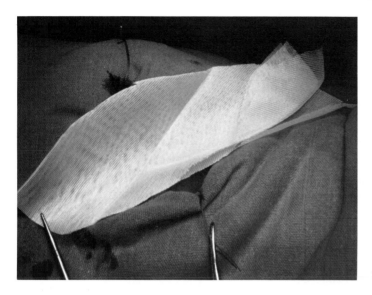

FIGURE 19.1 Resorbable polyglactin 910 (Vicryl) mesh used in layers.

the surrounding rigid wall, the meshes seal the pleural cavity efficiently.

The main advantage is probably its slow resorption within 40 to 60 days as it is replaced by a rigid fibrous ingrowth of tissue without residual foreign material.

MUSCLE FLAP

In our experience, the indications for using a muscle flap are (1) to supply soft tissue to fill a small defect and provide airtight parietal reconstruction or (2) to provide coverage of a prosthesis when full-thickness resection has been performed. Omental transposition[17] must be reserved as a backup procedure, for use if muscle transposition fails.

CHEST AND PARIETAL DRAINAGE

Pleural cavity drainage is performed in the usual way, using two large-diameter chest tubes connected to an underwater suction system. The average duration of drainage is 36 hours until lung expansion is complete and fluid drainage stops.

The space between the chest wall prosthesis and the muscle is drained for 3 or 4 days with a device called a Redon catheter (Uniredon Fandre Laboratory, Ludres, France). One or two catheters are used (Fig. 19.2). Each catheter is connected to a small glass bottle in which a strong (700 mm Hg) negative pressure is created.[18] The drainage must be cultured daily.

Prophylactic antibiotics are administered

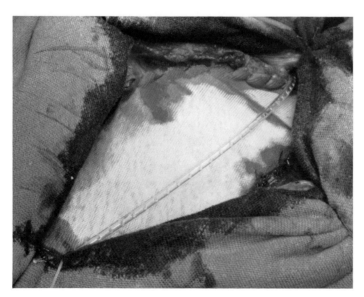

FIGURE 19.2 Drainage between chest wall prosthesis and muscle with Redon catheter.

systematically in all cases, during and after operation.

SPECIAL LOCATIONS

Primary chest wall tumors involving the superior sulcus may invade the neurovascular bundle of the thoracic outlet. Resection of the first rib is the key to approach these structures. An ultrasonic surgical aspirator (Surgitron) facilitates the dissection and reduces postoperative pain and neurological damage related to lesions of the brachial plexus.

Lower rib tumors are usually associated with diaphragmatic involvement. In most cases, the diaphragm can be easily reattached, either to the costal margin (up to the fourth rib), to the chest wall prosthesis, or to the large thoracoabdominal muscles. After more extended diaphragmatic resections, a prosthetic reconstruction using an airtight material (polytetrafluoroethylene [PTFE], Marlex mesh or Goretex) is mandatory.

Extension to the spine may require resection of the transverse process or lateral resection of the vertebral body. Limited extension into the foramen can be adequately removed by using the Surgitron.

Primary involvement of the sternum or extension of a rib neoplasm originating at the anterior arch is rare.[13] We did not encounter any in our experience. However, as in adults, complete sternal resections require a rigid reconstruction using a sandwich of mesh (Marlex) and methyl methacrylate.[15]

A defect after limited resection can be filled with mesh (Marlex) or a patch (Goretex).

POSTOPERATIVE COMPLICATIONS

Early postoperative complications are rare. In our experience all patients were immediately extubated.

Nonspecific complications include prolonged air leaks, intrathoracic bleeding, and incomplete lung expansion with postresectional residual space. They are routinely prevented by adequate hemostasis, airtight sutures, and correct chest tube drainage.

Parietal infections are rare. Preventive measures are aseptic operative techniques, adequate chest wall drainage, and prophylactic antibiotherapy. Prosthetic infection did not occur in our experience. It is reported to be more common after aggressive chemotherapy or irradiation.[19]

LATE COMPLICATIONS

Besides local recurrence or metastatic spread of the disease, local complications include respiratory insufficiency, scoliosis, and chest wall deformities.

The development of respiratory insufficiency has many causes, combining the effects of lung irradiation and chest wall resection. Since childhood is a period of rapid lung growth, the effects of therapeutic irradiation include the loss of a number of preexisting alveoli and a limitation of development of new alveoli. Skeletal and muscular growth are both reduced by resection and irradiation.[20,21]

In older children functional lung testing shows significant reduction in lung volumes. The magnitude of this reduction is further increased when reconstruction has been achieved by means of a rigid prosthesis.

Among five patients alive without evidence of disease at least 4 years after operation, four had been irradiated, before or after surgery. All demonstrate functional testing disorders, and in four, there was a significant reduction in lung volume. Two patients experienced mild functional impairment.

Scoliosis

Both surgical and irradiation factors play a role in the occurrence of scoliosis.

Unilateral growth of the chest wall is secondary to skeletal and muscular resection, including removal of intercostal neurovascular bundles. Lower spine irradiation[2,16,20,21] probably alters subsequent linear growth.

In our experience 2 patients of 24 developed scoliosis with severe disability but not requiring orthopedic management.

Chest Wall Deformities

Cosmetic deformities are related to the extent of the chest wall resection, with special concerns after full-thickness resection and related prosthetic fibrosis.

In our experience it was not a major problem in any patient. Plastic surgery of the breast was indicated only in one female teenager, who complained of a breast hypoplasia secondary to irradiation.

Material and Patients

Between 1970 and 1988, 24 children (16 boys and 8 girls) were referred to us for surgical management of a primary chest wall tumor. Ages ranged from 1.5 to 16 years (average 11 years) at the time of surgery.

Two neoplasms were benign (one lipoma and one angioma) and 22 were malignant. They included 12 Ewing's sarcomas, 4 Askin's tumors, 3 neuroblastomas, and one each of osteosarcoma, chondrosarcoma, and malignant mesenchynoma.

Among 22 patients referred for malignant tumors, 20 had received preoperative therapy; there was significant reduction of the bulky tumor in 19.

Surgical approach was a posterolateral thoracotomy in 20, an anterolateral thoracotomy in 2, and bilateral synchronous thoracotomies in 2.

Twelve patients had a single rib removed; the other had two or three ribs resected.

Combined resections were as follows: full-thickness (rib and muscle) in three patients, diaphragm in three, and lung in five, including four wedge resections and one regular lobectomy. Synchronous metastases were removed from the opposite lung of two patients.

Reconstruction of the chest wall carried out in 14 patients included three muscle flaps and 11 prostheses. Mesh (Marlex) was used in one patient, who had an anterior resection of three ribs. In all others the reconstruction was performed with a polyglactin 910 mesh.

Among 20 malignant neoplasms that had had preoperative therapy, 5 showed complete tumor sterilization in the operative specimen.

Resection was considered complete in 22 patients. Of 2 patients having residual tumor in the resection margins, surgery was repeated in 1 to ensure radical resection.

Among 22 patients who had surgery for malignant neoplasms, 7 died of progression of the disease between the 3rd and the 29th months after surgery and 2 of complications of postoperative therapy without evidence of disease.

One patient suddenly died, without evidence of disease 2 years later.

Among 12 patients who survived, 1 was lost to follow-up study at 2 and a half years without evidence of disease, and in another patient an extrathoracic recurrence occurred; it was successfully treated with chemotherapy.

The remaining 10 patients are all alive and have no evidence of disease from 12 months up to 10 years after operation (Table 19.1).

COMMENTS

Primary chest wall neoplasms are rare in childhood. The majority of these lesions are malignant and have traditionally been classified either as Ewing's sarcoma (with primary rib involvement) or as Askin's tumor with neuroectodermal differentiation.

However, Ewing's sarcoma may have neuroectodermal differentiation without primary rib involvement[12,19] and Askin's tumor may primarily involve the rib.[4,12,19] Ewing's sarcoma is associated with a high rate of metastases and Askin's tumors are reported to occur more often in female teenagers[4] and to recur locally. Distinguishing between them can be difficult and, as in recent publications, we tend to classify these two entities as "malignant small round cell tumors." The management is similar: it includes aggressive local therapy and adjuvant chemotherapy to prevent distal metastases.

Other histological types of soft tissue sarcoma involving the chest wall are exceedingly rare.

All malignant chest wall neoplasms require aggressive combined therapy, the aim of which is to achieve (1) local control of the tumor by means of chemotherapy, irradiation, or both, and complete surgical resection with immediate reconstruction, and (2) prevention of local recurrence and metastases.

For malignant small round cell tumors (MSRTs) we provide local control by preoperative chemotherapy and complete removal of the residual tumor. The initial bulky mass is usually greatly reduced after chemotherapy (Fig. 19.3A and B). This reduction facilitates a radical resection and adequate assessment of the resection margin, which must be tumor-free, as indicated microscopically.

Up to 1984, the drug association vincristin actinomycin D cyclophosphamid and vincristine adriamycin (VAC-Vad)[22] (see Table 9.1) had been commonly used, combined with resection, postoperative radiotherapy (30–50 Gy), and chemotherapy.

Between 1984 and 1987, ifosfamide was favored instead of cyclophosphamide.[23] Since 1987, most teams have followed the chemotherapy protocol developed by Hayes et al[24] for management of local and metastatic tumors.

During initial chemotherapy, five identical courses of cyclophosphamide and doxorubicin hydrochloride (Adriamycin) are given, maintaining white blood cell (WBC) counts above $2–10^3/mm^3$, and neutrophil counts above $500/mm^3$. All patients demonstrating a significant decrease of neoplasm are candidates for surgical resection.

Postresectional therapy includes maintenance chemotherapy (vincristine and actinomycin followed by cyclophosphamide and Adriamycin) and local irradiation. The dose is 30 Gy if resection has been microscopically complete; otherwise, irradiation is increased to 50 Gy.

TABLE 19.1 Clinical Findings and Treatment in 22 Patients (Malignant Tumors)

Case	Age Sex	Diagnosis	Preoperative Treatment RT	Preoperative Treatment Chemo	Operation	Postoperative Treatment RT	Postoperative Treatment Chemo	Results	Duration of Survival
1	13,5/M	ES	50 Gy	VAC-Vad	Resection R.R. 3		VAC-Vad	Died Pulmonary Mets	2 yr
2	13/M	ES	50 Gy		Resection R.R. 12		VAC	Alive. NED	10,5 yr
3	4,6/M	Askin's tumor		VAC-Vad	Resection L.R. 4.5.6 and Wedge		VAC-Vad	Died. METS	2,5 yr
4	12,5/M	ES		VAC-Vad	Resection R.R.9 en Bloc Chest Wall and Diaphragm	45 Gy	VAC-Vad	Died. METS	2,7 yr
5	14/M	ES		VAC-Vad	Resection R.R. 12	20 Gy	VAC	Left Inferior Lobectomy for METS Alive. NED	10 yr
6	11/M	Chondrosarcoma			Resection L.R. 9.10	40 Gy	V Metho	Died. METS	6 mo
7	14/M	Mesenchymal Sarcoma		VAC-Vad	Resection L.R. 1.2.3	45 Gy		Alive. NED	Lost to Follow-up Study at 2,5 yr
8	7,5/M	N.B		VAC-Vad	Resection R.R. 10 and Diaphragm	45 Gy	VAC-Vad	Alive. NED	7 yr
9	8/M	ES		VAC-Vad	Resection R.R. 1.2	40 Gy	VAC-Vad	Died. Recurrent Disease	6 mo
10	7/M	ES		VAC	Resection L.R. 2		IVA	Right Pulmonary Wedge for METS Alive. NED	6 yr

					Gy			
11	15/F	ES	VAC-Vad	Resection L.R. 5.6 and Diaphragm	40 Gy	VAC-Vad	Died. METS	10 mo
12	12/F	ES	VAC-Vad	Resection L.R. 2 and Wedge		IVad	Died. Recurrent Disease	3 mo
13	14/M	ES	IVA-IVad	Resection R.R. 8	45 Gy	Vad	Alive. NED Pleural Abrasion	4 yr
14	5/M	N.B	VAC-Vad	Resection L.R. 4.5 en Bloc Chest Wall and Left Upper Lobectomy	30 Gy		Died. Recurrent Disease	5 mo
15	11/F	ES	IVA-IVad	Resection R.R.6 and Wedge	45 Gy	IVA	Died	2,3 yr
16	12/F	Askin's Tumor	IVA-IVad	Resection R.R. 4.5.6. and Wedge		BCNU	Alive on CHEMO with Disease	2 yr
17	2/M	Askin's Tumor	IVA-IVad	Resection R.R. 10.11.12. en Bloc Chest Wall and Diaphragm		IVA	Died. Recurrent Disease	5 mo
18	12/F	ES	VAC-Vad	Resection R.R.3	50 Gy	VAC-Vad	Alive. NED	18 mo
19	5/F	Osteogenic Sarcoma		Resection R.R. 3.4.5		Cad	Alive. NED	16 mo
20	2,6/M	ES	Cad	Resection L.R. 5.6	35 Gy	VA-Cad	Alive. NED	15 mo
21	3/M	N.B	Cad	Resection L.R. 10	35 Gy	VA-Cad	Alive. NED	15 mo
22	16/F	Askin's Tumor	Cad	Resection R.R. 6.7	50 Gy	VA-Cad	Alive. NED	12 mo

ES = Ewing's sarcoma, N.B = Neuroblastoma, RT = Radiation therapy, GY = Grays, CHEMO = Chemotherapy, V = Vincristine, A = Actinomycin D, ad = Adriamycin, C = Cyclophosphamide, I = Ifosfamide, METHO = Methotrexate, R.R = Right rib, L.R = Left rib, METS = Metastases, NED = No evidence of disease, VAC-Vad = (vincristine, actinomycin D, cyclophosphamide) and (vincristine, Adriamycin).

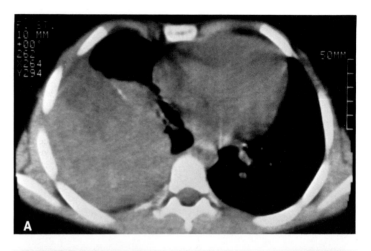

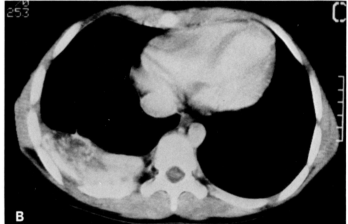

FIGURE 19.3 A. Ewing's sarcoma before and after chemotherapy (in preoperative period). **A.** Before chemotherapy. **B.** After chemotherapy.

Complete tumor resection is the key to successful management. Wide resection must include all of the involved ribs with the corresponding anterior arch and posterior disarticulation, as well as all attached structures, such as lung, diaphragm, and large chest wall muscles. A reasonable margin of normal tissue is advisable on all sides, demonstrated to be tumor-free on frozen sections.

Many surgeons repair chest wall defects with rigid materials that provide adequate chest stability, such as mesh (Marlex) or PTFE patch. We favor an absorbable prosthesis of polyglactin 910 (Vicryl) because chest wall stability has been adequate in all patients, and none has developed prosthesis infection or adverse reactions. Resorbable material is useful in the prevention of local complications in patients submitted to aggressive postoperative therapy leading to severe immunosuppression.

We believe that fibrosis after resorption is adequate to provide chest wall stability and to produce an acceptable cosmetic result. We believe that the effects of a resorbable prosthesis on chest wall development in young patients are preferable to the nonresorbable prosthesis.

This small series does not permit definite conclusions regarding the influence of potential prognostic factors. Five patients (four with malignant small cell tumor (MSCT) and one with osteochondrosarcoma) showed a resectional specimen free of tumor after preoperative chemotherapy. Among these, two patients died within a year and three patients (cases 2, 10, 22, Table 19.1) are alive without evidence of disease at 1, 6, and 10 years.

Synchronous metastases should not preclude resection when the tumor has demonstrated a response to chemotherapy.[19] Four patients, in our experience, had synchronous metastases. In two, pulmonary resection was performed. Three patients are alive without evidence of disease 2 years after resection and combined therapy.

CONCLUSION

The prognosis of malignant chest wall neoplasms in infants and children has been dramatically improved during the last decade with the development of efficient multidrug chemotherapy. Achievement of extended disease-free survival in patients is now a consistent observation.

Further progress is required and expected so that aggressive combined therapy may provide a reasonable likelihood of survival.

REFERENCES

1. Kumar APM, Green A, Smith JW, et al: Combined therapy for malignant tumors of the chest wall in children. *J Pediatr Surg* 1977;12:991–999.
2. Henderson ED, Dahlin DC: Chondrosarcoma of bone: A study of 288 cases. *J Bone Joint Surg* 1963;45:1450.
3. Raney BR, Ragab AH, Ruymann FB, et al: Soft-tissue sarcoma of the trunk in childhood: Results of the intergroup rhabdomyosarcoma study. *Cancer* 1982;49:2612–2616.
4. Ewing S: Diffuse endothelioma of bone. *Proc NY Pathol Soc* 1921;21:17–24.
5. Askin FB, Rosai J, Sibley RK, et al: Malignant small cell tumor of the thoracopulmonary region in childhood. *Cancer* 1979;43:2438–2451.
6. Berard JS, Jaubert de Beaujeu M, Valla JS: Les tumeurs primitives de côtes chez l'enfant et l'adolescent: A propos de 15 cas. *Chir Pediatr* 1982;23:387–392.
7. Sabanathan S, Salama FD, Morgan WE: Primary chest wall tumors. *Ann Thorac Surg* 1985;39:4–15.
8. Shawker TH, Nilprabhassorn P, Dennis JM: Benign intrathoracic lipoma with rib erosion in an infant. *Radiology* 1972;104:111–112.
9. Brand T, Hatch EI, Schaller RT, et al: Surgical management of the infant with mesenchymal hamartoma of the chest wall. *J Pediatr Surg* 1986;21:556–558.
10. Oakley RH, Carty H, Cudmore RE: Multiple benign mesenchymomata of the chest wall. *Pediatr Radiol* 1985;15:58–60.
11. Sato Y, Frey EE, Wicklund B, et al: Embolization therapy in the management of infantile hemangioma with Kasabach Merritt syndrome. *Pediatr Radiol* 1987;17:503–504.
12. Gonzales-Crussi F, Wolfson SL: Peripheral neuroectodermal tumors of the chest wall in childhood. *Cancer* 1984;54:2519–2527.
13. Pairolero PC, Arnod PG: Chest wall tumors: Experience with 100 consecutive patients. *J Thorac Cardiovasc Surg* 1985;90:367–372.
14. Grosfeld JL, Rescorla FJ, West KW, et al: Chest wall resection and reconstruction for malignant conditions in childhood. *J Pediatr Surg* 1988;23:667–673.
15. Eschapasse H, Gaillard J, Henry E, et al: Chest wall tumors: Surgical Management. In: *International Trends in General Thoracic Surgery: Major Challenges.* Philadelphia, Penn: WB Saunders Co, 1987;2. 292–307.
16. Malangoni MA, Ofstein LC, Grosfeld JL, et al: Survival and pulmonary function following chest wall resection and reconstruction in children. *J Pediatr Surg* 1980;15:906–912.
17. Kiricuta I: L'emploi du grand épiploon dans la chirurgie du sein cancéreux. *Presse Méd* 1963;71:1–5.
18. Durandy Y, Batisse A, Bourel P, et al: Mediastinal infections after cardiac operation: A simple closed technique. *J Thorac Cardiovasc Surg* 1989;97, 2:282–285.
19. Schamberger RC, Grier HE, Weinstein HJ, et al: Chest wall tumors in infancy and childhood. *Cancer* 1989;63:774–775.
20. Benoist MR, Lemerle J, Jean R, et al: Effects on pulmonary function of whole lung irradiation for Wilms' tumor in children. *Thorax* 1982;37:175–180.
21. Wohl MEB, Griscom T, Traggis DG, et al: Effects of therapeutic irradiation delivered in early childhood upon subsequent lung function. *Pediatrics* 1975;55, 4:507–516.
22. Demeocq F, Oberlin O, Brunat Mentigny M, et al: Primary chemotherapy and tumor resection in Ewing's sarcoma of the ribs: Report of the French society of Paediatric Oncology. *Eur Paediatr Haematol Oncol* 1984;1:245–250.
23. De Kracker J, Vouté PA, Hayes FA: Ifosfamide and vincristine in paediatric oncology. *Cancer Treat Rev* 1983;10(A):165–166.
24. Hayes FA, Thompson EI, Hustu HO, et al: The response of Ewing's sarcoma to sequential cyclophosphamide and adriamycin induction therapy. *J Clin Oncol* 1983;1:45–51.

DISCUSSION

Primary Chest Wall Tumors in Infancy and Childhood

Jay L. Grosfeld, MD

Primary tumors arising in the chest wall are relatively uncommon. The experience at any one center is often limited, and it is difficult to develop any valid conclusions regarding therapy unless a cooperative study among multiple pediatric institutions is undertaken. Dr Lemoine's chapter on chest wall tumors includes 22 malignant lesions, a reasonably large experience with these lesions. Twelve of the children had Ewing's sarcoma, 4 had Askin's tumor, 3 had neuroblastoma, and the rest had osteosarcoma, chondrosarcoma, and malignant mesenchymoma. The distribution of cases is somewhat similar to that of previous reports on the subject. It would be of interest to know whether the three children with neuroblastoma had been staged or whether any specific tumor markers of prognostic significance were obtained, such as the number of N-myc oncogene copies, deoxyribonucleic acid (DNA) flow cytometry, serum ferritin, or neuron specific enolase. Although the author "lumped" the small round cell tumors together, the prognosis may not be the same for all of them. Children with malignant peripheral neuroectodermal tumors (PNETs) that affect the chest wall seem to be less responsive to treatment than those with Ewing's sarcoma.

In regard to the surgical management of these cases, more than half the patients had only a single rib excised; this is somewhat less than one would consider an adequate cancer operation. Usually at least one rib above and one below the lesion is considered an appropriate excision. This may, however, reflect the utility of current preoperative chemotherapy programs in shrinking the primary lesion and making it possible to simply resect a single rib in some cases. The author recommends the use of an absorbable po-

lyglactin 910 (Vicryl) mesh as the prosthetic material of choice for chest wall reconstruction. Most previous reports regarding chest wall reconstruction have described the use of either mesh (Marlex) or patches (Goretex) to bridge the resulting surgically created defect. The fact that only two of the patients under Dr Lemoine's care developed scoliosis is an admirable result. Although early results indicate a low incidence of postoperative scoliosis, with growth, survivors in our study of 14 children with chest wall tumors often developed asymmetrical chest wall growth, including scoliosis.[1] Marlex and Goretex are permanent synthetic materials and may produce severe fibrous changes and rigidity that prevent adequate chest wall growth, interfere with intercostal expansion, and may also be associated with restrictive pulmonary changes documented by pulmonary function tests. Whether Vicryl mesh prevents these late effects of reconstruction remains to be seen; however, Dr Lemoine's early observations are promising. Irradiation therapy may also have an adverse effect on chest wall and spine development as well as pulmonary function. Patients receiving irradiation of more than 1800 R to the lung fields are at risk for developing radiation pneumonitis and fibrosis. In the National Wilms' Tumor study 13% of patients treated with pulmonary irradiation for lung metastases developed this complication of tumor therapy. The use of radioenhancing drugs such as actinomycin D and doxorubicin hydrochloride (Adriamycin) may augment chest wall fibrosis and pulmonary injury. Both of these agents were used in the cases described by Dr Lemoine.

The author indicates that there are 10 survivors of the patients in the study with malignant tumors. The duration of follow-up study unfortunately is less than 2 years in 6 of these cases, which is obviously too short a time to assess the efficacy of treatment and the subsequent incidence of postresectional and therapeutic complications accurately.

Current Topics in General Thoracic Surgery:
An International Series

246

Although the author emphasizes the importance of preoperative chemotherapy and irradiation, he also states that chest wall resection and reconstruction are essential to cure the child of the malignancy. Previous reports by Shamberger and colleagues at the Children's Hospital Medical Center in Boston and our group at the J. W. Riley Hospital for Children in Indianapolis would agree with this extirpative surgical approach.[1,2] However, a report by Rao and co-workers from St Jude's Children's Hospital in Memphis challenges this long-established concept.[3] These authors report similarly good results (86% survival) in the management of malignant Ewing's sarcoma of the rib in 14 children using multimodal (four-drug) chemotherapy and delayed resection of the involved rib without the necessity of extensive chest wall resection. The latter report also suggested that more intense chemotherapy may obviate the use of irradiation in these cases and reduce the incidence of adverse late effects. Only 2 of the 14 cases required radiotherapy. If the St Jude's data hold up with time, extensive chest wall resection and reconstruction for Ewing's sarcoma may be of historical interest only. On the other hand, these procedures will remain an important component of the surgeon's management of chondrosarcoma, malignant mesenchymal tumors, rhabdomyosaroma of the chest wall, osteosarcoma of the rib, PNET lesions, and those instances of Ewing's sarcoma unresponsive to chemotherapy.

REFERENCES

1. Grosfeld JL, Rescorla FJ, West KW, et al: Chest wall resection and reconstruction for malignant conditions in childhood. *J Pediatr Surg* 1988;23:667–673.
2. Shamberger RC, Grier HE, Weinstein HJ, et al: Chest wall tumors in infancy and childhood. *Cancer* 1989;63:774–775.
3. Rao BN, Hayes FA, Thompson EI, et al: Chest wall resection for Ewing's sarcoma of rib: An unnecessary procedure. *Ann Thorac Surg* 1988;46:40–44.

Chapter 20

Tumors of the Bronchus, Lung, and Pleura in Childhood

Daniel M. Hays, MD and Hiroyuki Shimada, MD, DMS

PRIMARY TUMORS

The "Bronchial Adenoma" Tumor Group

The bronchial adenoma tumors are clearly the most frequently encountered category of primary tumors of the pulmonary system in childhood, usually classified by histological features as carcinoid, mucoepidermoid carcinoma, and adenoid cystic carcinoma. The predominant histological type is carcinoid[1]; it is estimated that 10% of all carcinoid tumors found in childhood are in the bronchi. These patients usually have hemoptysis and cough or pneumonia. The diagnosis in this group of tumors is routinely made with an endoscope, but endoscopic tumor resection is frequently followed by local recurrence. Children with "bronchial adenomas" are usually successfully treated by local bronchial resection at thoracotomy, but lobectomy may be required. Metastases occur in 10% to 15% of children with carcinoid tumors. Most mucoepidermoid carcinomas are low-grade and do not metastasize, whereas the rarer cystic carcinoma variant is associated with higher rates of relapse. One functionally active carcinoid tumor of the bronchus has been reported.[2]

Pulmonary Blastoma of Childhood

The pulmonary blastoma of childhood, also known as pleuropulmonary blastoma,[3] may be primary in the lung, mediastinum, or pleura. There is a preference for subpleural sites. The

major histological feature is the presence of small primitive cells with blastematous characteristics, separated by uncommitted stromal cells. Histological studies, including electron microscopy and immunohistochemistry, have demonstrated focal differentiation toward rhabdomyosarcomatous, chondrosarcomatous, and liposarcomatous elements (Fig. 20.1). Epithelial and mesothelial components or both types in the childhood disease are always benign and show simply an "entrapped" appearance. The histology of childhood pleuropulmonary blastoma is clearly different from that of the "pulmonary blastoma" seen in adults, which is defined as carcinosarcoma, with both epithelial and mesenchymal malignant components.

Approximately 25% of all patients with pulmonary blastomas are children, and many have a history of previously recognized congenital cystic disease of the lung or some form of bronchopulmonary dysplasia. Frequently, blastomas have been discovered incidental to surgery carried out for these benign conditions.[4,5] The male/female patient ratio is 2:1.

Three infants with pleuropulmonary blastoma have been reported and a minimum of 15 others below 15 years of age. The usual symptoms are cough, fever, and chest pain. Complete opacification of a hemithorax is a common initial finding. Pleural effusions and hydropneumothorax are common. In the largest series of pediatric patients with pleuropulmonary blastomas, half of the tumors were confined to mediastinal and pleural surfaces and had no pulmonary involvement.[3] In the remainder, the pleura was involved in addition to the pulmonary parenchyma. Only 1 of 11 had no connection with the pleura. On the other hand, all the "pulmonary blastomas" in adults have an anatomical origin

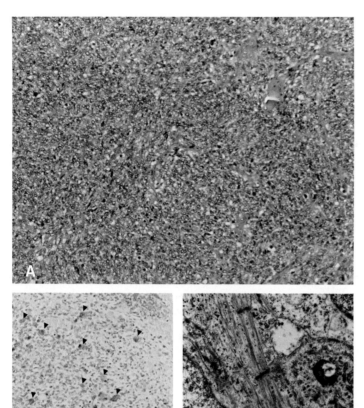

FIGURE 20.1 Pulmonary blastoma. **A.** Diffuse growth of primitive (blastematous) cells. **B.** Focal areas of rhabdomyosarcomatous differentiation identified by desmin-positive cells are indicated by triangles. These are scattered among the primitive sarcoma cells. Also note the entrapped benign epithelial lining cells, indicated by arrows. **C.** The well-organized thick and thin filaments with Z-disc formation are seen in the same tumor, again illustrating myogenic differentiation (electron microscopy × 1100).

in the pulmonary parenchyma, rather than the pleura.

The diagnosis of this condition is ordinarily made at surgery after an excision attempt, with or without lobectomy. Complete excision is usually not feasible. In recent years, almost all of these patients have been treated with radiotherapy and adjuvant chemotherapy including VAC with or without doxorubicin, 5-Florouracil, and/or cisplatin. In the largest series from a single institution, 7/11 patients have had lethal tumor relapse. Among 18 patients collected from the literature, only 7 were alive more than 4 months after the onset of therapy.[3]

The prognosis in patients with pleuropulmonary blastoma is grave, and recurrence after resection, common. Both irradiation and chemotherapy have been employed with inconsistent results.

Bronchogenic Carcinoma

Approximately 50 cases of primary bronchogenic carcinoma have been described in patients less than 16 years of age. The histological subtypes seen in adults (squamous cell carcinoma, adenocarcinoma, small cell and large cell undifferentiated carcinoma) are all represented. The incidence of squamous cell carcinoma is far lower in children than in adults.[6] The mean survival duration after diagnosis among children treated in the 1970s was estimated to be 6.1 months.

Other Primary Bronchopulmonary Neoplasms

Several mesotheliomas of the pleura have been described in childhood,[7] but an association between these lesions in pediatric patients and asbestos exposure has not been established. Hartman and Shochat have described nine cases of primary rhabdomyosarcoma of the lung, although lung is not recognized as a primary site for this histological tumor type by the Intergroup Rhabdomyosarcoma Study Committee. These cases may be examples of monodirectional (myogenic) differentiation of pleuropulmonary blastoma. Other primary sarcomas found in pleura or lung include fibrosarcoma, leiomyosarcoma, and fibroleiomyosarcoma of myofibroblastic origin. These tumors in children tend to behave less aggressively than their counterparts in adults.[8] Adenocarcinoma resembling fetal lung (pulmonary endodermal tumor) is a rare tumor with a peculiar morphology similar to that of developing lung tissue in the pseudoglandular stage (22 to 24 weeks of gestation).[9] Children with this tumor have a high relapse rate.

METASTATIC TUMORS OF LUNG

Excision of metastatic tumor nodules in lung has been performed since 1939 and has included examples of almost all childhood tumors that may result in pulmonary metastasis. Among pediatric patients, excision of pulmonary nephroblastoma (Wilms' tumor) has been carried out for more than 30 years and was, at one time, the principal form of management for pulmonary dissemination of this tumor. Series of patients undergoing excisional procedures for pulmonary metastasis have now been reported in a wide variety of tumors, including children with Ewing's sarcoma, rhabdomyosarcoma, synovial sarcoma, liposarcoma, yolk sac testicular tumors, renal adenocarcinoma, papillary thyroid carcinoma, leiomyosarcoma, fibrosarcoma, and chondrosarcoma, in addition to the larger groups of children with metastatic osteosarcoma and nephroblastoma.[10–17]

Osteogenic Sarcoma

By the mid-1960s, it was recognized that an aggressive surgical approach to pulmonary metastatic disease was particularly appropriate in osteosarcoma. Recurrence, in more than 85% of patients in which it occurred, was localized to lung. Development of nonpulmonary metastasis after resection of pulmonary metastatic nodules was uncommon. Surgery without the use of irradiation or adjuvant chemotherapy could be curative, whereas pulmonary metastatic disease was rarely, if ever, cured by chemotherapy alone. Early in the development of this concept, surgery was usually performed for "late" solitary metastasis, which is currently a rare indication for thoracotomy. During the 1970s, in many centers, only peripheral lesions were considered appropriate for resection.[18] Indications for surgery in patients with metastatic pulmonary osteosarcoma have been progressively extended as an increasingly favorable outcome after these procedures has been recognized.

Currently, in some clinics, all patients with pulmonary metastatic lesions are considered candidates for excisional surgery, including those with relatively short tumor-free intervals and bilateral disease.[19] Others have found the presence of an excessive number of visible nodules on preoperative full-lung tomography an indication that resection will not be helpful.[20] Large bilateral or recurrent hilar masses and presence of extrapulmonary disease are widely recognized as contraindications to surgery. When all gross tumor cannot be resected at surgery, the results are decidedly inferior in all sizable series.[18,21] Multiple thoracotomies have been carried out in all large series with a maximum of 10 and a mean of more than 2 procedures per patient in several.

Survival data for these procedures are described by institution, as methods of reporting vary. At the Children's Orthopedic Hospital, Seattle, 17 patients underwent 34 thoracotomies (1964–1980); 41% of these patients were alive and disease-free in 1981. No patient with pulmonary metastatic disease, without surgical resection, survived during the same interval.[18]

The Surgery Branch of the National Cancer Institute conducted a prospective trial, including 43 patients with pulmonary metastatic disease, 39 of whom had one or more thoracotomies (1975–1982). Actuarial 5-year survival in the total group was 40%.[20]

At the Mayo Clinic, 57 patients less than 21 years of age underwent 111 thoracotomies for metastatic disease during a 6-year period (1974–1980). Twenty-six of these patients were free of disease in 1981, with an actuarial curve predicting 5-year survival in approximately 40%.[22] At the Dana-Farber Cancer Institute, Boston, among 32 patients with relapse in lung (only), 26 had thoracotomy (1972–1981). In 11 of these, apparent complete resection of all metastatic disease was possible. Nine of these 11 patients were free of disease in 1984 with a median duration of survival of 42 months (range 3–72 months).[21] At the M. D. Anderson Hospital and Tumor Institute, Houston, 56 patients with metastatic osteogenic sarcoma were treated by resection with a cumulative percentage surviving for 5 years of 50.7%.[23]

In a series with a longer follow-up period reported from Memorial Sloan-Kettering Cancer Center, New York City, 6 of 22 patients treated by resection had survived for 10 to 15 years after surgery.[17]

It would appear that approximately one third of the patients treated surgically for pulmonary metastatic disease of any extent are relatively long-range survivors; the majority of these have had complete resection of all visible tumor at one or more thoracotomies. Almost all authorities recognized wedge resection as the most appropriate form of surgical resection, with lobectomy and even pneumonectomy occasionally performed. Adjuvant chemotherapy after resection of pulmonary metastatic disease is employed currently in most series.

The pulmonary metastatic nodules of osteosarcoma may be soft and hemorrhagic or may demonstrate a bonelike appearance. Histological examination of pulmonary nodules from a known osteosarcoma patient may demonstrate mature osseous tissue unaccompanied by obvious sarcoma cells. This type of lesion is currently interpreted as metastatic osteosarcoma, though its biological behavior is unknown.[24]

Nephroblastoma (Wilms' Tumor)

The general use of computerized axial tomography (CAT) has created a new category of Wilms' tumor patients with pulmonary metastasis, that is, those who have positive CAT findings but negative conventional roentgenogram results. The prognosis in this group is still uncertain,[25] and surgery is probably not indicated.

At present, most patients with metastatic pulmonary nephroblastoma are treated by chemotherapy alone. This is supplemented with complete lung irradiation in some institutions, and isolated chemotherapy-resistant nodules are treated with small-field radiotherapy in others. Surgical resection remains the recommended approach to chemotherapy-resistant nodules in many centers.[26] Surgery may be performed (1) as first treatment, followed by chemotherapy; (2) as a complement to radiation therapy; and (3) after failure of all forms of management.[16] Wedge resection is the most widely employed technique,[11] although more extensive resection such as lobectomy must be considered more frequently in patients with nephroblastoma than in those with metastatic osteosarcoma. This reflects a characteristic of metastatic Wilms' tumor that is rarely seen in osteosarcoma: the development of one or several large metastatic lesions, at times late in the course.

More than 50% of children with pulmonary metastatic disease (alone) survive.[27,28] This includes patients who have received nonintensive forms of chemotherapy initially. Among patients in the National Wilms' Tumor Study (NWTS), those with pulmonary metastasis at diagnosis

arising from tumors with "favorable" histological features (approximately 89% of all Wilms' tumors) had a survival rate of 71% at 2 years during the interval 1968–1974, which rose to 91% during the interval 1980–1985.[29] This was presumably the result of more intensive chemotherapy. In the "unfavorable" histological categories, survival rate among patients with pulmonary disease ranged from 10% to 20%.

Although the results of an initial surgical approach to metastatic nephroblastoma have been excellent with an 82% relapse-free survival in NWTS-1 and NWTS-2,[30] the current study (NWTS-4) recommends initial irradiation after pulmonary relapse on chemotherapy, with surgery reserved for demonstrated radiotherapy-resistant nodules.

REFERENCES

1. Andrassy RJ, Feldtman RW, Stanford W: Bronchial carcinoid tumors in children and adolescents. *J Pediatr Surg* 1977;12:513–517.
2. Ward PS, Mott MG, Smith J, Hartog M: Cushing's syndrome and bronchial carcinoid tumour. *Arch Dis Child* 1984;59:375.
3. Manivel JC, Priest JR, Watterson J, et al: Pleuropulmonary blastoma. *Cancer* 1988;62:1516–1526.
4. Weinblatt ME, Siegel SE, Isaacs H: Pulmonary blastoma associated with cystic lung disease. *Cancer* 1982;49:669–671.
5. Holland-Moritz RM, Heyn RM: Pulmonary blastoma associated with cystic lesions in children. *Med Pediatr Oncol* 1984;12:85–88.
6. Shelley BE, Lorenzo RL: Primary squamous cell carcinoma of the lung in childhood. *Pediatr Radiol* 1983;13:92.
7. Kaufman SK, Stout AP: Mesothelioma in children. *Cancer* 1964;17:539–544.
8. Guccion JG, Rosen SH: Bronchopulmonary leiomyosarcoma and fibrosarcoma: A study of 32 cases and review of the literature. *Cancer* 1972;30:836.
9. Kodama T, Shimosato Y, Watanabe S, et al: Six cases of well-differentiated adenocarcinoma simulating fetal lung tubules in pseudoglandular stage: Comparison with pulmonary blastoma. *Am J Surg Pathol* 1984;8:735.
10. Kilman JW, Kronenberg MW, O'Neill JA, Klassen KP: Surgical resection for pulmonary metastases in children. *Arch Surg* 1969;99:158–165.
11. Ballentine TVN, Wiseman NE, Filler RM: Assessment of pulmonary wedge resection for the treatment of lung metastases. *J Pediatr Surg* 1975;10:671–676.
12. Stauffer UG, Pluss HJ: Chirurgische exzision von lungenmetastasen bei kindern mit malignen tumoren: indikationen, resultate. *Z Kinderchir* 1977;20:237–246.
13. Rogers BM, Talbert JL, Alexander JA: Pulmonary metastases in childhood sarcoma. *Ann Thorac Surg* 1980;29:410–414.
14. Roth H, Bolkenius M, Daum R, et al: Surgery of lung metastases in childhood. *Z Kinderchir* 1981;32:47–51.
15. Frenckner B, Lannergren K, Soderlund S: Results of

surgical treatment of lung metastases in children. *Scand J Thorac Cardiovasc Surg* 1982;16:201–204.

16. Baldeyrou P, Lemoine G, Zucker JM, Schweisguth O: Pulmonary metastases in children: The place of surgery: A study of 134 patients. *J Pediatr Surg* 1984;19:121–125.

17. Beattie EJ Jr: Surgical treatment of pulmonary metastases. *Cancer* 1984;54:2729–2731.

18. Shaller RT, Haas J, Schaller J, et al: Improved survival in children with osteosarcoma following resection of pulmonary metastases. *J Pediatr Surg* 1982;17:546–550.

19. Telander RL, Pairolero PC, Pritchard DJ, et al: Resection of pulmonary metastatic osteogenic sarcoma in children. *Surgery* 1978;84:335–341.

20. Putnam JB, Roth JA, Wesley MN, et al: Survival following aggressive resection of pulmonary metastases from osteogenic sarcoma: Analysis of prognostic factors. *Ann Thorac Surg* 1983;36:516–523.

21. Goorin AM, Delorey MJ, Lack EE, et al: Prognostic significance of complete surgical resection of pulmonary metastases in patients with osteogenic sarcoma: Analysis of 32 patients. *J Clin Oncol* 1984;2:425–431.

22. Han MT, Telander RL, Pairolero PC, et al: Aggressive thoracotomy for pulmonary metastatic osteogenic sarcoma in children and young adolescents. *J Pediatr Surg* 1981;16:928–933.

23. Mountain CF, McMurtrey MJ, Hermes KE: Surgery for pulmonary metastasis: A 20-year experience. *Ann Thoracic Surg* 1984;38:323–330.

24. Dunn D, Dehner LP: Metastatic osteosarcoma to lung: A clinicopathologic study of surgical biopsies and resections. *Cancer* 1977;40:3054.

25. Wilimas JA, Douglass EC, Magill HL, et al: Significance of pulmonary computed tomography at diagnosis in Wilms' tumor. *J Clin Oncol* 1988;6:1144–1146.

26. Wilimas JA, Champion J, Douglass EC, et al: Relapsed Wilms' tumor: Factors affecting survival and cure. *Am J Clin Oncol* 1985;8:324–328.

27. Simone JV, Cassady JR, Filler RM: Cancers of childhood. In: DeVita VT Jr, Hellman S, Rosenberg SA, eds. *Cancer: Principles and Practice of Oncology.* Philadelphia: JB Lippincott Co, 1982;1254–1330.

28. Cassady JR, Tefft M, Filler RM, et al: Considerations in the radiation therapy of Wilms' tumor. *Cancer* 1973;32:598–608.

29. Breslow NE, Churchill G, Nesmith B, et al: Clinicopathologic features and prognosis for Wilms' tumor patients with metastases at diagnosis. *Cancer* 1986;58:2501–2511.

30. Green DM: The treatment of advanced or recurrent malignant genitourinary tumors in children. *Cancer* 1987;60:602–611.

Tumors of the Bronchus, Lung, and Pleura in Childhood

Georges Lemoine, MD and Michel Deneuville, MD

An excellent overview of clinicopathological features in tumors of the bronchus, lung, and pleura in childhood is presented in the chapter written by Professor Daniel Hays and Dr Hiruki Shimada. We certainly agree with Professor Hays and Dr Shimada in their discussion of clinical, pathological, and prognostic features in pulmonary blastomata of childhood.

In our experience such lesions have been exceedingly rare. During a 25-year period, 10 patients (7 male, 3 female) have been referred to us for surgical management. Ages ranged from 3 to 14 years. Different clinical presentations are reported. Some patients referred for surgical resection of residual tumor after a massive neoplasm involving an entire hemithorax have demonstrated a significant response to chemotherapy. The remaining patients are referred for pulmonary coin lesions.

Four patients had a rhabdomyosarcoma, originating in the parietal pleura in two, in the visceral pleura in one, and within the lung in one. Among three with massive pleuropulmonary neoplasms with pleural effusion, two were first treated with chemotherapy, followed by surgical resection of residual tumor and combined with postoperative chemotherapy. Complete tumor necrosis was noted at specimen examination. En bloc resection included extrapleural dissection and lung wedge resection. All patients are alive without evidence of disease 2 and 3 years later. The remaining patient, without preoperative chemotherapy, had a complete resection. Despite irradiation and postoperative chemotherapy, he died from recurrence 8 months after surgery. In another patient with intrapulmonary neoplasms involving the left auricle, a pneumonectomy combined with auricular wall resection was performed, using cardiopulmonary bypass.

He is alive at 21 months with no evidence of disease.

Three patients had a pulmonary blastoma. The first patient, who had undifferentiated blastoma, underwent en bloc resection of lung and diaphragm with prosthetic reconstruction. Resection margins yielded positive findings, and he died from recurrence 18 months after resection. The two other patients had chondrosarcoma differentiation and underwent potentially curative resections. Both are alive 5 years after postoperative chemotherapy using etoposid (VP16) and cisplatin. One is suffering a myeloblastic leukemia. One patient was referred for life-threatening tracheal obstruction. Endobronchial tumor involving the proximal right main stem bronchus was identified, and a right pneumonectomy with lateral resection of tracheal wall was performed. Histological findings were consistent with a malignant fibrous histiocytoma. The patient is alive with no evidence of disease at 12 years. The latter two patients had plasma cell granuloma of the lung identified at specimen examination of isolated lung nodules (lobectomy).

We did not observe any bronchogenic tumors in our series. Bronchogenic tumors are divided into a broad spectrum of histological types. Tumors arising from the bronchial mucosa are more frequently encountered. Those tumors include carcinoid, mucoepidermoid, and adenoid cystic carcinoma, all demonstrating a low-grade malignancy. They may involve the main stem bronchus or the carina and can recur many years after previous resection.[1] Various neoplasms originating at the submucosal level from connective tissue (chondroma, leiomyoma, and so on) are less common.

METASTATIC LUNG DISEASE

Metastatic lung disease (MLD) is by far the most common pulmonary neoplasm found in childhood and infancy (97% in our experience). We completely agree with the principles of therapeutic management given by Professor Hays and Dr Shimada in their overview of the literature. However, in the light of our extensive experience, we would like to stress several points that remain controversial, with special regard to surgical procedures and selection of patients, and report our survival results.

Various histological types of primary tumors are encountered, demonstrating a broad spectrum of biological behavior.

Pediatric oncologists are now well acquainted with the natural history of most primary tumors, and efficient chemotherapy is available for several histological types. Combined therapy is accepted practice in the management of pulmonary metastases in children, and surgery remains an effective method of removing all residual tumor. One must await the response to chemotherapy and spare as much functional tissue as possible.

SURGICAL PROCEDURES

The operative approach for patients with MLD remains controversial.[2-4] Our series stresses the excellent tolerance of bilateral staged thoracotomies that children demonstrate and we continue to favor the transthoracic lateral approach rather than median sternotomy.

The following arguments support this choice:

Recurrence after previous metastasectomy, in children with apparent unilateral disease revealed by CAT scan, was confined to the same lung in 76% of patients. Furthermore, the benefit from early detection of occult bilateral metastases remains unclear.[4]

Posterior and lower lobe metastases are inadequately exposed through a sternal split incision. Removal of large metastases in the posterior mediastinum may be hazardous or incomplete.

Multiple bilateral resections may lead to severe contusion of both lungs and may require mechanical ventilation. Increased morbidity, caused by prolonged air leaks and infection, could delay hospital discharge.[3]

Therefore, since 1986, we have used median sternotomy only to remove bilateral and superficial small metastases that are anteriorly located.

The following findings should preclude sternal split incision:

Open or infected wounds remaining after the treatment of the primary tumor

Intensive postoperative chemotherapy with aplasia

Previous mediastinal irradiation

Synchronous bilateral axillary thoracotomies can be considered as a reasonable alternative.

A vast majority of patients are routinely explored through a posterolateral thoracotomy preserving the anterior serratus muscle. Careful examination of the entire exposed and deflated lung is made to detect all nodules. The thoracic cavity, including mediastinum and hilar nodes, is systematically explored. Transdiaphragmatic liver palpation is routinely performed.

Wedge resection is the standard excision procedure. During resection, the electrocautery is used to remove a small margin of normal tissue surrounding the nodules. We do not favor automatic stapling devices (except the GIA device for large wedge resections) because they preserve less tissue and risk both tumor violation and postoperative adhesions to chest wall and mediastinum. Lung defects after wedge resection are closed by interrupted deep sutures and superficial running sutures using absorbable monofilament 5-0 (polydioxanome). Fibrin glue is useful for providing airtight sutures. More extended resections (lobectomy or segmentectomy) are performed in the removal of large, deep, or multiple metastases located in the same area.

SELECTION OF PATIENTS

During the last decade, indication for surgery in the management of MLD has changed.[4-6]

Metastatic nephroblastoma is now uncommon, and chemotherapy alone provides a fair likelihood of cure.

At present, the vast majority of patients referred for surgical resection have been submitted to intensive multidrug chemotherapy. Most have highly aggressive tumors including osteogenic and soft tissue sarcoma and round cell tumors. In some cases, either metastases are chemotherapy resistant, or all forms of management have failed. The aim of resection, then, is to remove all residual tumor while sparing as much functional lung tissue as possible.

According to our experience,[7] the following points should be emphasized:

1. No preoperative prognostic criteria proved to be discriminating enough to select patients who would not benefit from surgical resection. Numerous nodules found at preoperative CAT scan should not preclude the surgical procedure. In our study, individual long-term survival was observed in patients having up to 50

metastases removed from a single lung. Therefore, an aggressive effort should be made to resect all pulmonary nodules regardless of their bilateral location and multiplicity.

2. Surgery should not be ruled out in the presence of synchronous lung metastasis if there is potential control of the primary tumor. The incidence of unresectable tumor was similar to that of other patients, and resection provided a reasonable 52% 5-year survival rate in our experience.

3. Reoperations for tumor recurrence must be considered in all patients demonstrating disease confined to the chest, and particulary for osteogenic and soft tissue sarcoma.

4. Further investigations are required to determine the value as predictive criteria of microscopic findings including the degree of tumor necrosis after chemotherapy, tumor microfoci, and visceral pleura invasion. This could define the population with a high risk of recurrence.

MATERIAL AND COMMENTS

From 1962 to 1986, 258 children with metastatic lung disease (147 boys, 111 girls) were referred from oncological pediatric departments for surgical management. Age ranged from 2 months to 15 years (mean 7.7 years).

Primary tumors were as follows: Wilms' tumor, 124 (48%); osteogenic sarcoma, 68 (26%); Ewing's sarcoma, 26 (10%); miscellaneous, 40 (16%), including a majority of soft tissue sarcoma (Fig. D20.1).

Metastatic nephroblastoma was most frequently encountered before 1974, whereas most of the osteogenic and soft tissue sarcoma was referred since 1976. Patients considered for surgical resection met the following criteria:

Effective control of primary tumor

Evidence of disease confined to the chest

Potential for complete operative resection

Expectation of sufficient functional reserve, particularly in patients undergoing serial thoracotomies or after previous lung irradiation

Since 1980, CAT scan was routinely used to detect lung metastases at follow-up observation.

The median disease-free interval was 12.8 months (ranging from 1 to 89 months). A total of 390 thoracotomies were performed, ranging from 1 to 7 per patient. Thirty patients (12%) required three or more thoracotomies. Wedge resections, ranging from 1 to 80 per patient (mean 4.5), were preferentially performed.

Two hundred thirty-one patients had complete tumor removal at first surgical procedure (single thoracotomy or bilateral staged thoracotomies carried out in the same hospital admission), and 27 had unresectable tumors (10%). Reexplorations (one or more) were required in 57 patients (25%) with an average disease-free interval of 11.8 months. Postresectional recurrence was confined to the same lung in 66% of patients.

Postoperative mortality was 0.8%, and complications occurred in 5% of thoracotomies. These included prolonged air leaks (15 patients), reoperation for bleeding (3 patients), severe pneumonia (1 patient), and postpneumonectomy empyema (1 patient). No mechanical ventilation was required. Combined therapy (irradiation and/or chemotherapy) was used in most children before or after surgery or both, depending on histological findings, the chemotherapy protocol, and the available drug at time of treatment.

Actuarial survival after the last pulmonary resection was 62%; at 1 year, 46%; and at 10 years, 43% in 221 patients available for long-term follow-up (Fig. D20.2). The 5-year survival rate was 52% in Wilms' tumor patients, significantly higher than in osteogenic sarcoma (28%), in Ewing's sarcoma (24%), and in all others (27%) ($p < .001$) (Fig. D20.3A to D).

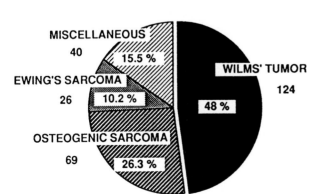

FIGURE D20.1 Distribution of pathological types of secondary tumor in lung.

256

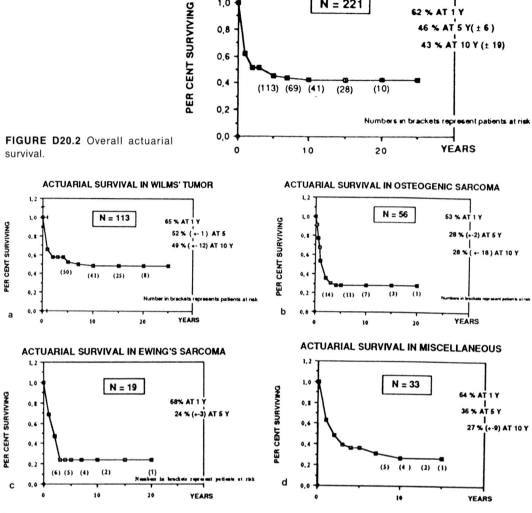

FIGURE D20.2 Overall actuarial survival.

FIGURE D20.3 A. Actuarial survival with Wilms' tumor. B. Actuarial survival in osteogenic sarcoma. C. Actuarial survival in Ewing's sarcoma. D. Actuarial survival in miscellaneous tumor.

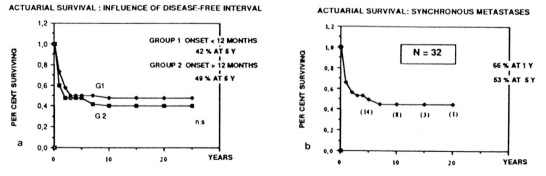

FIGURE D20.4 A. Actuarial survival: influence of disease-free interval. B. Actuarial survival: synchronous metastases.

ACTUARIAL SURVIVAL: INFLUENCE OF NUMBER OF METASTASES

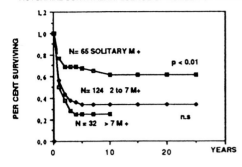

FIGURE D20.5 Actuarial survival: influence of number of metastases.

Various factors were analyzed for their potential influence on postresectional survival (log rank test). No significant difference was identified in two groups of patients with early (1–12 months) or late (more than 12 months) onset of metastases, nor in patients with synchronous lung metastases amenable to resection (32 patients, 49%, at 5 years) (Fig. D20.4A and B). Borderline significant difference was found in two groups having, respectively, two to seven and eight or more metastases removed. Patients with single metastasis did have significantly improved survival rates ($p < .001$) (Fig. D20.5). Statistically significant lower survival rates were obtained with patients requiring two or more surgical procedures ($p < .01$).

Microscopic lymphatic invasion of visceral pleura or alveolar extension (5% to 10%) or parietal involvement (7%) was related to a 75% mortality rate. Extrathoracic metastases or recurrences at the primary site had impaired survival results in 21% to 40% of patients, depending on histological type.

REFERENCES

1. Grillo HC: Carinal reconstruction. *Ann Thorac Surg* 1982;34(4):356–373.
2. Cooper JD, Nelers JM, Pearson PG, et al: Extended indications for median sternotomy in patients requiring pulmonary resection. *Ann Thorac Surg* 1978;26:413.
3. Johnston MR: Median sternotomy for resection of pulmonary metastases. *J Thorac Cardiovasc Surg* 1983;85:516–522.
4. Roth JA, Pass HI, Wesley MN, et al: Comparison of median sternotomy and thoracotomy for resection of pulmonary metastases in patients with adult soft tissue sarcoma. *Ann Thorac Surg* 1986;42(2):134–138.
5. Lanza LA, Miser JJ, Pass HI: The role of resection in the treatment of pulmonary metastases from Ewing's sarcoma. *J Thorac Cardiovasc Surg* 1987;94:181–187.
6. Roth JA, Putnam JB, Wesley MN: Differing determinants of prognosis following resection of pulmonary metastases from osteogenic and soft tissue sarcoma patients. *Cancer* 1985;55:1361–1366.
7. Deneuville M, Lemoine G, Baldeyrou P: Pulmonary metastases resection in children: A study of 258 cases. First International Congress on metastatic disease, Lyons, France, Oct 1988.

Chapter **21**

Mediastinal Tumors in Infancy and Childhood

Georges Lemoine, MD and Philippe Montupet, MD

A broad spectrum of malformations or neoplasms may develop in the mediastinum. Mediastinal disorders have been recognized since antiquity. Pietro Rubino first reported in 1810 an anatomico-clinical description of a dermoid cyst.[1] Hobert Hart, in 1889, published the first pathological textbook with significant attention to mediastinal disorders.[2]

Specific publications about mediastinal tumors in childhood were contributed in 1924 by Smith and Stone,[3] and in 1933 by Marquezy and Heraux.[4]

The mediastinum is a well-defined anatomical region. It is bounded on both sides by the mediastinal pleura, at the top by the thoracic inlet, at the bottom by the diaphragm, anteriorly by the sternocostal chest wall, and posteriorly by the spine.

The mediastinum is classically divided into three anatomicoradiological spaces in both vertical and sagittal planes.

The divisions into the vertical plane define

The upper mediastinum, bounded at the top by the thoracic inlet and by the aortic arch below

The lower mediastinum, ranging from the carina to the diaphragm

The middle mediastinum, situated between the former spaces and containing the tracheal bifurcation and the aortic arch

The divisions in the sagittal plane define three compartments:

The anterior compartment ranges from the sternocostal wall to the anterior aspect of the trachea and pericardium.

The middle compartment contains the trachea and the paratracheal spaces.

The posterior compartment is located between the posterior aspect of the trachea and the spine. Paravertebral spaces classically are included in the posterior mediastinum.

The location of a tumor in one of the anatomical divisions is an important guideline to diagnosis (Table 21.1).

About 50% of the neoplasms are asymptomatic and discovered on a routine chest roentgenogram. In symptomatic neoplasms presenting complaints are usually chest discomfort, respiratory manifestations, or signs of compression of vital vascular or neurological structures.

New tools in medical imaging, percutaneous needle biopsy, and tumor markers have recently modified the diagnostic management of and the therapeutic strategy for these neoplasms.

1. Mediastinal tumors will be described in terms of decreasing frequency. Solid neurogenic tumors are the most commonly encountered, located in the posterior mediastinum.

2. Malignant lymphomas, located in the middle mediastinum, are equally frequent. However, lymphomas seldom represent an indication for surgical resection.

3. Primary germ cell tumors or mesenchymal tumors developing from muscles, fat tissue, or vascular structures commonly lie in the anterior mediastinum, as do the rare thymic tumors.

4. The last group of neoplasms comprises all other tumors wherever located. The pathological examination of the resection specimen usually ensures definite diagnosis.

Mediastinal congenital malformations (bronchogenic cysts, foregut duplications) are

TABLE 21.1 Mediastinal Masses in Children

Anterior	Middle	Posterior
Teratoma	Lymphoma	Neurogenic
Thymoma	Lymphadenopathies	Tumors
Thymic Cyst	Granulomatous	Foregut
Lymphangioma	Lymphadenitis	Duplications
Hemangioma	Bronchogenic Cyst	and Cysts
Connective		
Tissue		
Tumors		
Pericardial		
Cyst		

excluded from this study and are presented in Chapters 6 and 9.

NEUROGENIC TUMORS

Neurogenic tumors arise within the posterior paravertebral gutter from an intercostal nerve or the sympathetic chain.

Neurogenic tumors are grouped in the pathological entity described by Bolande[5] as neurocristopathies.

The most frequently encountered mediastinal tumors originate in the sympathetic system (Fig. 21.1). The thoracic location is the second location (second only to the abdominal area) for harboring such tumors in childhood and infancy.

Mediastinal tumors of the sympathetic chain are divided by histological features into neuroblastoma and ganglioneuroblastoma, formed from malignant embryonal cells, and ganglioneuroma, which is a benign tumor.

Malignant neurogenic cells have the ability to secrete catecholamines, a high serum level of which is therefore a useful guide to diagnosis.

Biological and histocytological refinements as well as new tools in medical imaging currently provide a precise assessment of the lesion and its local extension.

In the last decade, major improvements in chemotherapy have basically changed therapeutic strategy and prognosis of malignant neurogenic tumors.

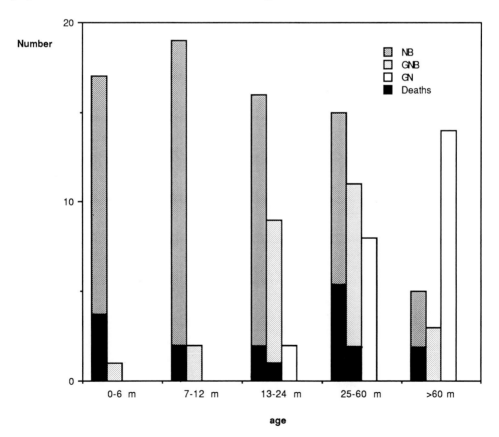

NB=neuroblastoma, GNB= ganglioneuroblastoma, GN= ganglioneuroma

FIGURE 21.1 Sympathetic tumors. Breakdown by age and histological type.

The great majority of neuroblastomata are reported to occur during early childhood; 93% of the patients are less than 6 years old. The male to female patient ratio does not reveal a sex-linked predilection. Ganglioneuromas are very rare in infancy.[6]

The exact cause of these tumors remains to be clearly elucidated.

Pathological Findings

Neuroblastoma is a soft solid tumor, of grayish color, variegated in appearance on cross section, with areas of both hemorrhage and necrosis.

Intratumoral calcifications are found in 50% of cases. The size of the tumor is variable, ranging from small to bulky neoplasm invading the entire pleural cavity. The neoplasm may be encapsulated or grossly invasive into connective tissue and adjacent structures.

Microscopically neuroblastoma is a lobulated tumor made of small tumor cells, with small round nuclei and much cytoplasm. Tumor cells can link together in rosette formation, the center of which contains cystoplasmic pseudopods. In more differentiated subtypes, larger tumor cells appear.

Combination in the same tumor of areas containing neuroblastoma cells with areas having more differentiated ganglioneural cells characterizes the ganglioneuroblastoma.[6]

Completely mature ganglioneuroma demonstrates only normal ganglioneural cells and spindle cells (Schwann's cells).

According to Shimada[7] the prognosis in malignant neurogenic tumors is related to the degree of differentiation and the mitotic index.

Before the age of 1 year, the prognosis is more favorable whatever the degree of differentiation, although the only histopathological factor influencing outcome is the mitotic index.

Between 1 and 5 years of age, both differentiation and number of mitosis must be considered. Beyond 5 years, prognosis is dismal.

Clinical Features

Clinical modes of presentation are variable. Table 21.2 summarizes initial complaints in our experience of 122 patients. Although signs and/or symptoms are due to compression of adjacent organs, in more than 50% of cases the mass is asymptomatic and detected on routine roentgenogram. Chest roentgenogram usually demonstrates a round or oval mass located lateral to the spine. Intercostal spaces adjacent to the tumor are commonly enlarged with rib erosions. The mass projects into the posterior compartment of the mediastinum (Fig. 21.2A and B).

TABLE 21.2 Mediastinal Neuroblastoma/Ganglioneuroma*

Respiratory	14
Spinal Cord Compression	12
Horner's Syndrome	12
Cervical Adenopathies	8
Supraclavicular Neck Mass	7
Opsomyoclony	4
Severe Secretory Diarrhea	4
Pleurisy	2

* One hundred twenty-two cases presenting symptoms. Of the patients 50% were diagnosed on a routine chest roentgenogram. Some exhibited signs related to more than one system.

In metastatic disease, initial complaints include weight loss, fever, and diffuse or localized skeletal pain. Spontaneous orbital hematoma (Hutchinson's syndrome) is a strong indication of metastatic neuroblastoma.

Nodular liver enlargement is the predominant sign of Pepper's syndrome and is usually encountered in infancy. Sometimes there are associated subcutaneous metastatic nodules.

Lymph node metastases rarely lead to the diagnosis.

Spinal cord compression by direct extension of a paraspinal mass through an intervertebral foramen (hourglass) may occur, and the clinical features are predominantly neurological dysfunctions. A sudden paraplegia may even occur. Unfortunately recognition of cord compression in the infant can be very difficult.

Associated Syndromes

The following associated syndromes are rare. (1) Watery diarrhea, characterized by chronicity and resistance to all forms of treatment, is related to secretion of vasoactive intestinal peptides by tumor cells. Tumor removal provides complete remission of the diarrhea.[8] (2) The opsomyoclonic syndrome combines fast, clonic movements of eyes and limbs, a cerebellar syndrome, and muscle hypotonia. This is uncommonly associated with malignant neurogenic tumors.[6]

Biology

A high urinary level of catecholamines and their derivatives, vanillylmandelic acid (VMA), homovanillic acid (HVA), and dopamine, is a useful guide to diagnosis.[9] The sensitivity reaches 90% in secreting tumors.[6] The highest level of tumor markers is usually associated with distant metastases (stages IV and IV S in Evan's Classification[10] Table 21.3).

Repeated evaluation of tumor markers is important in the follow-up of the disease. However,

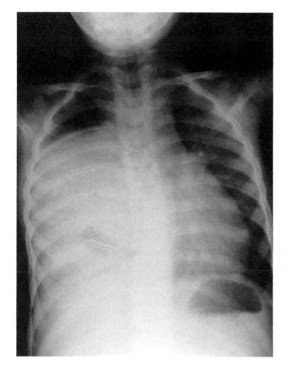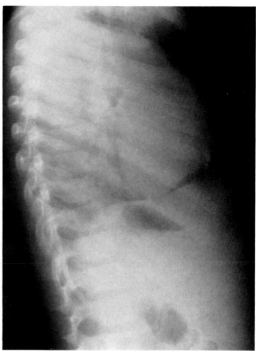

FIGURE 21.2 A. Chest roentgenogram of a thoracic sympathetic tumor. **B.** The mass projects in the posterior compartment of the mediastinum.

the urinary level of catecholamines is not a strict reflection of progression of the disease, and a return to normal level is not always associated with complete remission.[9]

Vasoactive intestinal peptides (VIPs) are occasionally excreted by these tumors and are responsible for watery diarrhea. A more favorable prognosis seems to be associated in cases with high VIP levels.[8]

Most neuroblastic cells are characterized by their ability to bind with false neuromediators such as metaiodobenzylguanidin (M-IBG) marked with radioactive iodine 125 or 131.[11] This is the physiological basis for the isotopic scanning used at present.

TABLE 21.3 Staging Proposed by Evans and Associates

Stage I	Tumors limited to the organ of origin
Stage II	Regional spread that does not cross the midline
Stage III	Tumors extending over the midline
Stage IV	Metastases to distant lymph nodes, bone, brain, or lung
Stage IV S	Small primary tumors and distant metastases limited to liver, skin, bone marrow, or all without radiologic evidence of bony metastases

The neuron-specific enolase (NSE) is a specific factor secreted in unusual amounts by neuroblastic or neuroectodermal cells.[12] As with the other markers, the highest plasma levels are observed in stages III and IV. In a complete remission the NSE plasma level always returns to normal.

Chromosomal examination of neurogenic tumors is a subject of basic research. The N-myc oncogene seems to be an important factor, which warrants further investigation.[13]

In summary, the diagnosis of neurogenic tumor is, in most cases, based on clinical and biological findings. Percutaneous needle biopsy remains very difficult to interpret.[14]

Tumor Assessment

Major improvement in medical imaging tools has fundamentally changed the approach to diagnosis, assessment, and follow-up study of the neoplasm.

Progress in transthoracic echography now reveals highly sophisticated information, including tumor size and measurements, and demonstrates any encroachment on adjacent organs.

Computerized axial tomography (CAT) scan is mandatory before any decision to operate. It provides visualization of the mediastinal mass (containing calcifications in 50% of cases) and identifies tumor extension into adjacent organs, intercostal spaces, and intervertebral foramina, as well as lymph node enlargement. CAT scan is now an efficient alternative to myelography, in the investigation of paraspinal soft tissue and extradural extensions. Angioscans demonstrate the vascularity and degree of necrosis of the neoplasm, mainly after chemotherapy.

Magnetic resonance imaging (MRI) provides a three-dimensional analysis of the tumor and is helpful in determining encroachment on versus invasion of vital intrathoracic structures with special regard to the extradural space extension.

Bone marrow aspiration at multiple sites and osteomedullary biopsy are systematically performed to detect bone marrow involvement.[15] Total body scintigraphy with 131 or 125 I metaiodobenzylguanidine is a major improvement in the detection of distant metastases. Sensitivity of the examination approaches 90%. The absence of isotopic fixation after treatment indicates a complete remission of metastatic disease.[16]

Summary of Surgical Treatment

Anesthetic management is based on techniques normally used in thoracic surgery, including appropriate monitoring and use of large-bore venous catheters.

The aim of surgery is to ensure a complete resection of the neoplasm. However, en bloc resection may be difficult or dangerous in bulky tumors, in certain locations, or when there is massive invasion of adjacent vital structures. Therefore, tumor division must not be regarded as a technical mistake and may facilitate safer resection.[17,18]

Surgical Approach

Posterolateral thoracotomy is advisable in a great majority of cases. For tumors in the upper mediastinum or involving the thoracic inlet, the pleural cavity is entered in the second or third intercostal space. A combined supraclavicular approach is seldom required to ensure a complete resection. Extension into the thoracic inlet is usually removed through the thoracic approach.

For tumors arising in the middle or lower mediastinum, the level at which the pleural space is entered must be guided by the radiological projection of the middle part of the neoplasm.

In bulky tumors, it may be necessary to perform a second thoracotomy two or three spaces below, through the same skin incision.

Tumor dissection is performed in the extra-pleural plane. In bulky tumors, dissection and proximal control of the aorta, esophagus, azygos vein, and phrenic and pneumogastric nerves are mandatory distant from the tumor. These organs may be encroached on or invaded by neoplasm, and their dissection without initial control can be hazardous. Progressive mobilization of the neoplasm follows the intercostal spaces involved by the tumor. All intercostal neurovascular bundles must be carefully ligated and transected as proximally as possible. Tumor extension into intervertebral foramina must be resected.

Since 1986 we have favored use of the Surgitron (ultrasonic surgical system aspirator) as described by Loe and co-workers.[19] It provides a major advance in radical resection of neurogenic tumors. Dissection of neurovascular bundles, major intrathoracic vessels, and intercostal nerves is greatly facilitated. On occasion apparently involved intercostal vessels and nerves may be spared.

Special Locations

Tumors arising from the upper and posterior mediastinum usually enter the thoracic inlet and involve the subclavian artery, the C8-D1 nerve roots, the right recurrent laryngeal nerve, and the lower cervical sympathetic ganglia. Careful dissection performed in the adventitial plane using the Surgitron usually allows complete freeing up of the subclavian artery. In the same way, the phrenic and pneumogastric nerves can usually be spared. In contrast, the sympathetic chain, including the cervical node, is transected in all cases. These tumors can be huge and may lead to tracheobronchial compression, which can require emergency surgery.

Although lower tumors may extend through the diaphragmatic foramen into the inframediastinal space, complete resection is usually possible through the transthoracic approach. However, the aorta, esophagus, and thoracic duct must be carefully located before tumor mobilization.

Extradural involvement, consisting of small tumor extensions into the intervertebral foramina is easy to remove using the Surgitron. However, deeper invasion into the spinal canal requires neurosurgical involvement.

Bilateral tumors (Fig. 21.3A and B) may extend from one paraspinal space to the contralateral and may involve or compress the aorta and esophagus. Complete resection through a single thoracotomy may be difficult and dangerous. In our series, we have favored contralateral thoracotomy 7 days later to ensure complete removal of the tumor.

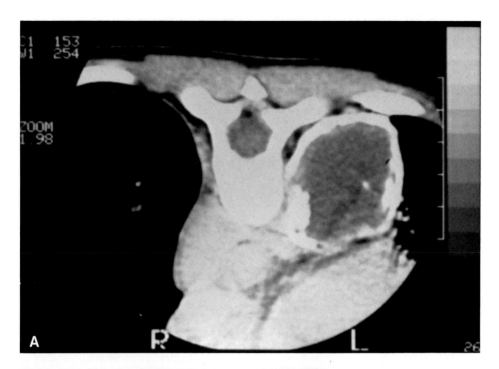

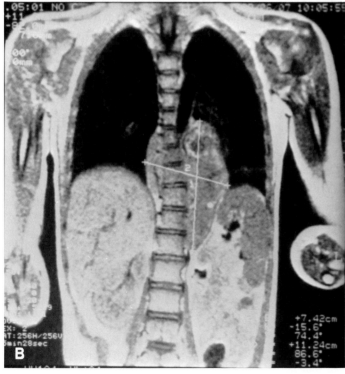

FIGURE 21.3 A. Bilateral sympathetic tumor (CAT scan). **B.** Bilateral sympathetic tumor (MRI).

Combined Therapy

Radiotherapy

Radiosensitivity of the neuroblastoma is accepted by most authors. However, the use of radiation must be tempered by the complications of growth disturbance and pulmonary fibrosis, particularly in children less than 5 years of age.

Radiotherapy, in small doses (25 to 35 Gy) according to the age, using high-energy proton irradiation, provides optimum results. We limit radiotherapy to the postoperative period with the aim of local control of residual microscopic tumor.

In disease that is locally advanced, radiotherapy is sometimes indicated after chemotherapy and surgical resection.

Chemotherapy

Despite various chemotherapeutic trials during the last two decades it has not been demonstrated that neuroblastoma can be cured by chemotherapy alone. However, the development of effective chemotherapy has dramatically improved the outlook of patients with neuroblastoma. Multidrug chemotherapy is now commonly recommended, using a combination of three or four cytotoxic agents from the following: cyclophosphamide, doxorubicin, vincristine, cisplatin, epidophyllotoxine.[20] These agents have proved to be consistently effective, with a rate of response ranging from 25% to 67%.[20] The most significant results are observed after aggressive chemotherapy using high doses and frequent cycles.

In our series, chemotherapy evolved with time. A conservative schedule with alternating vincristine and cyclophosphamide was followed until 1974. Then a combination of high doses of cyclophosphamide with vincristine and adriamycin was given alternatively, either as a primary treatment for disseminated disease or as adjuvant therapy after operation.[21]

Comments

Between 1960 and 1988, 122 tumors of the sympathetic system were surgically resected: 24 tumors were benign and 98 malignant (neuroblastoma and ganglioneuroblastoma). There was no sex predilection and tumors were observed at an equal rate on both sides of the chest. Figure 21.1 breaks down the author's series by histological types and by age.

Before the age of 2 years only one ganglioneuroma was encountered. Between 2 and 5 years of age, malignant tumors are three times as frequent as benign ones. After 5 years of age the absolute number of malignant neoplasms

gradually decreases but the degree of malignancy rises. The prognoses for neuroblastoma and ganglioneuroblastoma were similar. The histological subtyping did not influence therapeutic management in our experience.[21]

Since 1964, tumor marker assays have been systematically determined, except in chronic diarrhea. In this subgroup of four patients, VIP radioimmunological assays were performed in one child only. The serum concentration was very elevated but declined rapidly with effective treatment, which was also associated with regression of the diarrhea.

Preoperative assessment of the neoplasm before the use of computerized axial tomography led to misdiagnosis in three cases. At exploratory thoracotomy the mediastinal mass proved to be a teratoma in one case, a hemangiolymphangioma in another, and an aneurysm of the descending thoracic aorta in the third. The chief technical hazards during operation are related to local and regional extensions of the neoplasm.

Among 122 tumors of the sympathetic system, 49 involved the intervertebral foramina, 44 the intercostal muscles, 33 the thoracic inlet, and 7 the inframediastinal space. Nineteen patients had extradural involvement extending into the medullary canal and required emergency laminectomy. Resection of the thoracic portion of the neoplasm was performed after an 8- to 15-day interval. Twenty-four patients had a bulky tumor also involving the opposite hemithorax. In most cases, the esophagus and aorta were displaced or enclosed within the tumor. However, direct invasion of these organs is rare. Five patients had a synchronous abdominal tumor.

Results

No patients died during the early postoperative period. Four patients (3%) suffered postoperative complications, including two with chylothorax that subsided spontaneously and two with phrenic nerve palsy. One of these patients required a diaphragmatic plication.

Tumor resection was macroscopically complete in 89 patients. Among the other 33 patients, complete tumor removal could not be guaranteed because of extension into the foramina or the intercostal muscles or because of adherence to paraspinal ligaments. It is our belief that the recent use of the Surgitron has improved resectability rate. All 24 patients with ganglioneuroma have been cured after total surgical resection.

Among 98 patients with malignant tumor, 84 were followed for at least 24 months. Nineteen died from progression of the disease and 64 are alive without evidence of disease, including 33 patients who are 10-year survivors. In our experience, the influence of tumor staging on survival results is comparable to reports of others (Table 21.4).

Hourglass tumors seem to be associated with a less favorable prognosis and have a 34% mortality rate.

Late Postresectional Disorders

Late complications are observed after a majority of the hourglass tumor resections. Among 16 long-term survivors, 7 have mild to severe neurological deficit related to initial paraplegia.

Skeletal deformities have developed in 24 cases, after treatment of both benign and malignant neoplasms. Spinal deformities including kyphosis and scoliosis are most likely to occur when more than four intercostal neurovascular bundles have been transected or after decompression laminectomy.

However, after intraperiosteal laminectomy or when the articular processes are spared, there is a lower rate of spinal deformities. Postoperative irradiation of residual tumor plays a role in the genesis of such deformities.

Linear growth of the spine is usually limited, resulting in a dorsal kyphosis, or a scoliosis if the vertebral bodies are only partially involved. Therefore, all patients submitted to surgical resection of a neurogenic tumor require prolonged orthopedic surveillance.

Horner's syndrome secondary to resection of a cervicothoracic neoplasm usually does not improve.

Breast aplasia and general disturbances in growth are rare complications with modern radiation techniques.

Scheme of Therapeutic Management

The current therapeutic approach in tumors of the sympathetic system is guided by the age of

the patient and the extent of the disease at diagnosis.

Prognosis of neuroblastoma is significantly improved before the age of 1 year. Local control of the primary tumor is the aim of surgical resection.

During the last decade, therapeutic indications have been clarified. Our current approach can be summarized as follows:

1. Benign tumors (ganglioneuromas) are virtually cured after a complete surgical resection. However, technical difficulties such as large tumor size, local spread, or adhesions may necessitate extensive dissection.

2. For malignant tumors therapeutic indications depend on the stage of the neoplasm.

   a. *Metastatic disease* (stages IV and IV S) is usually managed by chemotherapy. Patients demonstrating a significant response at both primary and metastatic levels may be eligible for surgical resection.

   b. *Nonmetastatic disease.* Before the age of 1 year, primary surgical resection is our current approach in all patients regardless of the neoplasm, because initial aggressive chemotherapy is not well tolerated.

   After the age of 1 year, bulky tumors (stages II and III) are first treated by preoperative chemotherapy, using three to six combination cycles of the following agents: vincristine, cyclophosphamide, doxorubicin, cysplatinum, Etoposide (Vp 16), or Tenifoside (VM 26). Chemotherapy is usually effective in a majority of cases with very significant reduction in size of the neoplasm. Commonly the residual tumor is limited to a simple thickening of the mediastinal border, detectable only by CAT or MRI. The aim of surgical treatment is radical removal of the residual tumor.

In our experience, however, frozen section examination of the operative specimen has shown in all cases that tumor cells were present in residual tissue.

On unusual occasions the neoplasm fails to respond to primary chemotherapy. In spite of this, surgical resection may be considered after six chemotherapy cycles.

Postoperative Treatment

Indications for postoperative treatment depend on whether the surgical resection can be considered complete or not. After radical resection, with the tumor margin free of malignant cells at specimen examination and no lymph node involvement, no additional treatment is needed. However, clinical, radiological, and biological

TABLE 21.4 Staging and Mortality: Neuroblastomas and Ganglioneuroblastomas[a]

Stage	Cases	Mortality
I	15	0
II	25	2
III	26	4
IV	13	12
IV S	5	1
	84	19 (22%)

[a] Eighty-four cases.

follow-up study is mandatory. In all other cases, combination chemotherapy (six to eight cycles) is required. Irradiation is reserved for patients in whom the tumor was not completely removed.

In hourglass tumors with medullary compression, emergency decompression laminectomy is required. Resection of the thoracic portion of the tumor is performed later, after the chemotherapy protocol already mentioned. In tumors with asymptomatic extradural extension, primary chemotherapy may be considered after careful neurosurgical assessment.

Other Neurogenic Tumors

The other neurogenic tumors are rare and are essentially neurofibroma and pheochromocytoma.

Neurofibromas arise from the nerve sheath or nerve fibers and are associated with von Recklinghausen's disease. The combination of sympathetic tumors with von Recklinghausen's disease is reported with an unusual frequency.[6] In such situations, the detection of a tumor arising from the posterior mediastinum leads to a difficult diagnostic and management problem. High urinary levels of tumor markers and MIBG scintigraphy represent major tools to differentiate a simple neurofibroma from a neuroblastoma.

Pheochromocytoma may occur as a primary lesion, and we have seen one case. The diagnosis can be made by measurement of elevated catecholamines in the blood.

MEDIASTINAL LYMPHADENOPATHIES

Mediastinal lymph node enlargements secondary to neoplasm or inflammation are frequent. Lymphadenopathies are the most common tumors involving the middle mediastinum in childhood.

Lymphomas

Lymphatic tumors, including the well-recognized entities of Hodgkin's disease and non-Hodgkin's lymphoma, represent the most frequent malignant mediastinal tumors. However, surgical resection is very seldom required in these lesions. Surgery may contribute to diagnosis by providing large samples of neoplastic tissue, using either anterior mediastinoscopy or thoracotomy when percutaneous needle biopsy guided by CAT scanner has failed. Indications for resection are rare. The wide majority of Hodgkin's and non-Hodgkin's lymphomas receive multidrug chemotherapy combined with irradiation.

On rare occasions, a residual mass may be detectable at staging with CAT scan or MRI. Surgical resection of such a localized mass and histological examination may be required to differentiate postchemotherapy fibrosis from residual tumor tissue. Histological findings guide in the assessment of treatment effectiveness and in modifying that treatment. During the last 4 years, six patients were referred to us for a residual mass localized in the mediastinum. Their ages ranged from 10 months to 15 years. Four lymphomas were classified T cell type and two B cell type. Three T lymphomas and one B lymphoma demonstrated complete tumor sterilization at specimen examination.

Granulomatous Lymphadenitis and Inflammatory Nodes

In the large group of granulomatous lymphadenitis and inflammatory nodes only two disorders may require surgical resection.

Angiofollicular lymph node hyperplasia (Castleman's disease) was described in 1956 as a form of benign lymph node hyperplasia simulating thymoma.[22] Seventy percent are found within the mediastinum, predominantly in the anterior portion. Patients are usually asymptomatic, although they may have fever, anemia, signs of mediastinal compression, or all these symptoms. Angiography demonstrates the vascularity of the lesion. As in the experience of others, we have removed a tumor identified as Castleman's disease in a 5-year-old girl, because of diagnostic uncertainty (thymoma suspected).

Mediastinal or hilar lymphadenopathy secondary to infection by *Mycobacterium tuberculosis* is common in children with primary tuberculosis and may be manifested as a mediastinal mass. However, this disorder is at present uncommon except in recent immigrants. In a minority of cases, surgical excision or drainage is required to prevent fistulization into the trachea or the bronchus. We have not encountered any such cases in the last 10 years.

GERM CELL TUMORS

Primary germ cell tumors may occasionally arise in extragonadal areas from primordial germ cells of the nephrogenic ridge persisting after embryogenesis. These tumors may develop anywhere from the sacrococcygeal area to the base of the skull. The anterosuperior mediastinum is the most common location, but occasionally they occur within the posterior mediastinum,[23] the pericardial sac,[24] or, rarely, within the lung.[25] Intrathoracic locations have been reported to comprise 7% of all gonadal and extragonadal germ cell tumors in childhood.[26]

Pathological and Biological Definitions

"The two oldest schools of thought attribute the origin of teratomas to germ cells and to undifferentiated embryonic cells respectively. Out of these differing histogenic concepts have arisen disparities in classification that persist to our day."[27]

We have used the WHO classification:[28]

Seminoma (or dysgerminoma): thoracic localization is very rare in childhood.

Nonseminomatous germ cell tumors are of the following subgroups:

α-Fetoprotein- (AFP-) secreting yolk sac tumors (YSTs) have many different tissue types, such as vesicular, labyrinthic, papillary or angioid,[29] which are found in varying proportions within the same tumor. Schiller-Duval corpuscles and hyalin globules are not specific but aid in the diagnosis.

Chorionic gonadotropic hormone (β-human chorionic gonadotropin [BHCG]) secreting choriocarcinomas are characterized by association of cytotrophoblastic clear cells and syncytiotrophoblastic giant cells.

Embryonal carcinomatas (ECs) with an epithelial or cord component do not secrete AFP or β-HCG.[30]

Teratomata: When the tissues are well differentiated and organoid, that is, corresponding to mature tissues (bone, nerve), the teratoma is mature and benign (dermoid cyst). When the differentiation is not complete, the tumor is considered immature and malignant. The two forms are often combined within the same tumor. The mature teratoma would appear to be the final outcome of the immature teratoma.[31]

These different subgroups are often associated in the same tumor. It is never possible to be sure that the teratoma is fully mature; a minimal embryonal component may be present. Detection of AFP or β-HCG on immunohistochemical slides confirms the presence of malignancy.

Biology

The yolk sac tumor component secretes AFP,[29] which can be detected by radioimmunology or immunoenzymologic assay. Trophoblastic tissue secretes HCG, of which the Beta component is specific. Abnormally high levels of AFP or BHCG confirm the presence of these components in the tumor.

Clinical Features

A variable proportion of benign germ cell tumors (mature teratoma) are asymptomatic, although signs or symptoms referable to the presence of a mediastinal mass are frequent in teratoma (tracheal or pleuropulmonary compression). Klinefelter's syndrome appears to predispose to the development of germ cell tumors, especially nonseminomatous tumors.[30] Intrapericardial teratomas have a higher incidence in infancy. They are an important subset of mediastinal germ cell tumors to recognize. If there is a significant delay in diagnosis and treatment, they can be fatal because of compression of the heart and great vessels. Furthermore, intrapericardial teratomatas are found to be consistently benign.[27] Symptoms are related to cardiac tamponade and pericardial effusion. Cardiac ultrasonography usually demonstrates a displacement of cardiac structures.

On chest roentgenogram, CAT scan, or MRI, the mediastinal mass is usually in the anterosuperior compartment, and generally asymmetrical, with extension into one hemithorax or the other (Fig. 21.4). In rare instances, the mass occupies the entire anterosuperior plane of the chest. The presence of intratumoral or peritumoral calcifications is not rare. A high level of tumor markers—β-HCG and α-fetoprotein—is correlated with the presence of malignant components. They decline rapidly with effective treatment. Determination of tumor marker assays can lead to the biological diagnosis of malignant nonseminomatous tumor in nearly 75% of cases.[31]

Surgical Approach

Mediastinal germ cell tumors are best approached through a sternal-splitting incision. In rare instances, asymmetrical growth of the neoplasm into one hemithorax requires a lateral thoracotomy. In bulky tumors extending bilaterally into both hemithoraxes, we favor a bilateral anterior thoracotomy combined with a transverse section of the sternal body. This extensive approach provides a large exposure and control of both hilar vessels, superior vena cava, aorta, and phrenic nerves. Benign teratomas are commonly encapsulated, and dissection from the pericardial sac and the great vessels is usually easily performed. In malignant teratomas, multiple encroachments or adherence to adjacent organs requires combined en bloc resection of lung and a portion of the diaphragm or anterior pericardial sac. As in neurogenic tumors, dissection from vital structures is facilitated by the use of the ultrasonic dissection system aspirator (Surgi-

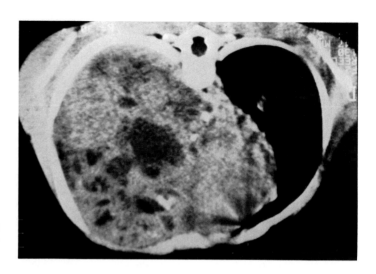

FIGURE 21.4 CAT scan of a bulky teratoma with intratumoral calcification.

tron). When there is adherence to thymic tissue, resection of a thymic lobe is easy to perform.

For an intrapericardial teratoma, the surgical approach must be guided by the location of the neoplasm at ultrasonography. Most of these tumors arise from one side of the heart and are rarely circumferential.[27] In such a case a lateral thoracotomy is better than a sternotomy. The chief technical hazard of operation is inadvertent injury to the coronary vessel that usually lies close to the margin of the neoplasm.

Comments

Between 1967 and 1988, 12 children (10 boys and 2 girls) were referred to us for surgical management of a mediastinal germ cell tumor. Their ages ranged from 2 months to 10 years. Four tumors were benign and eight malignant.

Among the four benign tumors, two were situated in the anterosuperior mediastinum. Acute tracheal compression in one of these patients required intubation, emergency surgery, and postoperative mechanical ventilation. He was the only patient not immediately extubated in our experience. Another patient had a posterior mediastinal mass, suspected to be a neurogenic tumor. The fourth one, two months of age, had a tumor located in the pericardium. The neoplasm was easily dissected free of the heart after careful exposure of the left coronary artery.

During the same period of time, eight patients (seven male and one female) were referred for malignant germ cell tumor (Table 21.5).

Dyspnea and chest pain were the most common complaints. Calcifications were obvious on chest roentgenograms in 30% of cases. In six cases, the mediastinal neoplasm was associated with a dysgonadic or endocrine syndrome. Association with Klinefelter's syndrome is a consistant observation.[32–34] Male hypogonadism combined with an XXY karyotype was encountered in three patients in early puberty: two lacked the XXY karyotype and Cushing's syndrome was encountered in the only female patient of this series. In her, hypercorticism declined following tumor resection.

The neoplasm ranged in weight from 250 to 1500 g. Gross morphological findings revealed lobulation and variegation with both solid and cystic areas.[24,34,35,36] Cerebroid portions were strongly suggestive of sarcomatous or malignant yolk sac components at gross inspection when they were present. The microscopic structure was often difficult to assess.[36] In toto sampling of the primary tumor was mandatory to exclude the presence of frankly malignant elements. The malignant component was not initially detected in two of our patients because it involved a minor portion of the tumor (cases 1 and 4). High serum levels of α-fetoprotein later demonstrated the presence of a yolk sac component. Among eight patients, six had complex and mixed immature teratomata, one an embryonal carcinoma, and one a pure immature teratoma. In this latter patient, a complete resection was performed and the patient is alive without evidence of disease.

Current Approach in Therapeutic Management

In mediastinal tumors associated with a significant level of tumor markers, primary chemotherapy is required. Chemotherapy usually consists of alternate courses of actinomycin D, cyclophosphamide, and vincristine, bleomycin, doxorubicin (Adriblastin), or cisplatin. In our se-

TABLE 21.5 Malignant Germ Cell Tumors

Case	Age/Sex	Symptoms	Tumor Histology	Preoperative Treatment	Operation	Postoperative Treatment	Results	Duration of Survival
1	5Y/M	Pleurisy, Sexual Precocity	YST TM		CSE	RT CHEMO	Dead Metastases	15 mo
2	2,5Y/F	Pleurisy, Cushing's Syndrome	CC TM		CSE	RT CHEMO	Dead Metastases	7 mo
3	6Y/M	Klinefelter's Syndrome	YST CC		CSE	CHEMO	Alive NED	17 yr
4	10Y/M	Chest Pain, Respiratory Distress	YST CC		CSE	RT	Dead Local Recurrence	3 yr
5	2,5Y/M	Pleurisy	EC		ISE	CHEMO	Dead Local Recurrence	2 yr
6	10Y/M	Chest Pain, Klinefelter's Syndrome	EC YST	CHEMO	CSE	CHEMO	Alive NED	12 yr
7	10Y/M	Klinefelter's Syndrome	TI		CSE	CHEMO	Alive NED	9 yr
8	11Y/M	Sexual Precocity	YST CC	CHEMO	CSE	CHEMO	Alive NED	4 yr

EC = embryonal carcinoma, YST = yolk sac tumor, CC = choriocarcinoma, TI = teratoma immature, TM = teratoma mature, RT = radiation therapy, CHEMO = chemotherapy, CSE = complete surgical excision, ISE = incomplete surgical excision, NED = no evidence of disease.

ries, despite the usual effectiveness of this treatment, mediastinal tumors rarely demonstrated a complete response. Surgery was always indicated, in order to resect the residual tumor, which was still bulky in some instances.

After complete surgical excision, no combined therapy is needed. Follow-up study of the tumor marker level (α-fetoprotein and β-HCG) is mandatory. Postoperative chemotherapy is instituted when the level, which initially declines with treatment, does not reach normal values within 4 months of surgical removal.

For patients in whom the mediastinal germ cell tumor is not completely removed (debulking operation) intermittent combination chemotherapy seems the most beneficial regimen to date.

In mediastinal neoplasms without elevated levels of β-HCG or α-fetoprotein, a surgical approach is required in all cases. It provides adequate sampling of the primary tumor, which is unresectable at initial operation or allows complete tumor removal. For patients in whom the neoplasm is unresectable at initial operation, cytoreductive adjuvant therapy may permit a subsequent operation with an attempt at debulking or perhaps complete resection. For all others in whom a complete resection has been performed no combined therapy is needed except for those harboring an embryonal carcinoma for whom chemotherapy is recommended.

The therapeutic management of recurrent tumors depends on the level of tumor markers. With elevated markers, chemotherapy is required before reassessment of the tumor. In all others surgical resection should be considered if staging demonstrates the potential for complete tumor removal.

MESENCHYMAL TUMORS
Tumors of Vascular Origin

Lymphangiomas (hygromas) mainly occur in childhood. They comprise a variety of malformations in which embryonal lymphatic vessels have not connected with the lymphatic or venous network at embryogenesis. This results in the formation of dilatations and cysts. Lymphangiomas are usually localized in the anterior mediastinum but may extend as far as into the neck region or cause considerable signs of displacement. They appear as cavernous or cystic tumors. Commonly these tumors cause no symptoms and are detected on a routine roentgenogram. On rare occasions, patients with mediastinal lymphangioma exhibit acute symptoms because of complications such as inflammation, intracystic bleeding, or chylothorax. At ultrasonography and CAT scan, lymphangiomas display the characteristics of a water-filled mass. Lymphangiomas are usually associated with a venous element, which establishes the diagnosis of hemolymphangioma.

Phleboliths within the mass may indicate such a lesion. CAT scan with contrast reveals the vascularity of this tumor.

Pure hemangiomas of the mediastinum are rare neoplasms.[37] At CAT scan they are solid masses of variable shape, surrounded by a connective tissue capsule, and may be multiple. They are usually localized to the posterior mediastinum. Angiography helps to identify the collecting venous network.

Both lymphangiomas and hemangiomas require surgical resection. Technical difficulties may be encountered because of encroachment on major mediastinal organs, including the superior vena cava, esophagus, or phrenic nerve. Furthermore, recurrence related to incomplete resection is a consistent observation. However, in diffuse and multiple lymphangiomas with dense adherence to adjacent organs that presents considerable surgical hazard, part of the capsule may be left in place. After surgical excision of a lymphangioma located in the lower anterior mediastinum, further lymphatic dilatations may develop, resulting in chylothorax, pulmonary edema, or pericardial effusion.[38]

Thoracic hemangiomas are usually easily removed without the severe postoperative blood loss reported in other locations. The tumor is surrounded by a connective tissue capsule that is safely dissected free of the adjacent tissue. Postoperative irradiation is of no value in this neoplasm, and no malignant transformation has been reported.

We have encountered six cystic lymphangiomas and one mediastinal hemangioma in children whose ages ranged from 3 months to 10 years. For the lymphangiomas, 50% of the surgical resections were incomplete and one patient required reoperation to remove a cervical extension. Postoperatively, one patient displayed phrenic palsy and another Horner's syndrome.

All other neoplasms of vascular origin (including hemangiopericytoma and hemangioendothelioma) are far less frequent than the two previously described tumors.

Other Mesenchymal Tumors

Other mesenchymal tumors found in childhood include neoplasms arising from fibrous tissue, adipose tissue, and smooth or striated muscles.

Pericardial cysts are rare and arise from persistence of the distal portion of a ventral parietal recess of the pericardium. These are frequently located at the right pericardiophrenic junction. Diagnosis is easily made by echocardiography or CAT scan. The pericardial cyst is frequently asymptomatic and always benign. Local resection is indicated only with a bulky mass. We did not encounter any of these lesions in children below the age of 16 years.

Mediastinal lipomas are exceedingly rare.[39] Despite their intrinsic benignity, these tumors are clinically very important because they tend to grow to enormous proportions and cause life-threatening compression. Total extirpation is essential because this tumor has a tendency to recur.

Liposarcomas are also very rarely encountered.[40] A combination of surgical resection, irradiation, and chemotherapy seems to be the most effective treatment.

Lipoblastoma is a neoplasm found in infancy arising from the fetal adipose tissue. The postresectional course is consistently benign.[41,42]

Rhabdomyosarcomas are malignant tumors of striated muscle origin. They are the most frequent soft tissue sarcoma in children, yet they are seldom encountered as primary mediastinal neoplasms.[43] We have observed only one case.

OTHER RARE TUMORS

Among all other rare mediastinal tumors encountered in childhood, thymic lesions must be identified. Cysts and hyperplasia are the predominant pathological findings.

Thymic hyperplasia (typical thymic shadow) in asymptomatic infants up to 4 years old must not be regarded as a tumor, and involution can be expected. Unless associated with myasthenia gravis, thymic hyperplasia below the age of 4 years requires only careful observation and annual chest roentgenograms. In the older child who is asymptomatic and has typical roentgenographic features of thymic enlargement, surgical resection is debatable.[44] The main risk is failing to treat a thymoma or an intrathymic teratoma without elevated markers.

Thymic cysts[45] and thymolipomas[46] occurring in childhood display specific features at ultrasonography and CAT scan. These lesions are safely removed and resection results in cure.

Thymomas

Although the term *thymoma* has been applied in the literature to indicate any type of tumor that originates in the thymus, it should be restricted to tumors originating in thymic epithelium.[47] These thymic lesions are not common in childhood and account for only 5% of mediastinal masses in children.[48] Symptoms caused by compression and invasion are frequent because thymoma is usually aggressive and quickly growing. Association with a variety of syndromes (myasthenia gravis, leukemia, and so on) is rarely reported.

In the vast majority of cases, percutaneous fine needle biopsy provides the diagnosis. We have encountered four patients with invasive thymomata referred for surgical resection. Stage I disease (intracapsular growth only) was not observed in any of our patients. All but one died within 6 months of progression of the disease. The remaining patient is alive without evidence of disease at 8 years. In this patient, reductive chemotherapy of a bulky neoplasm was first used and the residual mass was then successfully removed.

In treating an invasive thymoma aggressive surgical staging and total excision should be attempted. The best results in both children and adults are reported after complete removal, chemotherapy, and complementary irradiation.[44]

Among the other mediastinal tumors, endocrine tumors such as thyroid or parathyroid are exceedingly rare in childhood. We have encountered none.

REFERENCES

1. Rubino P: *Giornale Sc Med* 1810;7–297.
2. Hart H: *Pathological Anatomy, Clinical Study and Diagnosis of Mediastinal Diseases.* Philadelphia: Blakston, 1889.
3. Smith B, Stone J: Mediastinal tumors in children. *Ann Surg* 1924;79:687–709.
4. Marquezy, Heraux: Les tumeurs du médiastin chez l'enfant. *Gaz Med Fr* 1933;97–102.
5. Bolande RP: The neurocristopathies. *Hum Biol* 1974;5:409.
6. Schweisguth O: *Tumeurs solides de l'enfant.* Paris: Flammarion, 1979.
7. Shimada H, Chatten J, Newton WA, et al: Histopathologic prognostic factors in neuroblastic tumors. *J Natl Cancer Inst* 1984;73:405–416.
8. Kemshead JT, Pritchard J: Neuroblastoma: Recent development and current challenges. *Cancer Surveys* 1984;3:691–708.
9. La brosse EH, Comoy E, Buhuon C, et al: Catecholamine metabolism in neuroblastoma. *J Natl Cancer Inst* 1976;57:433–438.
10. Evans A, D'Angio GJ, Randolph: A proposed staging for children with neuroblastoma. *Cancer* 1971;27:374–378.
11. Buck J, Bruchet C, Girbert R, et al: Specific uptake of m-125 Iodobenzylguanidine in the human neuroblastoma cell like SK-H-NH. *Cancer Res* 1985;45:6366–6370.
12. Zeltzer PM, Marangos PJ, Evans AE, et al: Serum neuron specific enolase in children with neuroblastoma. *Cancer* 1986;57:1230–1234.
13. Seeger RC, Brodeur GM, Stather H: Association of multiple copies of the N-myc oncogene with rapid progression of neuroblastomas. *N Engl J Med* 1985;313:111–116.
14. Couanet D, Caillaud JM, Geoffray A, et al: Ponction biopsie percutanée à l'aiguille fine des masses tumorales de l'enfant. *Ann Radiol* 1986;29:293–300.
15. Baylec C, Hartmann O, Garre S: The value of bone marrow aspirates in 10 sites for detection of bone marrow involvement in neuroblastoma. 17th SIOP Meeting, Barcelona 1984;238–239.
16. Hoefnager CA, Vouté PA, De Kraker J: Total body scintigraphy with 131 I meta-iodobenzylguanidine for detection of neuroblastoma. *Diagn Imag Clin Med* 1985;54:21–27.
17. Catacano PW, Newton WA, Willima TE, et al: Reasonable surgery for thoracic neuroblastoma in infants and children. *J Cardiothorac Surg* 1978; 76:459–463.
18. Lemoine G, Montupet P, Baldeyrou P: Tumeurs neurogènes intrathoraciques: A propos de 78 cas. *Ann Chir Thorac Cardiovasc,* 1981;3:227–231.
19. Loe R, Applebaum H, Takasugi J, et al: Resection of advanced stage neuroblastoma with the Cavitron ultrasonic surgical aspiration. *J Pediatr Surg* 1988;23:1135–1138.
20. Carli M, Pastore G, Perilongo G, et al: The role of chemotherapy in neuroblastoma. In: Raybaud E, et al, eds. *Pediatric Oncology.* Amsterdam: Excerpta Medica 1982;151–160.
21. Hartmann O, Scopinaro M, Tournade MF: Neuroblastomes traités à l'Institut Gustave Roussy de 1975 à 1979 (173 cas). *Arch Fr Pediatr* 1983;40:15–21.
22. Castelman B, Iverson L, Menendez V: Localized mediastinal lymph node hyperplasia resembling thymoma. *Cancer* 1956;9:822–830.
23. Karl ST, Dunn J: Posterior mediastinal teratomas. *J Pediatr Surg* 1985;20:508–510.
24. Summer TE, Crowe JE, Klein A: Intrapericardial teratomas. *Pediatr Radiol* 1980;10:51–53.
25. Lack EE, Weinstein HJ, Welch KJ: Mediastinal germ cell tumors in childhood: A clinical pathological study of 21 cases. *J Thorac Cardiovasc Surg* 1985;89:826–835.
26. Dehner LP: Gonadal and extragonadal germ cell neoplasia of childhood. *Hum Pathol* 1983;14:493–511.
27. Gonzalez C: *Extragonadal Teratomas: Atlas of Tumor Pathology.* Washington: AFIP, 1982.
28. Mostofi FK, Sobin LH: *International Histological Classification of Tumors of Testis* (n 16). Geneva: World Health Organization, 1977.
29. Truong LD, Harris L, Mattioli C, et al: Endodermal sinus tumors of the mediastinum: A report of seven cases and review of the literature. *Cancer* 1986;58:730–739.
30. Manivel C, Wick MR, Abenoza P: The occurrence of sarcomatous components in primary mediastinal germ cell tumors. *Am J Surg Pathol* 1984;10:711–717.
31. Carter D, Dibro MC, Touloukian RJ: Benign clinical behavior of immature mediastinal teratoma in infancy and childhood: Report of two cases and review of the literature. *Cancer* 1982;49:398–402.
32. Chaussain JL, Lemerle J, Roger M, et al: Klinefelter syndrome, tumor and sexual precocity. *J Pediatr* 1980;97:607–609.
33. Flamant F, Bienayme J, Bargy F: Les tumeurs germinales malignes de l'enfant ou tératomes malins. *Arch Fr Pediatr* 1983;40:117–122.
34. Baldeyrou P, Andre-Bougaran J, Lemoine G: Les tu-

meurs germinales primitives du médiastin chez l'enfant. *Ann Chir Thorac Cardiovasc* 1986;40:578–589.

35. Wychulis AR, Payne WS, Clagette OT, et al: Surgical treatment of mediastinal tumors. *J Thorac Cardiovasc Surg* 1971;62:379–392.

36. Wolley MM: Malignant teratomas in infancy and childhood. *World J Surg* 1980;4:39–47.

37. Cohen AJ, Sbaschnig RJ, Hochholzer L, et al: Mediastinal hemangiomas. *Ann Thorac Surg* 1987;(43)6:656–659.

38. Johnson DW, Klazynski PT, Gondon WH, et al: Mediastinal lymphangioma and chylothorax: The role of radiotherapy. *Ann Thorac Surg* 1986;41(3):325–328.

39. Kleinhaus S, Ducharme JC: Mediastinal lipoma in children. *J Pediatr Surg* 1969;66:790–793.

40. Koster B, Bude U: Mediastinal liposarcoma in a 14 year old girl. *Monatsschr Keinderheilk* 1985;133:490–491.

41. Sancho-Cerquella V, Gil-Vernet JM, Caceres F, et al: Lipoblastomatose médiastinale bénigne. *Chir Pediatr* 1985;26(6):379–381.

42. Stringel G, Shandling B, Mancer K, et al: Lipoblastoma in infants and children. *J Pediatr Surg* 1982;17:277–280.

43. Enziger FM, Weiss SW: *Soft Tissue Tumors.* St. Louis, Mo.: CV Mosby Co, 1983.

44. Lake EE: Thymic hyperplasia with massive enlargement: Report of two cases with review of diagnosis criteria. *J Thorac Cardiovasc Surg* 1981;81:741–746.

45. Welch KJ, Tapper D, Vawter GP: Surgical treatment of thymic cystis and neoplasms in children. *J Pediatr Surg* 1979;14(6):691–698.

46. Tazi M, Barahiout M, Assem A, et al: Un nouveau cas de thymolipome chez l'enfant. *Chir Pediatr* 1984;25:233–335.

47. Snover DC, Levine GD, Rosai J: Thymic carcinoma: Five distinct histological variants. *Am J Surg Pathol* 1982;6:451–470.

48. Dehner LP, Martin SA, Summer HW: Thymus related tumors and tumor like lesions in childhood with rapid clinical progression and death. *Hum Pathol* 1977;37:953–957.

Mediastinal Tumors in Infancy and Childhood

Arvin I. Philippart, MD

This chapter by Drs Lemoine and Montupet includes experience very similar to that in large pediatric surgical departments in North America. This commentary will largely follow the organization used by the authors for ease of reading.

Division of the mediastinum into anatomical regions is highly useful in differential diagnosis and appropriate selection of preoperative studies. Subdivision into superior/anterior, middle, and posterior mediastinal regions appears most useful. Masses in the superior mediastinum are largely lymphatic in origin. Anterior mediastinal lesions are most commonly teratomatous. Middle mediastinal lesions include a heterogenous group of vascular, lymphatic, and enterogenous masses. Posterior mediastinal masses are largely neurogenic. Although large-mass lesions may transgress these artificial boundaries, few processes are truly integral to multiple such regions. Those processes that may involve several subdivisions include lymphangioma/hemangioma, fibromatosis, or neurofibromatosis. Additional refinement of differential diagnosis can be obtained by using age at presentation. In general, mass lesions in younger children are more likely to be developmental anomalies than malignant neoplasms.

Such pattern recognition is most valuable in providing economies of time and cost, most important in the child who has a compromised airway. Many diagnostic modalities are now available for the evaluation of such mass lesions, but not all need to be used for prompt diagnosis and initiation of therapy.

NEUROBLASTOMA

The spectrum of neuroblastoma/ganglioneuroma of the posterior mediastinum has always been associated with excellent patient salvage originally

attributed to site and now attributed to lower primary tumor (T), regional node (N), metastasis (M) (TNM) classification. The initial clinical presentation is most commonly the result of serendipitous recognition of a mass lesion on a chest roentgenogram done for other indications. Symptoms, when present, are more commonly cord compression and, less frequently, opsoclonus-polymyoclonus. Rarely is the initial presentation the result of metastatic disease.

Preoperative evaluation in North America has followed cooperative tumor protocols for many years. Of the numerous studies on tissue and body fluids, not all have yet clearly demonstrated differential sensitivities and specificities. A number are unavailable to the clinician at the time of decision making. They are of greater value in the study of tumor biology and longitudinal follow-up evaluation of the individual patient. In initial assessment, the chest film, computerized axial tomography (CAT) scan, and magnetic resonance imaging (MRI), as well as a vanillylmandelic acid (VMA) screen supplemented by bone marrow aspirate is most valuable. Except in the very occasional circumstance of a lytic bone lesion with negative bone marrow aspirate findings, we limit bone biopsy to the rib obtained extraperiosteally at the time of thoracotomy. This has the additional advantage of increasing exposure and minimizing the need for a second intercostal incision. Although the majority of these lesions can be resected intact by enucleation of foraminal extensions, we agree that tumor division necessitated by safety does not appear to compromise prognosis when staging is considered.

The management of extradural intraspinal disease remains incompletely defined. For the patient with symptomatic cord compression, decompressive laminectomy with interval thoracotomy and removal of the primary tumor is the obvious therapeutic strategy. Less clear is the role of surgery in the removal of asymptomatic residual intraspinal disease after resection of the primary tumor. Some have advocated simultaneous resection of the primary tumor and intraspinal mass by resection of pedicles and lamina as an extension of the thoracotomy. We have not used that approach; nor do we consider it necessary in terms of the biology of the disease because of concern about later kyphoscoliosis. For the same reason we have ceased our earlier use of postoperative irradiation in all children and currently use postoperative chemotherapy as the only adjunct to thoracotomy. We have not used preoperative chemotherapy for thoracic lesions with the rare exception of a stage IV initial presentation with a thoracic primary tumor.

Our series of patients is similar in number to that reported by the authors except that ours has a lesser percentage of stage IV lesions and a cure rate greater than 90% for all patients. All tumors with malignant elements are TNM staged and treated with chemotherapy for residual disease. Because of the frequently good prognosis, and because of the minimal benefit of second-look procedures in the abdomen, we have not employed second look operations for thoracic primary lesions. Although there is no objection to staged bilateral thoracotomies for bulky disease, we have not used that approach.

LYMPHOMA

Lymphomas of Hodgkin's or non-Hodgkin's type generally are manifested as either clinically apparent cervical adenopathy with mediastinal involvement on the chest roentgenogram or as airway obstruction with or without adenopathy. Among other studies, metastatic bone surveys are performed for all. Where possible by clinical assessment, a tissue diagnosis is obtained by node biopsy. In Hodgkin's disease, any lytic lesion in bone receives biopsy examination because a positive biopsy result precludes need for abdominal staging procedures. Despite the reports of others, when the diagnosis can only be established by biopsy of the mediastinum, we have used a limited anterior thoracotomy for biopsy to provide adequate tissue for both cell culture and histological examination. Needle biopsy is not uniformly successful, and mediastinoscopy

is frequently precluded, in our view, by a concomitant superior vena caval syndrome. In severe airway obstruction, we have occasionally used a steroid pulse for lympholysis before biopsy without limitation of the subsequent diagnosis.

LYMPHANGIOMA/HEMANGIOMA

Although both vascular elements are frequently present simultaneously in lymphangioma and hemangioma, the hygroma (lymphangioma) is the dominant element in the large majority. These lesions are not uncommon in our experience, and the clinical diagnosis is usually apparent from concomitant neck involvement. We believe strongly that a one-staged cervicomediastinal (via sternotomy) approach with a painstaking (if necessary) attempt at total excision is highly preferable to a staged approach. Secondary operations can be very difficult, often incomplete, and fraught with a higher complication rate. Results of one-stage excision have largely been very good, with the exception of a small subset of patients with diffuse hemangiolymphangioma with diffuse mediastinal involvement and osteolysis of the chest wall (Gorham's syndrome), for which any resection is incomplete, chylothorax is a serious problem, and late nonoperative mortality is significant.

THYMIC HYPERPLASIA

Symmetrical thymic enlargement in an infant is a nonsurgical lesion to be observed in the presence of normal peripheral blood count and bone marrow aspirate results. We have operated on several children with markedly asymmetrical thymic enlargement; findings in individual cases have been unilobar cysts, lipomata, or nodular hyperplasia in patients in whom the opposite lobe was grossly and histologically normal. Thymic lobectomy with biopsy of the opposite normal lobe has had good results. The diagnosis of normality is confirmed by (thymus-) T- and (bursa-) B-cell culture findings, as we have also shown in Castleman's disease.

PART VIII

Chest Injuries

Chapter 22

The Child with Thoracic Trauma

Kurt D. Newman, MD and Martin R. Eichelberger, MD

Trauma is the leading killer of children in North America. Thoracic injuries make up a small but lethal subset of pediatric trauma. The mortality rate of children with a thoracic injury is 26% at Children's National Medical Center (CNMC), a regional pediatric trauma center in Washington, DC.[1] This compares to an overall mortality rate of 2.2% in all injured children. Awareness of the patterns of thoracic injury in children, combined with prompt recognition and expeditious treatment, is the cornerstone of efforts to improve survival.

The incidence of thoracic injury in children differs by geographic region and by size of the study population. Velcek noted a 27.7% incidence in a series of children who died before receiving medical treatment.[2] Mayer reported that 25% of their pediatric patients sustained a thoracic injury.[3] Sinclair and Moore identified thoracic injuries in 15% of children admitted with trauma.[4] In contrast, at CNMC, thoracic injury occurred in 4.4% of 2400 consecutive children admitted for traumatic injury during a 36-month period.[5]

Though rare in children, thoracic injury has a high combined mortality rate, much higher than the rates reported in many adult series.[6,7] The mortality rate associated with chest injury varies directly with the number of anatomical systems affected. Isolated chest injury results in a mortality rate of 5.3%; if two body systems are injured, as assessed by the Abbreviated Injury Scale (AIS), the mortality rate increases to 28.6%; for injuries to three body regions, the mortality rate is 33%. Combined injuries to the head, chest, and abdomen produce a mortality of 38%. Clearly, multisystem injury involving the chest heralds a potentially lethal outcome.

Pediatric thoracic injury usually results from blunt trauma: the incidence is 78% at CNMC. The most common mechanisms are pedestrian injury (37%), presence during motor vehicle crashes (32%), penetrating injury (12%), falls (10%), and child abuse (8%). Occasionally chest trauma is associated with a burn or caustic ingestion. The distribution of causes of injury varies according to the setting: more penetrating injuries in urban areas and more farm vehicle injuries in rural areas. The mortality rate is highest for victims of child abuse.

The high mortality rates are not the only data documenting the severe nature of pediatric chest trauma. Children with thoracic trauma have a lower mean trauma score (TS) than those without thoracic involvement. The mean injury severity score (ISS) is also much higher for children with thoracic injury. These measurements document significant physiological compromise, as well as serious anatomical injuries. TRISS analysis confirms this by showing a much lower probability of survival ($p_s > .701$) in children with chest injury than in those without ($p_s > .977$). Another indicator of severity is the rate of admission to the ICU: 70% for those with thoracic injury compared to 19% in the group of children with no thoracic injury (Table 22.1).

The high mortality and indicators of physiological derangement compel early recognition and treatment of thoracic injury. The approach to the child considers the special differences in anatomy and physiology that require attention during resuscitation and diagnosis. The priorities during resuscitation are airway, breathing, and circulation (ABC).[8]

Provision of a patent and secure airway is the top priority.[9] Perform all airway maneuvers with concern for possible cervical spine injury until it is definitely excluded. This means manual maintenance of cervical in-line stabilization, ap-

TABLE 22.1 Differences in Measures of Injury Severity for Children With and Without Thoracic Injury

| Measurement | Thoracic Injury | | Significance (p Value) |
	Positive ($n = 104$)	Negative ($n = 1982$)	
Mortality Rate	26%	1.4%	<.0001
TRISS	.701	.977	<.107
Trauma Score	10.8	14.8	<.001
Injury Severity Score	26.7	7.3	<.001

plication of a rigid neck collar appropriate for size, or proper backboard immobilization. Suction the mouth to remove foreign material and secretions. The chin lift or jaw thrust maneuver helps open the airway and provides better gas exchange. Oxygen (100%) by face mask is given at all times. If the airway is tenuous or if mask-assisted ventilation fails, endotracheal intubation establishes a secure airway. Head injury and altered consciousness are additional indications for intubation to prevent aspiration and poor ventilation.

The anatomy of the airway of the child frequently makes intubation difficult.[10] The oropharynx is small, thus creating difficulty in visualization and instrumentation of the larynx. Enlarged or inflamed adenoids and tonsils, which are common in children, block the view of the vocal cords, making precise tube placement a challenge. Esophageal intubation is a hazard because of the relatively anterior and cephalad location of the larynx. The vocal cords are more prone to injury than those of adults because the structure is more cartilaginous and distensible. The tongue is relatively large and easily obstructs the small airway.

Since the trachea of the child is short, bronchial intubation or perforation results when a tube is placed too deeply. Use a smaller and shorter endotracheal tube tailored to the size of the child.[11] Employ uncuffed endotracheal tubes to prevent pressure necrosis of the sensitive trachea, which may result in subglottic stenosis. Tolerance of a small leak around the tube helps prevent tracheal injury. Check the tube position immediately by auscultation of breath sounds and confirm by chest roentgenogram. Secure the tube carefully to prevent dislodgment.

Needle cricothyroidotomy is rarely necessary in children but is a safe alternative when facial or oropharyngeal trauma makes intubation difficult. Incise the skin over the cricothyroid membrane, which is palpable just below the thy-roid cartilage. A 14-gauge needle is inserted through the cricothyroid membrane. After several breaths, extend the incision through the membrane and insert a narrow tracheostomy tube. In the smaller child the cricothyroid cartilage readily sustains injury, which may result in an unstable upper airway. Tracheostomy is difficult under emergency conditions; performance is best in the controlled environment of the operating room.

Once the airway is secure, assess the adequacy of ventilation. Hyperventilation (Pco_2 = 28–30 mm Hg) with 100% oxygen is the initial treatment. Alveolar rupture and pneumothorax result from high inspiratory pressures during ventilation, especially in infants or children with noncompliant lungs. Serial, arterial blood gas determination confirms the ability to ventilate and oxygenate the child. Placement of a nasogastric tube decompresses the stomach, which is often distended as a result of aerophagia. Gastric dilatation can reduce diaphragmatic excursion necessary for proper ventilation. Similarly, needle aspiration of the abdomen is lifesaving when massive pneumoperitoneum is present, especially in infants.

Assessment of circulatory status and prevention of shock are the next priorities. Recognition of shock is difficult in the child. An elevated pulse rate (>130 beats/min) and prolonged capillary refill (>2 s) help to suggest the diagnosis of decreased tissue perfusion; a weak and thready peripheral pulse is characteristic since cardiac output decreases with loss of blood. Altered mental status and mottling are often present. Systolic blood pressure (<80 mm Hg) is a relatively poor sign since loss of more than 20% of blood volume is necessary to produce a fall in blood pressure in a child.[12]

Pulse rate and quality, capillary refill, urine output (1 mL/kg/h), and blood pressure are guides to adequacy of resuscitation. While controlling major external bleeding with direct pressure, obtain venous access with at least two large-bore catheters via percutaneous puncture or cutdown exposure of extremity veins. Surgical isolation of the vein is useful, especially in infants and smaller children, when percutaneous access is difficult. The saphenous vein at the ankle or groin is a reliable location for venous cannulation. Resuscitation is most effective through peripheral catheters in children since central venous catheter insertion can cause hemothorax or subclavian artery laceration. Intraosseous infusion is an effective alternative in infants when attempts at other sites fail.

The blood volume of infants and children is approximately 80 mL/kg. Loss of a relatively small volume causes tissue hypoperfusion, shock, and hypotension. Begin resuscitation with the infusion of 20 mL/kg of a crystalloid solution of Ringer's lactate solution and reassess vital signs. If signs do not improve, infuse another 20-mL/kg bolus of fluid. Begin transfusion of packed red blood cells (10 mL/kg) if hypoperfusion persists; repeat if the response is inadequate. Use universal donor blood until type-specific or crossmatched blood becomes available. Blood warmers are useful to prevent hypothermia. If the heart fails, begin external cardiac massage, endotracheal ventilation, insertion of chest tubes bilaterally, and pericardiocentesis as a last maneuver.

Resuscitation of the child with chest trauma begins with a survey for immediate life-threatening injury using inspection, palpation, and auscultation. Recognition of decreased breath sounds, tympany to percussion, and hypotension suggests tension pneumothorax. Perform needle aspiration of the pleura in the fourth intercostal space in the midaxillary line to relieve the compressed air and to establish a diagnosis. Insert a thoracostomy tube in the midaxillary line if air or blood is noted in the pleural space (12 French in infants and 20–24 French in larger children). Use sterile petroleum jelly- (Vaseline)-impregnated gauze to cover an open chest wound that communicates with the pleura.

Needle aspiration of the pericardial space is lifesaving when tamponade is present. If the child responds and is stable, delay thoracotomy until transfer to the operating room. If there is no response, perform an emergency room thoracotomy, especially in the presence of a penetrating injury.

Indications for urgent thoracotomy are as follows:

1. Penetrating wound of the heart or great vessels
2. Massive or continuous intrapleural hemorrhage
3. Open pneumothorax with major chest wall defect
4. Aortogram confirming aortic transection
5. Massive pleural air leak suggestive of bronchial or tracheal disruption
6. Cardiac tamponade after pericardiocentesis
7. Rupture of the esophagus
8. Diaphragmatic rupture
9. No palpable pulse despite cardiac massage

The physiological status of the child determines the timing and location of the thoracotomy; however, the need for emergency room thoracotomy is rare.[13] The most common indication

is failure of the child to respond promptly to resuscitation after a penetrating wound in the area of the midsternum or left sternal border. Emergency room thoracotomy for blunt thoracic trauma is rarely successful.

INJURIES TO THE THORAX

Trauma to the thorax of children produces a wide spectrum of injuries. The severity varies according to the mechanism, amount, and location of force applied and the response of the involved organs. The thorax of the child is quite compliant because of the elasticity of the ribs that results from their greater cartilage content. This compliance diffuses the force of impact, leading to fewer rib fractures than in adults. Diagnosis of rib fracture is by roentgenogram or bone scan in the chronic case observed in abused children.[14] Oral analgesic agents are usually sufficient to control pain; however, intercostal nerve block by local anesthetic instillation provides effective relief for severe pain. Though splinting from the discomfort is common in children, atelectasis rarely occurs. Healing of the rib fracture is usually complete at 6 weeks. Multiple fractures should raise the suspicion of child abuse.

The incidence of rib fracture is 1.6% (33) of 2400 children admitted for trauma to CNMC.[15] Thirty-two percent (32%) of the children with thoracic injury had a rib fracture. There were no deaths in those children with a single rib fracture. The mortality is 42% when a rib fracture is present, an indication of the severe nature of the striking force required to produce a fracture. The average number of fractures was 3.5; multiple rib fractures portend high mortality. All of the rib fractures were produced by blunt trauma, most commonly in pedestrian car crash victims (47%). Child abuse is another significant mechanism. All children with four or more rib fractures had additional concomitant thoracic injuries.[11]

Rib fractures often result in intrapleural injury. Children with rib fractures are twice as likely to have pneumothorax or hemothorax as those without. The sharp edges of the bony fragments tear the pleura and the lung, producing pneumothorax (12.5%), hemothorax (13.5%), or hemopneumothorax (14.5%). Penetrating trauma is another source of intrapleural injury.

Tension pneumothorax requires urgent treatment. Air that cannot escape accumulates in the pleural space after pulmonary parenchymal or bronchial injury. Since the mediastinum of a small child is quite flexible and mobile, the pressure shifts the mediastinum away from the involved side, compresses the contralateral lung, twists the great vessels, and impedes blood return to the right side of the heart. Needle aspiration of the pleura is lifesaving in the unstable child; thoracostomy tube placement is the definitive treatment.

The child with simple pneumothorax manifests tachypnea and oxygen desaturation of the circulating blood, both signs of respiratory compromise. Breath sounds are diminished on the involved side. If the child is stable, a chest roentgenogram confirms the diagnosis before chest tube placement. If the child is unstable, tube placement precedes radiological verification. The overall mortality of children with pneumothorax is 15.4% at CNMC; however, most children die of associated injuries.

Trauma to the chest may also produce a hemothorax, a result of bleeding into the pleural space.[16] Blood loss may be from injury to the intercostal vessels or lung, but bleeding from the heart and great vessels accounts for the mortality rate of 57% when hemothorax is present. Hemothorax is manifested as either hypotension or a hazy density on chest roentgenogram in the less acute case. Occult blood accumulates in the chest and causes hypotension and shock. Treatment of the injury requires restoration of intravascular volume and evacuation of the blood via a chest tube.

If the child is unstable, as manifested by a pulse rate of greater than 130 beats/min, systolic blood pressure of less than 80 mm Hg, pulse pressure less than 20 mm Hg, cyanosis, and slow response to resuscitation, perform emergency thoracotomy to control the bleeding. Continued bleeding through a chest tube is another indication for thoracotomy. A bleeding rate of 1–2 mL/kg/h is useful as a guideline for operative intervention. The physiological response of the child to volume resuscitation is the best guide in decision making. A prompt and sustained response to resuscitation precludes emergency thoracotomy. Persistent shock despite adequate resuscitation is an indication for exploration.

Blunt injury to the chest often produces pulmonary contusion, which was found in 48% of children with thoracic injury. The blunt force is transmitted to the lung parenchyma via the chest wall.[17] The kinetic energy produces a bruise of the lung with transudation of fluid and hemorrhage into the alveolar spaces. After appropriate resuscitation, restrict fluid infusion in the presence of pulmonary contusion to prevent progressive interstitial fluid accumulation. Supplemental oxygen is usually required, and in severe cases mechanical positive-pressure ventilation with positive end-expiratory pressure (PEEP) improves gas exchange. Most injuries heal with time, but complications can develop, especially in relation to nosocomial infection. Administration of steroids has little value, though culture-specific antibiotic administration is appropriate.

At CNMC children with pulmonary contusion had a mortality of 34%, higher when multiple lobes of the lung were involved. This poor outcome reflects the amount of force applied and the associated injuries caused when pulmonary contusion is produced. Improvement in diagnostic sensitivity may enhance treatment schemes. In the early phases of parenchyma injury the chest roentgenogram is often clear; radiological infiltrates become apparent over the subsequent days. A computerized axial tomography (CAT) scan is a more sensitive test for the early recognition of pulmonary injury. Routine chest roentgenogram missed or underestimated 38% of pulmonary injuries in a group of children with abdominal trauma.[18] CAT scan is indicated in children who manifest thoracic injury (Fig. 22.1).

In contrast to adults, children rarely have flail chest.[19] The flexibility of the chest wall usually averts the creation of a flail segment when multiple ribs are injured. A flail chest is identified when a portion of the chest wall moves paradoxically with breathing; on expiration, the flail segment moves outward though the rest of the chest is collapsing; on inspiration, the flail segment falls inward in response to the negative intrathoracic pressure. Ventilation worsens as a consequence of the commonly associated underlying pulmonary contusion. Direct treatment to limiting fluid infusion while enhancing gas exchange with positive-pressure mechanical ventilation.

Suspect tracheobronchial injury when crepitus or subcutaneous emphysema appears on physical examination of the child.[20] Air dissects through the mediastinum, neck, and chest wall after the trachea or bronchus is torn; respiratory distress is common. Diagnosis is most efficient by rigid bronchoscopy under anesthesia, although flexible fiberoptic bronchoscopy is useful in intubated children. Exercise caution with the cervical spine since associated injuries are common. Direct suture repair is necessary in major bronchial injury; however, lesser injury to the distal airway may heal spontaneously. Small and premature infants are especially prone to pneumothorax and pneumomediastinum as a result of barotrauma secondary to the high airway pressure required to ventilate poorly compliant lungs.

With pericardial tamponade the classic picture of bulging neck veins and pulsus paradoxus is rarely found in the acute situation. The scenario of a child in shock after penetrating trauma is more common. In children small amounts of blood in the pericardial space produce compres-

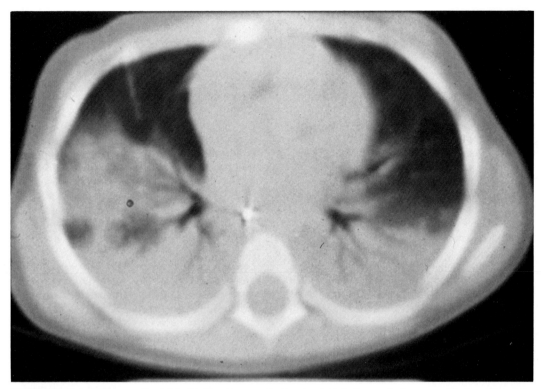

FIGURE 22.1 A CAT scan of a child with blunt trauma to the chest. Note the posterior consolidation bilaterally. The simultaneous chest roentgenogram was clear.

sion of the heart and a decrease in venous return to the right side of the heart with resultant hypotension. A low-velocity-missile or stab wound is the common mechanism of injury; blunt trauma is rarely the cause.[21] Pericardiocentesis is useful to make the diagnosis and may alleviate tamponade. Emergency room thoracotomy also relieves tamponade and allows control of cardiac injury in the unstable child. Exposure through an anterolateral incision in the fourth intercostal space is most effective. The pericardium is tense with accumulated blood; longitudinal incision of the pericardial membrane prevents injury to the phrenic nerve and relieves the pressure. Control lacerations of the heart with direct suture repair using pledgets. Prevent compromise of the coronary vessels by proper placement of myocardial sutures.

Injuries to the heart and great vessels from blunt trauma are rare in children but produce high mortality. Traumatic aortic rupture is infrequent and probably due to the greater flexibility of the mediastinum. A fall or car crash is the usual mechanism of injury. A widened mediastinum revealed by chest roentgenogram or CAT scan prompts an urgent aortogram to confirm the diagnosis. Though most children with an aortic rupture die immediately, a small number survive transport to reach the hospital; hypotension is common. Immediate surgical repair with an interposition graft is lifesaving. Analysis of 551 children who died of trauma revealed an incidence of 2.1% of aortic rupture; the mortality was 92% and pedestrian-auto crash was the mechanism in 46% of the ruptures.[22]

Direct, blunt trauma to the heart produces a spectrum of injuries. The mildest is myocardial contusion, which was present in 7.7% of selected children with multiple injuries.[23] Electrocardiographic (ECG) changes, creatine phosphokinase (CPK) isoenzyme patterns, echocardiography, and radionuclide cardiography detect the injury and define the extent. Most resolve spontaneously but require observation of cardiac rhythm for 24 hours. More severe injuries produced by blunt trauma include papillary muscle rupture, ventricular septum disruption, and rupture of the myocardium.[24] Early recognition with echocardiography and expeditious surgical intervention give the best chance for surviving these rare, lethal injuries.

Diaphragmatic injury occurs with blunt and

penetrating trauma.[25] Gunshot and stab wounds can easily lacerate the diaphragm. A blunt force to the torso may raise intraabdominal pressure, producing a tear of the diaphragm. Diagnosis is difficult, but a high index of suspicion helps improve recognition in the presence of an appropriate mechanism of injury. Repair through the abdomen is preferable. Reapproximation of the edges of the tear and placement of a chest tube are usually sufficient treatment.

Traumatic asphyxia results from severe blunt force to the chest or epigastrium.[26] The ensuing pressure on the inferior vena cava is transmitted cephalad toward the superior vena cava since there are no caval venous valves. The increased venous pressure disrupts the capillary bed and forces blood into the tissues along the distribution of the superior vena cava and brachiocephalic veins. Scleral hemorrhage and petechiae in the skin of the upper body give the child a frightening appearance. Treatment is expectant, since the features resolve spontaneously with time. Associated injuries to the liver, lungs, and heart are common.

Most esophageal injury results from iatrogenic manipulation with endoscopy or dilation. Penetrating wounds to the neck can also injure the esophagus. Keys to diagnosis are the history, presence of air in the mediastinum indicated by roentgenogram, and a finding of crepitus. Barium swallow and endoscopy may define the injury, but precise localization is often difficult. Adequate repair of the esophageal laceration and drainage are necessary for proper therapy. Proximal diversion of the esophagus by esophagostomy occasionally is useful in the management of a major disruption when distal esophageal repair is tenuous.

Caustic ingestion is another source of esophageal injury.[27] Alkaline agents cause a majority of the injuries, which occur most frequently in toddlers. Since the identification of oral burns does not correlate well with the presence of esophageal injury, all children who ingest alkaline agents require esophagoscopy. Endoscopy permits definition of the presence of a burn. To prevent perforation, terminate the endoscopic procedure at the level of the first severe burn. A radiological contrast study of the esophagus with barium helps define the depth and extent of severe injury. Children with deep and circumferential burns require gastrostomy for nutrition and placement of a string for eventual retrograde dilation. Reevaluate the child at 3 weeks with a contrast study and endoscopy since a stricture develops in approximately 15% of children. Most respond favorably to serial dilation. The role of steroid therapy in prevention of stricture is con-

troversial. Esophageal replacement reestablishes intestinal continuity in infants with intractable stricture. Disc batteries are an increasing source of localized injury to the esophagus in children.

Though most burns in children are caused by scald, flame burns commonly produce thoracic injury. Smoke inhalation and carbon monoxide poisoning are possible when examination reveals singed nasal hairs or a burn of the face or mouth. Inspection of the sputum may show charred material. Hypoxemia documented by arterial blood gas analysis and a serum carbon monoxide level greater than 10% indicate pulmonary injury. Chest roentgenograms often have normal results initially but progressively show diffuse infiltrates. Treatment focuses on respiratory support. Since edema of the neck and face may produce airway obstruction, early intubation is important. Positive-pressure ventilation is advantageous in severe cases. In children with intense carbon monoxide poisoning and neurological findings, hyperbaric therapy is helpful. Escharotomy is necessary to allow chest wall expansion when a deep burn wound restricts the chest circumferentially.

Children are uniquely prone to foreign body aspiration. A history of choking in a toddler is enough to suggest injury. Small toys, peanuts, and candy are common causative objects. Physical examination and roentgenograms may not be helpful. Inspiratory and expiratory chest roentgenograms may show hyperinflation of the involved side. Rigid bronchoscopy under anesthesia allows accurate diagnosis and retrieval of the foreign body. Failure to remove a foreign body results in eventual alveolar collapse, parenchymal consolidation, and bronchiectasis, which often requires pulmonary resection.

Thoracic injury in children is rare but produces high mortality. Since isolated injury is infrequent, improvement in survival rate depends on a coordinated multisystem treatment scheme. Protocols provide a systematic approach that accommodates the unique characteristics of anatomy, physiology, behavior, and mechanism of injury found in children. Though the best strategy is prevention, early diagnosis and appropriate resuscitation are essential to achieving improvement in outcome when thoracic injury occurs in children.

REFERENCES

1. Peclet MH, Newman KD, Eichelberger MR, et al: Patterns of injury in children. *J Pediatr Surg,* 1990;25:85–91.
2. Velcek FT, Weiss AD, DiMaio D, et al: Traumatic death in urban children. *J Pediatr Surg* 1977;12:375–384.

3. Mayer T, Matlak M, Johnson D, et al: The modified injury severity scale in pediatric multiple trauma patients. *J Pediatr Surg* 1980;15:422.
4. Sinclair MC, Moore T: Major surgery for abdominal and thoracic trauma in childhood and adolescence. *J Pediatr Surg* 1974;9:155.
5. Peclet MH, Newman KN, Eichelberger MR: Thoracic trauma in children: An indicator of increased mortality. *J Pediatr Surg* 1990;25:961–966.
6. Smyth BT: Chest trauma in children. *J Pediatr Surg* 1979;14:41–47.
7. Shorr RM, Crittenden M, Indeck M, et al: Blunt thoracic trauma. *Ann Surg* 1987;206:200–205.
8. American College of Surgeons Committee on Trauma: *Advanced Trauma Life Support Course Manual.* Chicago: American College of Surgeons, 1989;215–231.
9. Haller JA: Thoracic injuries. In: Welch K, ed. *Pediatric Surgery,* Chicago: Yearbook Medical Publishers, 1986;143–154.
10. McGill WA: Airway management. In: Eichelberger MR, ed. *Pediatric Trauma Care.* Rockville, Md: Aspen Publishers, 1988;51–57.
11. Howell CG, Ziegler MM: Acute management of major trauma and burns. In: Ludwig S, ed. *Pediatric Emergencies.* New York: Churchill Livingstone, 1985;79–105.
12. O'Neill JA: Emergency management of the injured child. In: Welch K ed. *Pediatric Surgery.* Chicago: Yearbook Medical Publishers, 1986;135–143.
13. Eichelberger MR, Randolph JG: Thoracic trauma in children. *Surg Clin North Am* 1981;6:1181–1197.
14. Schwab P, Fleisher G: Rib fractures in children. *Pediatr Emerg Care* 1985;1:187–189.
15. Garcia VF, Gotschall CS, Eichelberger MR: Rib fracture in children: A marker of severe trauma. *J Trauma* 1990;30:695–701.
16. Meller JL, Little AG, Shermeta DW: Thoracic trauma in children. *Pediatrics* 1984;74:813–819.
17. Bonadiro WA, Hellmich T: Post-traumatic pulmonary contusion in children. *Ann Emerg Med* 1989;1050–1052.
18. Sivit CJ, Taylor GA, Eichelberger MR: Chest injury in children with blunt abdominal trauma: Evaluation with CT. *Radiology* 1989;171:815–818.
19. Nakayama DK, Ramenoksky ML, Rowe MI: Chest injuries in childhood. *Ann Surg* 1989;210(6):770–775.
20. Deslauriers J, Bussieres J: Bronchial rupture. In: Grillo HC, Austen WG, Wilkins EW, et al, eds. *Current Therapy in Cardiovascular Surgery.* Toronto: BC Decker, 1989,42–45.
21. Barlow B, Niemirski M, Gonhi R: Ten years experience with pediatric gunshot wounds. *J Pediatr Surg* 1982;17:927–932.
22. Eddy AC, Rusch VW, Fligner C: Traumatic rupture of the thoracic aorta in pediatric patients. *J Trauma* 1990;30:989–992.
23. Tellez DW, Hardin WD, Takehashi M, et al: Blunt cardiac injury in children. *J Pediatr Surg* 1987;22:1123–1128.
24. Golladay ES, Donahoo JS, Haller JA: Special problems of cardiac injuries in infants and children. *J Trauma* 1979;19:526–531.
25. Adeymi SD, Stephens CA: Traumatic diaphragmatic hernia in children. *Can J Surg* 1981;24:355.
26. Haller JA, Donahoo JS: Traumatic asphyxia in children: Pathophysiology and management. *J Trauma* 1971;11:453.
27. Leape LL: Chemical injury of the esophagus. In Ashcraft KW, Holder TM, eds. *Pediatric Esophageal Surgery,* Orlando, Fla: Grune and Stratton, 1986;73–89.

The Child with Thoracic Trauma

David E. Wesson, MD, FRCS(C)

This chapter reflects the experience and practice of the Children's Hospital National Medical Center (CNMC), one of the largest and best organized pediatric trauma units in North America. The authors correctly point out that the incidence of thoracic trauma and the spectrum of injury vary with the geographic region and the size of the study population. They report a 22% incidence of penetrating injury, which is far higher than my own experience and that of Nakayama et al[1] at the Children's Hospital of Pittsburgh, who encountered only three penetrating chest injuries in a series of 105 cases over a 7-year period. The rising incidence of penetrating injury at CNMC is typical of the experience at major urban centers in the United States.

Newman and Eichelberger state that patients with thoracic injuries have worse physiological scores and a lower probability of survival than those without such injuries. This reflects the fact that high-energy transfers are required to produce thoracic injuries, especially in children, who have compliant and resilient thoracic structures.

The authors present the section on initial resuscitation in the usual airway, breathing, circulation (ABC) format. They rightly point out that endotracheal intubation is the most reliable way to establish a secure airway, but they gloss over the pros and cons of orotracheal versus nasotracheal intubation. In my own experience orotracheal intubation is quicker and more reliable and, in an emergency, is preferable to nasotracheal intubation in children.

Injuries such as tension pneumothorax that impair the mechanics of breathing must be diagnosed and treated at the time of the primary survey, but it should be noted that physical examination of the chest is not very reliable and that all children with multiple trauma should have a chest roentgenogram.

The section on circulation and shock is clear and concise, although I would take exception to the statement that recognition of shock is difficult. My own view is that any injured child with cool extremities, weak peripheral pulses, tachycardia, or hypotension should be presumed to be hypovolemic and should be treated as such with a bolus of 20 mL/kg of isotonic crystalloid (normal saline or Ringer's lactate solution).

The section on specific injuries follows the ABCs. I would add hemoptysis, persistent pneumothorax with a chest drain in place, and extensive atelectasis in association with a pneumothorax to the signs of tracheobronchial injury. I would also mention the use of echocardiography as a diagnostic tool when cardiac tamponade is suspected.

Rib fractures and pulmonary contusions are of less clinical significance in children than in adults not just because they are less common but also because they cause fewer problems. In fact, adult respiratory distress syndrome (ARDS) is much less common among injured children. This is supported by Nakayama's experience[1] that chest injuries produce a relatively mild compromise of respiratory function. Nakayama reported that pneumothorax and hemothorax prolonged hospitalization, whereas pulmonary contusion and rib fractures did not. Posttraumatic pneumatoceles are uncommon and most resolve spontaneously without treatment.

Burrington has published a table of priorities in the treatment of chest injuries[2]:

1. Establish patent airway
2. Occlude sucking wounds
3. Stop bleeding
4. Expand lungs
5. Stabilize chest wall
6. Drain pleural space

© 1991 Elsevier Science Publishing Co., Inc.
655 Avenue of the Americas, New York, NY 10010
Current Topics in General Thoracic Surgery:
An International Series

7. Restore circulation

8. Evaluate ventilation (blood gases)

Nakayama et al[1] found 41 immediately life-threatening injuries in 105 children with chest trauma. In decreasing order of frequency these were: obstructed airway (15), massive hemothorax (14), tension pneumothorax (9), cardiac tamponade (2), flail chest (1), and aortic transection (1).

In summary, thoracic injuries result from high energy transfer and are associated with a high rate of morbidity and mortality. Most can be treated with simple measures, including endo-tracheal intubation and intercostal drains. Careful evaluation of the history, physical examination, and plain roentgenograms leads to the diagnosis of the rare but treatable life-threatening injuries such as tracheobronchial rupture, great vessel injury, cardiac tamponade, and direct injury to the heart.

REFERENCES

1. Nakayama DK, Ramenovsky ML, Rowe MI: Chest injuries in childhood. *Ann Surg* 1989;210(6):770–775.
2. Burrington JD: Chest injuries in children. *Can J Surg* 1984;27(6):446–449.

PART IX

Chest Infections

Chapter 23

Open Lung Biopsy and Bronchoalveolar Lavage

Ann M. Kosloske, MD, MPH

Special techniques are necessary for the diagnosis of certain pulmonary infiltrates in children. The scenario is usually as follows: an immunosuppressed child develops a febrile respiratory illness, with bilateral spreading pulmonary infiltrates. Antibiotic therapy for bacterial pneumonia has no effect, and respiratory failure is impending. The differential diagnosis includes several obscure pulmonary infections, such as pneumocystis pneumonia and viral or fungal pneumonitis, and a neoplastic pulmonary infiltrate. Because effective therapies depend on accurate microbiological and histological diagnosis, direct sampling of lung tissue is considered necessary. In children as well as adults, the gold standard of diagnostic procedures in this situation is open lung biopsy.[1,2] Other diagnostic techniques, for example, percutaneous aspiration needle, cutting needle, and transbronchial biopsy, are of limited value in children. The role of bronchoalveolar lavage in the management of pulmonary diseases in children has yet to be established.[3]

OPEN LUNG BIOPSY

History

The original report was by Klassen and associates from the Ohio State University College of Medicine in 1949.[4] Fifty patients underwent diagnostic open lung biopsy under general anesthesia. A short submammary incision was made in the anterior fourth interspace. Carmalt clamps were placed on the lung, and a wedge of tissue was removed for histological evaluation and appro-

priate cultures. The lung margin was oversewn with 3-0 chromic suture. The safety and efficacy of the procedure were documented by Klassen and Andrews's cumulative series (which included a few pediatric patients[5]) of 270 open lung biopsies, published in 1967.[6] Diagnoses were obtained in all but 1 of the 270 cases. Complications, primarily pneumothorax, subcutaneous emphysema, and hemothorax, occurred in 7.8%. Two deaths in the series (0.7%) were a direct result of biopsy, one from aspirated food and one from empyema. From 1968 to 1974, several centers reported experience with open lung biopsies in children,[7–11] establishing the safety and efficacy of the procedure in pediatric patients. At Columbus Children's Hospital, open lung biopsy was compared to needle biopsy of the lung.[7] The diagnostic accuracy of open biopsy was superior (100% vs 60%) and the complication rate was lower (4.3% vs 24%). By the mid-1970s, open lung biopsy was established as the diagnostic procedure of choice in children with persistent diffuse pulmonary lesions.

Preoperative Considerations

Children who undergo open lung biopsy are often poor candidates for anesthesia and operation because of immunosuppression, spreading pulmonary infiltrates, and impending respiratory failure. Open lung biopsy should be carried out early in the disease process, rather than after respiratory failure has supervened and the child is dependent on a ventilator. Biopsy becomes a necessity if the respiratory status is deteriorating. Leijala and co-workers in 1982 outlined the policy of the Children's Hospital of Helsinki, Finland, where emergency open lung biopsy is performed on the day of admission if pneumocystis pneumonia is suspected.[12] The procedure should be conducted expeditiously. Operating time should never exceed 45 minutes, and anesthesia time should not exceed 1 hour. Careful preoperative review of chest roentgenograms must be carried out to identify the areas of heavy infiltrate, which are optimal sites for biopsy.[13]

Technique

Under general endotracheal anesthesia, an anterolateral thoracotomy is performed in the right or left fourth or fifth intercostal space. This incision provides access to the middle lobe or lingula, areas that are usually involved in diffuse pneumonitis. The margin of the lung is mobilized, extruded through the incision, and palpated, and a generous biopsy specimen is taken to include an abnormal area. The technique with the stapler is shown in Fig. 23.1 and Fig. 23.2. We[13] and others[14–16] prefer the stapler because of its speed and the low incidence of postoperative air leaks.

The biopsy specimen is divided into two portions and handed in sterile containers to the pathologist. One portion is submitted for touch imprints and routine processing and staining. Most special stains and immunohistochemical studies can be performed on routinely processed tissue. A part of the fresh specimen may also be frozen and saved if electron microscopy or deoxyribonucleic acid (DNA) marker studies are anticipated. The second portion is subdivided for cultures, including aerobic and anaerobic bacteria, fungi, mycobacteria, cytomegalovirus, and other suspected microbial pathogens. Good communication among the surgeon, pediatrician, and pathologist is essential to ensure that all appropriate studies are made.

Results

The results of open lung biopsy in several pediatric series from the 1970s and 1980s are summarized in Table 23.1. In experienced hands, the procedure entails low morbidity and virtually no mortality in spite of the patient population.[1,14,16,17] Biopsies in the 1970s typically identified a specific bacterial pneumonitis[7] or pneumocystis pneumonia,[14,17] which permitted institution of specific, often lifesaving antimicrobial therapy. In the Mayo Clinic series of 31 children who had 33 open lung biopsies, a tissue diagnosis was established in all but 1 (3%) case, influencing subsequent therapy in 91%.[16] The preoperative diagnosis was confirmed in 61% and corrected in 36%. Morbidity of the procedure, usually due to pneumothorax, ranged from 4% to 27% but was manageable by judicious handling of chest tubes. Mortality directly attributable to the procedure approached zero, although some children subsequently died of the underlying disease; in the 1970s that underlying disease was usually leu-

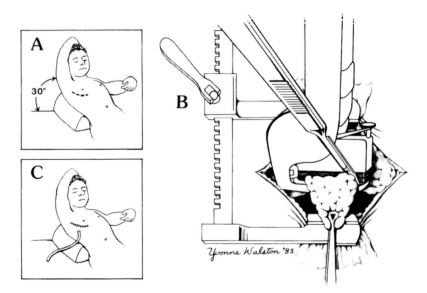

FIGURE 23.1 Technique of open lung biopsy. **A.** Anterolateral thoracotomy. **B.** Application of the stapler (TA-30 or TA-55) across a margin of lung that is involved in disease process. Alternatively, wedge application of the stapler may be used. Oversewing the staple line is usually not necessary. **C.** Chest tube drawn out through a lower intercostal space. Air leaks are uncommon unless the patient is being ventilated with very high pressures. The chest tube is left in place a minimum of 48–72 hours after any air leaks appear to be sealed. *Reproduced from Kosloske,[13] with permission.*

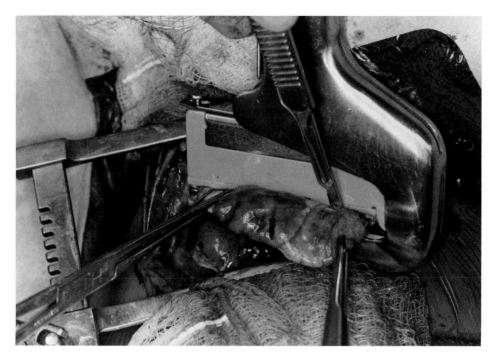

FIGURE 23.2 Operative photograph of open lung biopsy in a child with diffuse interstitial pneumonitis.

kemia. Ten percent (10%) of children died of *Pneumocystis carinii* pneumonia within a month of operation; overall mortality was 25%.[17,18]

Current Concepts

Recently there has been a tempering of enthusiasm for open lung biopsy as a diagnostic procedure, both in children[19–21] and in adults.[22,23] The patient population has changed since 1980. Pneumonia due to *Pneumocystis carinii* is now far less common in children under treatment for acute lymphocytic leukemia because of the general use and effectiveness of prophylaxis with trimethoprim-sulfamethoxazole (TMP-SMZ, Bactrim).[24,25] At Children's Memorial Hospital in Chicago emergency lung biopsy was reappraised as "friend or foe of the immunosuppressed child."[19] Patient benefit from the procedure was defined as follows: (1) the biopsy indicated a cause that necessitated a change of treatment, (2) the child survived. In spite of excellent diagnostic accuracy of open lung biopsy in 56 immunosuppressed children, only 13 (23%) derived benefit by these criteria. A specific infectious cause was diagnosed in 39 (69%) patients, but only 10 (18%) of these children survived after an appropriate change in therapy. Since 8 of the 10 patients had *P carinii,* the authors suggested that children with interstitial pneumonitis receive an empirical

course of therapy with TMP-SMZ and broad-spectrum antibiotics, limiting open lung biopsy to children who fail to respond to this empirical therapy. Although others[20,23] have reported a similar experience and have endorsed empirical treatment with TMP-SMZ and antibiotics, Grosfeld[26] and McElvein[27] cautioned against "carte blanche treatment with Bactrim," which might lead to delays in appropriate therapy for children whose infiltrates are secondary to neoplasm and other treatable causes. The opportunistic pathogen, *P carinii,* was until recently considered to be a protozoan, but ribosomal ribonucleic acid (RNA) sequence has now shown this organism to be one of the fungi.[28]

An emerging group of immunocompromised patients who are candidates for open lung biopsy are recipients of bone marrow transplants, in 41% of whom pneumonia develops.[29] In a report from the Children's Hospital of Philadelphia,[21] 14 of 22 open lung biopsies in marrow transplant recipients showed no causative microorganism. The authors considered open lung biopsy of limited value in this patient population. In contrast, a recent report by Foglia and associates found open lung biopsy of considerable value in a series of 26 immunocompromised children, more than half of whom had either bone marrow transplants or immunodeficiency syndromes.[30] An infectious cause was found in 65% of their cases. The largest

TABLE 23.1 Results of Open Lung Biopsy in Children

Author	Year	Center	No. of Patients	Most Common Diagnoses (No.)	Diagnostic Accuracy	Morbidity from Procedure	Mortality From Procedure	Mortality From Disease
Stringer[9]	1968	Los Angeles	16	Pulmonary Fibrosis (5) Interstitial Pneumonitis (5)	100%	0	0[a]	19%
Kilman[7]	1974	Columbus, Ohio	23	Chronic Pneumonitis (8)	100%	4.3%	0	0
Ballantine[17]	1977	Indianapolis	38	Pneumocystis Pneumonia (23)	100%	21%	0	10.5%
Adeyemi[14]	1979	Toronto	36	Pneumocystis Pneumonia (9)	97%	14%	0	NS
Stillwell[16]	1981	Mayo Clinic	31	Interstitial Pneumonitis (10)	97%	27%	0[b]	10%
Imoke[20]	1983	Johns Hopkins	34	Pneumocystis Pneumonia (11)	70%	6%	3%	15%
Doolin[19]	1986	Chicago	56	Pneumocystis Pneumonia (19)	82%	21%	NS	34%
Shorter[21]	1988	Philadelphia	21	Nonspecific Interstitial Pneumonitis (13)	41%	NS	0	62%
Foglia[30]	1989	UCLA	26	Viral Pneumonitis (9) Nonspecific Interstitial Pneumonitis (9)	65%	27%	0	54%

[a] 3 deaths (19%) may have been hastened by the biopsy procedure.
[b] One death (3%) may have been hastened by the biopsy procedure.
NS = not stated.

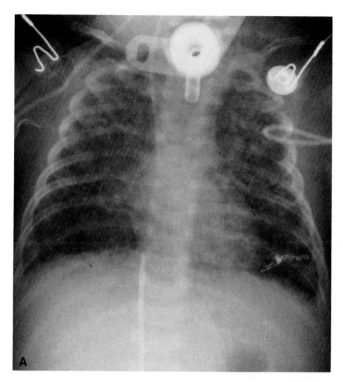

FIGURE 23.3 Interstitial pneumonitis in a 2-month-old boy. **A.** Chest roentgenogram shows diffuse severe infiltrates. Staples mark biopsy site in lingula. Note tracheostomy tube, two central venous lines, and other paraphernalia of intensive care. **B.** Biopsy shows flattened, simplified alveoli with fibroblastic proliferation in septa (hematoxylin-eosin ×100). Although the histological result was nonspecific, cultures of lavage fluid grew *Ureaplasma urealyticum*, and the pneumonitis cleared completely with specific therapy.

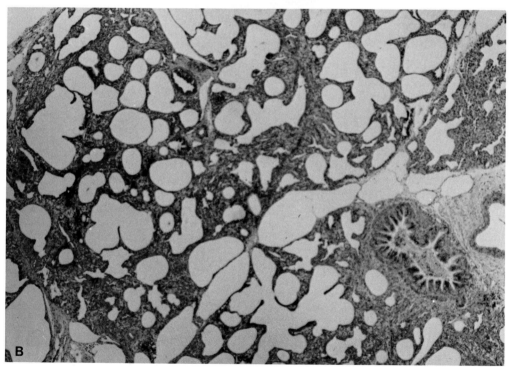

group had viral pneumonitis, which appeared to benefit from treatment with antiviral agents (DHPG for cytomegalovirus, [Ribivarin] for respiratory syncytial virus).[30] In spite of the controversies, the consensus regarding open lung biopsy was summarized in a review by Rivkin and Aronoff, who described open lung biopsy as "the most reliable diagnostic procedure available for the evaluation of pneumonia in the immunosuppressed (pediatric) patient."[31] They recommend that it be performed in instances when noninvasive studies have failed to yield a diagnosis. One of our recent patients (1989), whose open lung biopsy yielded a specific diagnosis amenable to therapy, is shown in Fig. 23.3.

Patients with acquired immunodeficiency syndrome (AIDS) may be considered for open lung biopsy. A prospective study of adults with AIDS compared bronchial washing, alveolar lavage, transbronchial lung biopsy, and open lung biopsy. A diagnostic yield of 85% for combined transbronchial lung biopsy and alveolar lavage was comparable to that of open lung biopsy (88%).[32] However, open lung biopsy was the only procedure that diagnosed Kaposi's sarcoma in lung.[32] In children with AIDS, although alveolar lavage may yield microbial pathogens, the diagnosis of lymphocytic interstitial pneumonitis (LIP), a pathognomonic finding in 28% of children with AIDS,[33] requires open biopsy. With the advent of steroid therapy for LIP, open biopsy remains essential for these patients.[33]

The future utility of open lung biopsy will depend on which diseases predominate in the pediatric population with interstitial lung disease. The procedure is safe, is technically simple, and provides an excellent sample of tissue for histological and microbiological studies. If institution of specific treatment for the future disease(s) has a reasonably good outcome, open lung biopsy should remain useful to the pediatric surgeon for years to come.

OTHER BIOPSY TECHNIQUES

Burt et al evaluated four diagnostic biopsy techniques in 20 patients with undiagnosed pulmonary infiltrates: aspiration needle, cutting needle, transbronchial, and open lung biopsy.[34] Diagnostic yields ranged from 29% for aspiration needle to 94% for open lung biopsy. Only two minor complications occurred among the 20 patients. The complication of pneumothorax was not evaluated in this report, as the needle and transbronchial biopsies were performed in the operating room immediately before thoracotomy for open lung biopsy. Graeve and associates retrospectively compared the diagnostic accuracy of bronchoscopic biopsy and percutaneous biopsy to open biopsy in 99 adult patients.[35] Complications were few and rates were similar for the three different procedures. The overall diagnostic accuracy of open lung biopsy, however, was far superior: 100%, compared to 52% for bronchoscopic biopsy and 61% for percutaneous needle. The diagnostic yield of the other biopsy techniques improved in specific situations: 82% for transbronchial biopsy of diffuse pulmonary infiltrates, 73% for percutaneous needle biopsy of nodules.[35] Wall and colleagues, in a prospective study comparing transbronchial and open lung biopsies in adults,[36] found diagnostic accuracies of 38% for transbronchial and 92% for open biopsy. Transbronchial biopsy diagnoses were often unreliable and misleading. In children, these alternative methods of lung biopsy have never found widespread application, although at some centers percutaneous transthoracic needle aspiration of the lung was used effectively in the diagnosis of *P carinii* pneumonitis.[37]

BRONCHOALVEOLAR LAVAGE

Introduction

A technique of bronchoalveolar lavage, introduced by Reynolds and Newball in 1974,[38] permitted serial sampling of the fluid lining the epithelial surfaces of the lower respiratory tract in normal and diseased lung. In adults, bronchoalveolar lavage has contributed to an understanding of the cellular events involved in lung injury and repair.[3,39] The role of bronchoalveolar lavage in pediatric interstitial lung diseases was reviewed by Murphy.[3] It is a promising investigative tool, although its status as a clinical tool is not yet established.

Technique

The flexible fiberoptic bronchoscope is wedged into a segmental or subsegmental bronchus, usually in the middle lobe or lingula; sterile isotonic saline solution (without bacteriostatic agent) at neutral pH and room temperature is instilled in aliquots and each is almost immediately aspirated. In adults, a total volume of 100–300 mL, and even as much as 500 mL, may be instilled into a segment, at a rate of 5 mL/s, in aliquots of 20–40 mL.[40] In children, aliquots are 3–10 mL, and total volume depends on the size of the child. The return is usually about one-half the volume instilled.[41]

Lavage in pediatric patients is limited by instrumentation. Since the flexible 2.7-mm pediatric fiberoptic bronchoscope has no suction channel, standard bronchoalveolar lavage may be used only on larger children (more than about 5 kg), whose airways will admit the 3.5-mm pediatric fiberoptic bronchscope. Ogden and associates[42] described an alternative technique that was used in intubated premature infants. The infant was placed on the right side for sampling the right lung. A total of 5 mL of sterile saline solution was instilled into the endotracheal tube, in aliquots of 1 mL. Mean recovery of lavage fluid was 2.7 ± .1 mL. The yield of cell populations and chemical findings in control newborn infants was similar to that seen in lavage specimens from healthy, nonsmoking adults, calculated on a weight or body surface area basis.[42]

The cellular and soluble components of the lavage fluid are analyzed. Total cell count is determined by hemocytometer before centrifugation, and a differential count is made of 100 cells stained with Wright's stain and esterase stain. Millipore filter preparations stained with hematoxylin-eosin have been recommended for the most accurate differential count,[43] but cytocentrifuged, pooled lavage fluids are equally accurate.[44] Murphy and associates[45] used flow cytometry for analysis of lavage fluids, demonstrating the advantage of flow analysis, which is that thousands of cells can be analyzed in a few seconds, eliminating the error in small sampling that occurs when only 100 cells are counted by hand. The soluble constituents of the lavage fluid are analyzed by appropriate chemical and electrophoretic techniques.

Results

The cellular and soluble components of normal bronchoalveolar lavage fluid are listed in Table 23.2. Alveolar macrophages predominate, comprising 80% to 95% of total cells,[46] and lymphocytes constitute approximately 10%.[39] The soluble constituents include immunoglobulins, complement, proteases, antiproteases, fibronectin, and surfactant. All of these are proteins of molecular weight of less than 150,000 daltons. Larger molecules, which are not freely diffusible, are not found in normal lavage fluid. The major immunoglobulins are immunoglobulin A (IgA) and IgG. Because of its larger molecular weight, IgM is not recovered from normal lavage fluid.

Information from lavage has contributed to an understanding of normal lung defenses as well as the pathophysiology of interstitial lung diseases, including sarcoidosis, hypersensitivity pneumonitis, idiopathic pulmonary fibrosis, and histiocytosis X.[3,39] Bronchoalveolar lavage is currently under evaluation in the study of AIDS, both in children and in adults.[32]

The risks of bronchoalveolar lavage are those of the bronchoscopy procedure. Wood,[47]

TABLE 23.2 Constituents of Bronchoalveolar Lavage Fluid

Cells		
Total cells		$10–37 \times 10^6/100$ mL
Macrophages		84%–93%
Lymphocytes		7%–11%
T Lymphocytes	62%–73%	
Helper (T4)	46%	
Suppressor (T8)	25%	
B Lymphocytes	5%–15%	
Neutrophils		0%–1%
Eosinophils,		Normally not
Basophils		Present
Soluble Factors		
Albumin		5.7 mg/dL/kg
IgG, IgA		+
IgM		−
C4, C3, Factor B		+
C5		−

+ = present, − = not present.
(Adapted from Murphy,[3] Ogden et al,[42] and Daniele et al.[39])

in a series of 1095 pediatric flexible bronchoscopies, reported only 22 complications, of which 4 were major, including two pneumothoraxes, one lung abscess, and one laryngospasm. Minor complications included transient bradycardia, epistaxis, anesthetic problems, and laryngospasm. At the University of New Mexico, 138 lavages in 44 premature infants on ventilators and oxygen had no complications.[42]

Current Concepts

A variant of bronchoalveolar lavage for therapeutic purposes was employed by Rothmann et al in patients with cystic fibrosis at the Children's Hospital of Akron, Ohio.[48] Under a brief general anesthestic, a 4% solution of acetylcysteine was injected into the distal airways in 8-mL increments. Suctioning yielded a large volume of secretions, including bronchial casts. Improvement in lung compliance during the procedure was noted by the anesthesiologist and bronchoscopist. Improvement in clinical status over the next 72 hours was associated with effective cough and massive production of mucus. Pulmonary function studies showed an increase in vital capacity that averaged 19.5%. Subjective improvement included school and work attendance and often improvement of chest film findings. Most centers, however, have not used this procedure for patients with cystic fibrosis, because the respiratory improvement, although impressive, is transient.

Microbiological diagnoses based on culture of bronchoalveolar lavage fluid are problematic because passage of the bronchoscope through the nasopharynx and oropharynx contaminates the suction channel with the flora of these regions. Thus the finding of *Hemophilus influenzae, Streptococcus pneumoniae,* or *Staphylococcus aureus* in a patient with pulmonary infiltrates may be difficult to interpret.[41] The findings, however, of *Pneumocystis, Candida albicans,* or other microorganisms that are not members of the normal nasopharyngeal and oropharyngeal flora may be indicative of a pathogen, especially in an immunocompromised child. Leigh and associates described the diagnosis of *P carinii* using bronchoalveolar lavage in two immunocompromised pediatric patients.[49] Frankel and co-workers successfully used a lavage technique for identification of the pathogen (usually *Pneumocystis*) in six of seven immunocompromised children.[41] The current status of bronchoalveolar lavage in children remains that of an investigative tool of great potential. Further studies are necessary to establish its place in the diagnosis and routine management of pulmonary disease.

REFERENCES

1. Michaelis LL, Leight GS Jr, Powell RD Jr, DeVita VT: Pneumocystis pneumonia: The importance of early open lung biopsy, *Ann Surg* 1976;183:301–306.
2. Niguidula FN, Balsara RK, Cuasay RS: Lung biopsy. In: Laraya-Cuasay LR, Hughes WT, eds. *Interstitial Lung Diseases in Children.* Boca Raton, Fla: CRC Press, 1988;101–110.
3. Murphy S: Bronchoalveolar lavage. In: Laraya-Cuasay LR, Hughes WT, eds. *Interstitial Lung Diseases in Children.* Boca Raton, Fla: CRC Press, 1988;111–128.
4. Klassen KP, Anlyan AJ, Curtis GM: Biopsy of diffuse pulmonary lesions. *Arch Surg* 1949;59:694–704.
5. Andrews NC, Klassen KP: Eight years' experience with pulmonary biopsy. *JAMA* 1957;164:1061–1069.
6. Klassen KP, Andrews NC: Biopsy of diffuse pulmonary lesions—a 17 year experience. *Ann Thorac Surg* 1967;4:117–124.
7. Kilman JW, Clatworthy HW, Hering J, et al: Open pulmonary biopsy compared with needle biopsy in infants and children. *J Pediatr Surg* 1974;9:347–353.
8. Roback SA, Weintraub WH, Nesbit M, et al: Diagnostic open lung biopsy in the critically ill child. *Pediatrics* 1973;52:605–608.
9. Stringer RJ, Stiles QR, Lindesmith GG, et al: Use of lung biopsy in diagnosis of pulmonary lesions in children. *Am Surg* 1968;34:810–812.
10. Toyama WM, Reyes CN, Lawton BR, Sautter RD: Open lung biopsy in infants and children. *Arch Surg* 1971;103:195–198.
11. Weng T, Levison H, Wentworth P, et al: Open lung biopsy in children. *Am Rev Respir Dis* 1968;97:673–684.
12. Leijala M, Louhimo I, Lindfors EL: Open lung biopsy in children with diffuse pulmonary lesions. *Acta Paediatr Scand* 1982;71:717–720.
13. Kosloske AM: Infections of the lungs, pleura, and mediastinum. In: Welch KJ, Randolph JG, Ravitch MM et al, eds. *Pediatric Surgery*, 4th ed. Chicago: Year Book Medical Publishers, 1986;657–666.
14. Adeyemi SD, Ein SH, Simpson JS, Turner P: The value of emergency open lung biopsy in infants and children. *J Pediatr Surg* 1979;14:426–427.
15. Prober CG, Whyte H, Smith CR: Open lung biopsy in immunocompromised children with pulmonary infiltrates, *Am J Dis Child* 1984;138:60–63.
16. Stillwell PC, Cooney DR, Telander RL et al: Limited thoracotomy in the pediatric patient. *Mayo Clin Proc* 1981;56:673–677.
17. Ballantine TVN, Grosfeld JL, Knapek RM, Baehner RL: Interstitial pneumonitis in the immunologically suppressed child: An urgent surgical condition. *J Pediatr Surg* 1977;12:501–508.
18. Wolff LJ, Bartlett MS, Baehner RL, et al: The causes of interstitial pneumonitis in immunocompromised children: An aggressive systematic approach to diagnosis. *Pediatrics* 1977;60:41–45.
19. Doolin EJ, Luck SR, Sherman JO, Raffensperger JG: Emergency lung biopsy: Friend or foe of the immunosuppressed child? *J Pediatr Surg* 1986;21:485–487.
20. Imoke E, Dudgeon DL, Colombani P, et al: Open lung biopsy in the immunocompromised pediatric patient. *J Pediatr Surg* 1983;18:816–821.
21. Shorter NA, Ross AJ III, August C, et al: The usefulness of open-lung biopsy in the pediatric bone marrow transplant population. *J Pediatr Surg* 1988;23:533–537.
22. Hiatt JR, Gong H, Mulder DG, Ramming KP: The value of open lung biopsy in the immunosuppressed patient. *Surgery* 1982;92:285–291.
23. Potter D, Pass HI, Brower S, et al: Prospective randomized study of open lung biopsy versus empirical antibiotic therapy for acute pneumonitis in nonneutropenic cancer patients. *Ann Thorac Surg* 1985;40:422–428.
24. Hughes WT, McNabb PC, Makres TD, et al: Efficacy of trimethoprim and sulfamethoxazole in the prevention and treatment of *Pneumocystis carinii* pneumonitis. *Antimicrob Agents Chemother* 1974;5:289–293.
25. Morgan E: Decreased incidence of nonspecific interstitial pneumonitis in children with acute lymphocytic leukemia treated prophylactically with trimethoprim-sulfamethoxazole. *J Pediatr* 1981;99:807–810.
26. Grosfeld JL: Discussion of: Imoke E, Dudgeon DL, Colombani PL, et al: Open lung biopsy in the immunocompromised pediatric patient. *J Pediatr Surg* 1983;18:816–821.
27. McElvein RB: Open lung biopsy versus empirical antibiotic therapy in the immunosuppressed patient. *Ann Thorac Surg* 1985;40:419–420.
28. Edman JC, Kovacs JA, Masur H, et al: Ribosomal RNA sequence shows *Pneumocystis carinii* to be a member of the fungi. *Nature* 1988;334:519–522.
29. Meyers JD, Flournoy N, Thomas ED: Nonbacterial pneumonia after allogeneic marrow transplantation: A review of ten years' experience, *Rev Infect Dis* 1982;4:1119–1132.
30. Foglia RP, Shilyansky J, Fonkalsrud EW: Emergency lung biopsy in immunocompromised pediatric patients. *Ann Surg* 1989;210:90–92.
31. Rivkin MJ, Aronoff SC: Pulmonary infections in the

immunocompromised child. *Adv Pediatr Infect Dis* 1987;2:161–180.

32. McKenna RJ Jr, Campbell A, McMurtrey MJ, Mountain CF: Diagnosis for interstitial lung disease in patients with acquired immunodeficiency syndrome (AIDS): A prospective comparison of bronchial washing, alveolar lavage, transbronchial lung biopsy, and open-lung biopsy. *Ann Thorac Surg* 1986; 41:318–321.

33. Beaver BL, Hill JL, Vachon DA, et al: Surgical intervention in children with human immunodeficiency virus infection (HIV). *J Pediatr Surg,* in press.

34. Burt ME, Flye MW, Webber BL, et al: Prospective evaluation of aspiration needle, cutting needle, transbronchial, and open lung biopsy in patients with pulmonary infiltrates. *Ann Thorac Surg* 1981;32:146–153.

35. Graeve AH, Saul VA, Akl BF: Role of different methods of lung biopsy in the diagnosis of lung lesions. *Am J Surg* 1980;140:742–746.

36. Wall CP, Gaensler EA, Carrington CB, Hayes JA: Comparison of transbronchial and open biopsies in chronic infiltrative lung diseases. *Am Rev Respir Dis* 1981;123:280–285.

37. Chaudhary S, Hughes WT, Feldman S, et al: Percutaneous transthoracic needle aspiration of the lung. *Am J Dis Child* 1977;131:902–907.

38. Reynolds HY, Newball HH: Analysis of proteins and respiratory cells obtained from human lungs by bronchial lavage. *J Lab Clin Med* 1974;84:559–573.

39. Daniele RP, Ellas JA, Epstein PE, Rossman MD: Bronchoalveolar lavage: Role in the pathogenesis, diagnosis and management of interstitial lung disease. *Ann Intern Med* 1985;102:93–108.

40. Daniele RP, Dauber JH: Collection and enrichment of human alveolar macrophages. In: Herscowitz HB, Holden HT, Bellanti JA, Ghaffar A, eds. *Manual of Macrophage Methodology,* New York: Marcel Dekker, 1981;23.

41. Frankel LR, Smith DW, Lewiston NJ: Bronchoalveolar lavage for diagnosis of pneumonia in the immunocompromised child. *Pediatrics* 1988;81:785–788.

42. Ogden BE, Murphy SA, Saunders GC, et al: Neonatal lung neutrophils and elastase/proteinase inhibitor imbalance. *Am Rev Respir Dis* 1984;130:817–821.

43. Saltini C, Hance AJ, Ferrans VJ, et al: Accurate quantification of cells recovered by bronchoalveolar lavage. *Am Rev Respir Dis* 1984;130:650–658.

44. Willcox M, Kervitsky A, Walters L, King T: Quantification of cells recovered by bronchoalveolar lavage. *Am Rev Respir Dis* 1988;138:74–80.

45. Murphy SA, Steinkamp JA, Martinez E, Stewart C: Flow cytometry can quantitate lavage cell concentrations in lung injury. *Am Rev Respir Dis* 1983;127:182A.

46. Hunninghake GW, Gadek JE, Kawanami O, et al: Inflammatory and immune processes in the human lung in health and disease: Evaluation by bronchoalveolar lavage. *Am J Pathol* 1979;97:149–206.

47. Wood RE: Spelunking the pediatric airways: explorations with the flexible fiberoptic bronchoscope, *Pediatr Clin North Am* 1984;31:785–799.

48. Rothmann BF, Stone RT, Walker LH, Seguin FW: Bronchoscopic limited lavage for cystic fibrosis patients: An adjunct to therapy. *Ann Otol Rhinol Laryngol* 1982;91:641–642.

49. Leigh MW, Henshaw NG, Wood RE: Diagnosis of *Pneumocystis carinii* pneumonia in pediatric patients using bronchoscopic bronchoalveolar lavage. *Pediatr Infect Dis* 1985;4:408–410.

Open Lung Biopsy and Bronchoalveolar Lavage

A. Grimfeld, MD

The paper by Dr Ann Kosloske dealing with open lung biopsy and bronchoalveolar lavage has an undue surgical bias. Indeed, there are many fewer indications for open lung biopsy than in the past.

Open lung biopsy for the diagnosis of opportunistic infections of the lung in immunocompromised patients has been largely replaced by bronchoalveolar lavage, which is as effective in identifying the infectious agent as open biopsy, with the exception of cytomegalovirus infection, in which biopsy remains more effective. For patients receiving intensive care lavage is being used more often and can be repeated several times. Open biopsy is still the method of choice when there is suspicion of a medication-induced fibrosing process for which corticosteroid agents might be indicated. This remains the case because in the diagnosis of fibrosis alveolar, cytological and microbiological findings are not as useful as actual histopathological findings.

In some situations bronchoalveolar lavage provides a legitimate alternative to open biopsy in providing pathological diagnosis. Histiocytosis X and alveolar proteinosis are prime examples of this, as OKT6 lymphocytes or yellow periodic acid-Schiff-(PAS)-positive material obtained from lavage washings establish these respective diagnoses without the need to resort to open biopsy.

In the growing field of lung transplantation, transbronchial biopsy has replaced open lung biopsy in assessing lung rejection. An important advantage of transbronchial biopsy over open biopsy in following the graft-host reaction is the frequency with which transbronchial biopsy can

be safely repeated. In a recent study,[2] 60 transbronchial lung biopsies were performed in eight children after heart-lung transplantation. In the diagnosis of lung rejection the histological results obtained from transbronchial biopsies showed a sensitivity of 91% and a specificity of 69%. Complications consisted of three pneumothoraxes and two clinical episodes of hemorrhage.

In summary, bronchoalveolar lavage is an effective, routine investigative procedure to be used in children for the diagnosis of peripheral lung infections and in several specific pathological processes. It can be easily and safely repeated even in the seriously ill.

With careful selection of the bronchoscopic technique and customary safeguards such as arterial oxygen saturation monitoring, transbronchial lung biopsy is also safe in children and the results reproducible. It may prove valuable in the diagnosis of interstitial and/or diffuse alveolar or localized lung disease such as nonbacterial pneumonias, lymphomas or leukemic infiltrates. It may also be effective in establishing the diagnosis of opportunistic infections in immunocompromised patients.

In all these situations bronchoalveolar lavage and transbronchial biopsy should be considered before open lung biopsy is carried out.

SUGGESTED READINGS

1. De Blic J, McKelvie P, Le Bourgois M, et al: Value of bronchoalveolar lavage in the management of severe acute pneumonia and interstitial pneumonitis in the immunocompromised child. *Thorax* 1987;42:759–765.
2. Scott JP, Higenbottam TN, Smyth RL, et al: Transbronchial biopsies in children after heart lung transplantation. *Pediatrics* 1990;86:698–702.

Published 1991 by Elsevier Science Publishing Co., Inc.
655 Avenue of the Americas, New York, NY 10010
Current Topics in General Thoracic Surgery:
An International Series

Complications of Lower Respiratory Tract Infection: Empyema Complicating Pneumonia, Pneumatoceles, and Respiratory Embarrassment

Christopher R. Moir, MD and Robert L. Telander, MD

Although no longer commonplace, empyema and pneumatoceles are still major and life-threatening complications of childhood pneumonia. The frequency of surgical procedures for these once feared postpneumonic complications has decreased in recent years. Early aggressive antibiotic therapy has arrested the progression of pneumonia such that most cases resolve or show a salutory response to drainage alone. Nevertheless, there are still significant mortality and morbidity from childhood empyema and pneumatoceles that must always be carefully considered. Advanced techniques of drainage and irrigation have added tremendous benefits to the care of these children but have not supplanted the basic treatment principles. Timely surgery in selected patients is as appropriate today as it was in the time of Hippocrates.

With the decline of serious complications from these usually community-acquired infections, there has been an emergence of serious problems with the hospitalized and immunosuppressed patient. Intensive chemotherapy in children with malignancies and organ transplantation, combined with immunosuppressive therapy, have resulted in a group of immunosuppressed children who are at risk of infection with opportunistic organisms. These and other nosocomial infections of surgical patients pose our greatest challenge today.

THORACIC EMPYEMA

Empyema thoracis refers to a collection of purulent fluid, debris, and pus in the pleural space.[1] In children, most empyemas result from infection of a pleural effusion associated with pneumonia (parapneumonic effusion).[2-6] Considerable advances in specific antimicrobial therapy have reduced mortality rates in the postwar period,[7-10] but many infants and small children continue to die each year despite all therapeutic advances. In the past two decades, the average mortality from pediatric pleural empyema is 8%.[2,4,11-14]

History

The basic principles of treatment of empyema have remained unchanged since the teachings of Hippocrates. As chronicled by Paget,[15] Hippocrates washed the patient, listened for a succussion splash, and then opened the chest where the pain and swelling were most evident. After controlled evacuation of the pus to prevent rapid fluid loss and death, he packed the wound open with a strip of linen cloth that was changed each day. Twice-daily irrigations with warm wine and

© 1991 Elsevier Science Publishing Co., Inc.
655 Avenue of the Americas, New York, NY 10010
Current Topics in General Thoracic Surgery:
An International Series

oil cleansed the surface of the lung, and when healing was well established, progressively smaller metal rods were placed in the wound until it had entirely healed. This lucid concept of empyema treatment remains valid 2400 years later. Writing in 1897, Paget[15] was distressed that the efforts of Ambrose Pare, Guy deChauliac, and Laennec notwithstanding, he found "whole ages of neglect or perversion of the truth (such that) the Hippocratic treatment of empyema became hopelessly lost." Surgical drainage was abandoned in favor of repeated thoracenteses. M. Bouchut published a series of cases in 1872 in which one patient underwent 122 punctures in 11 months before a cure was effected. Paget comments, "And the worst of it all is that out of 48 patients thus tormented, only 6 were cured."[15,16]

After centuries of slow progress, Paget's period, the late 1800s, was one of surgical revolution. Many of the operations still performed today were described during this time. Estlander[17] and Schede[16] pioneered the concept of pleurostomy, which has been refined by Clagett[3] and Eloesser.[18] Decortication of the lung was popularized by George Fowler in 1893,[19] although Carl Beck had described this operation in New York some time before.[16] This procedure was of such importance that the previously popular Estandler and Schede operations were no longer necessary. Decortication has remained standard treatment since that time.

The influenza pandemic of 1918 provided a major advance in understanding the basic principles of empyema therapy. As members of the United States Army Empyema Commission, Graham and Bell concluded that acute empyema should no longer be drained by open pneumothorax, which had a mortality rate of 61.2%.[20] They began closed thoracic drainage, which decreased the mortality to 9.5% in less than 2 years after change of therapy. The introduction of sulfonamides and penicillin did not alter the therapeutic plan developed over the centuries, but it clearly reduced the incidence of postpneumonic empyema. Antibiotics have halted the progression of disease such that many of the well-conceived surgical techniques are now less frequently used.[3,6,14,21–24]

Etiology and Pathogenesis

Appropriate treatment of empyema requires careful consideration of the bacteria involved and the natural progression of the infection.

An analysis of 227 cases of empyema in children[4] aged 15 years or younger has shown that 71% of empyemas occurred in the infant or small child. Almost one half of these cases were in the 7- to 24-month age group. The three major pathogens, *Staphylococcus aureus*, *Streptococcus*, and *Hemophilus influenzae* group B, accounted for two thirds to three fourths of all bacteria isolated. The difficult-to-isolate anaerobic bacteria are now emerging as significant pathogens in children, not only in community-acquired infections but particularly in hospitalized or neurologically impaired older children.[9] In this setting, initial antimicrobial coverage must now consider anaerobes such as microaerophilic *Streptococcus*, *Bacteroides*, and *Eikenella corrodens*.[4,12,25–28]

Parapneumonic effusions may be seen in 50% to 90% of childhood pneumonia secondary to *Staphylococcus aureus*, *Streptococcus*, or *H influenzae*.[4,29–32] However, in a recent study of 3248 children with pneumonia, only 1 in 155 cases progressed to empyema.[12] This low incidence of progression attests to the power of specific antimicrobial therapy early in the course of childhood pneumonia.

The pleural cavity is strongly resistant to infection when the adjacent lung tissue is healthy. As long as there is normal expansion of the healthy lung, persistent infection of the pleural space is unlikely. Persistent sepsis of the pleural space is generally the result of ongoing, uncontrolled pulmonary sepsis.[33] Empyema, once established, exhibits three stages:[1]

1. An early exudative stage when the fluid is thin. This initially sterile fluid represents an alteration in the Starling forces acting on the pleural membranes. Inflammation from adjacent parenchymal infection causes vascular congestion, increased capillary permeability, and accumulation of proteinaceous fluid, favoring further fluid accumulation in excess of visceral pleural absorption.

2. The fibropurulent stage with bacterial invasion and accumulation of large numbers of polymorphonuclear cells and debris. Fibrin is formed and deposited over all affected pleural surfaces. The fluid thus becomes loculated and thick.

3. The organization stage of invasion of fibroblasts into the now very thick exudate and fibrinous peel present on the pleural surfaces. The empyema may be diffuse and involve the entire pleural space or it may be localized and encapsulated, assuming an interlobar, diaphragmatic, or paramediastinal location. Mixed empyemas can exist and are often far more toxic than those due to a single organism.[34] Anaerobic infections in particular are associated with the highest mortality and re-

quire a more vigorous approach to ensure total evacuation of the empyema.[24,34]

Diagnosis

In the young child, there is often a rather acute, short history of respiratory infection followed by respiratory distress, fever, cough, and, at times, profound respiratory embarrassment.[35] The physical findings of decreased air entry, dullness, and mediastinal shift support the diagnosis.[26] Many young children complain of abdominal pain and exhibit abdominal distention secondary to paralytic ileus.

The chest roentgenogram confirms the pneumonia and is useful in quantitating and following the parapneumonic effusions or empyema (Fig. 24.1A).[36] Staphylococcal pneumonia is suggested by the presence of pneumatoceles on chest roentgenogram.[37] Ultrasonography and chest computerized axial tomography (CAT) scan distinguish fluid from consolidation in patients

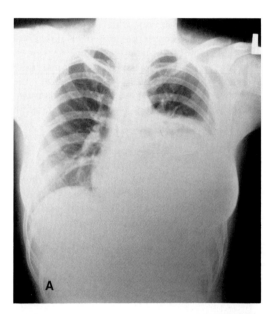

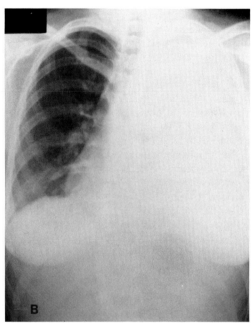

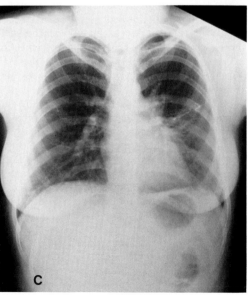

FIGURE 24.1 A. Upright chest roentgenogram demonstrating a left parapneumonic effusion and lingular pneumonia in a 13-year-old girl with a mediastinal teratoma. **B.** Progression of a left parapneumonic effusion to left empyema thoracis with compression of adjacent lung and mediastinal shift to right. **C.** Upright chest roentgenogram 3 months after decortication of left thoracic empyema and removal of mediastinal teratoma with adjacent abscess in left lingula.

with a "whiteout" of the hemothorax (Fig. 24.1B).[22] These scans have been particularly helpful in localizing loculated empyemas that may then be drained under radiological control.[38–41]

Thoracentesis of any identified fluid is essential to the diagnosis and early management of empyema. At times, fluoroscopy or ultrasound-guided needle aspiration may be necessary to maximize results.[40,42] The appearance of the aspirated fluid immediately differentiates an effusion from empyema and dictates further therapy.[36] The fluid is sent for Gram stain and culture, as well as determinations of pH, glucose level, cell count, lactic dehydrogenase (LDH), and amylase. Countercurrent immunoelectrophoresis for antigens to many of the gram-positive pathogens has been extremely useful in the management of childhood pneumonia.[43] Gas liquid chromatography for identification of volatile fatty acids of anaerobic bacteria is an experimental procedure that may aid in identification of the sometimes difficult-to-culture pleural effusions.

The diagnosis of empyema is often confirmed by appearance of the thoracentesis fluid alone, indicating immediate chest tube drainage. If the identification of empyema cannot be established by appearance of the fluid, immediate chest tube therapy drainage is indicated for fluid that has pH < 7.00, glucose level < 40 mg/dL, and LDH > 100 U/L.[36] These values are commonly found in fluid drawn from patients in the fibropurulent stage of empyema. Thin sterile fluid with a pH > 7.2 and glucose level > 40 mg/dL represents a parapneumonic effusion that has yet to progress to empyema. These patients usually respond to antibiotics without drainage.[26] The difficulty in obtaining a specific pathogen in many cases mandates blood culture as well as sputum culture in all children. Although it is difficult to tap the small effusion in the young child, thoracentesis is indicated for diagnostic and therapeutic purposes if the effusion is increasing in size or causing respiratory embarrassment.

Therapeutic Goals

The goal in eradicating the pleural space sepsis is complete evacuation of the purulent fluid and expansion of the underlying lung so that the pleural space is obliterated. The initial thoracentesis establishes the diagnosis, localizes a collection, and allows identification of the specific offending organisms. The appropriate antibiotic may be instilled into the pleural cavity if desired, although adequate antibiotic levels in pleural fluid are achieved with intravenous administration to patients with parapneumonic effusions.[32] If the purulent fluid is thick, closed drainage with an intercostal catheter is used, placing the tube in the most dependent aspect of the empyema cavity. This method of therapy has been very effective in treating an infant who has staphylococcal pneumonia.[35] Open drainage is indicated when tube drainage has been ineffective and expansion of the lung is needed to obliterate the cavity and relieve respiratory embarrassment.

In many children, as in adults, when the empyema cavity does not respond to repeated aspirations and closed tube drainage, decortication and empyemectomy should be considered.[44,45] This procedure, which has been used more commonly in adults, is extremely effective and allows full expansion of the lung under direct vision at the time of surgery.[6,21] This definitive procedure allows rapid recuperation and minimizes the morbidity of the empyema; the patient can usually be dismissed within 1 week after operation (Fig. 24.1C).[22,24,35]

Treatment

There is no question that children with pneumonia and parapneumonic effusions require early aggressive antibiotic treatment for the suspected pathogens discussed previously. Significant parapneumonic effusions are initially treated with thoracentesis, which may be repeated. Tube thoracostomy is indicated for large effusions causing respiratory embarrassment or when repeated thoracentesis is necessary. The timely placement of a chest tube is far superior to the discomfort and inefficiency of frequent aspiration in the distressed young child. There should be no fear that a carefully placed tube thoracostomy will suprainfect a pleural effusion; rather undrained proteinaceous fluid compressing the adjacent lung parenchyma poses the greatest threat to the child.

It is often difficult to detect clinically the transformation of a parapneumonic effusion to the fibropurulent stage of empyema. Recovery of pus with thoracentesis is the one essential proof of this stage, mandating immediate chest drainage. Most young children are adequately treated with closed chest drainage by large-bore tube thoracostomy. Clinical resolution with defervescence and return of white blood cell count to baseline is evident within 24–48 hours.[4,11,12,21] Despite these encouraging clinical signs, the radiographic appearance may lag well behind the patient's course. If the child is doing well, no further aggressive therapy is indicated.[22] The chest tube is removed in 1 to 2 weeks, and patients are generally discharged after 3 to 4 weeks of therapy. Radiographic evidence of pleural thickening may persist for several months but does not indicate chronic empyema.[22,24] Complete clinical and roentgenographic resolution is the rule.[46–48]

Once on specific antimicrobial therapy, the small number of patients who do not show significant signs of resolution within 2 days have an inadequately drained empyema. Choice of the next therapeutic step is a subject of considerable controversy. Many experienced pediatric surgeons have found it unnecessary to proceed with surgical drainage by thoracotomy or decortication.[22] Chest tube irrigation,[23] and use of streptokinase, thoracoscopy, and ultrasound guided drainage may have obviated the need for open drainage in these patients. Low rates of thoracotomy and decortication (0%–10%) in recent series support this conclusion.[2,4,10,12,14,49,50]

On the other hand, diligent assessment of the clinical progress of the child is of utmost importance. Undue reliance on antibiotics and repeated tube thoracostomy when the patient has not improved unnecessarily prolong the disease progress and increase the risk of permanent damage to the still growing lung. This statement is as true now as it was in Hippocrates' time. Although very few young children with gram-positive pneumonias require such treatment, it is especially important to consider early thoracotomy and decortication in older children or those hospitalized with other conditions, especially anaerobic infections.[24,34,35] Large series of very young patients with pneumonia show a very low decortication rate,[14,49] but other referral centers with a different patient population must resort to surgery more often. In our own series of 26 patients referred with empyema over the past 15 years, 15 patients (58%) required thoracotomy and decortication. These children were generally older (average age 8 years) and had had therapy for as long as 180 days before hospital admission. Ten of the 15 children requiring decortication or empyemectomy had specific underlying conditions that contributed to the chronicity of their infections. Three patients developed staphylococcal pneumonia in the postoperative period, two posttraumatic hypostatic pneumonia (both patients were paralyzed and ventilated), and one patient each had mediastinal teratoma, neutrophil chemotactic abnormality, diaphragmatic rupture of a subphrenic abscess, staphylococcal septic arthritis, and staphylococcal endocarditis. Our 58% decortication rate reflects the patient population more than a change in treatment philosophy. In fact, prolonged reliance on conservative therapy

in one patient resulted in the formation of an empyema necessitans before eventual decortication. Given the excellent initial care of pneumonia and effusions, referral centers may now experience a different spectrum of childhood empyemas that will benefit from earlier consideration of thoracotomy and decortication.

If thoracotomy and decortication are performed in the first month of empyema, the pleural rind has not become densely adherent to the pleura or lung and may be removed without the consequent blood loss and air leak associated with a chronic empyema. Kosloske and Foglia have reported excellent results with early decortication (within the first month) in unresponsive empyemas. There were no deaths, and patients were discharged home 7–10 days after the procedure. Decortication becomes particularly attractive when analyzing average hospital stay for more conservative therapy.[44] Lengthy hospital stays of 4 to 5 weeks are the rule rather than the exception for most children with empyema.[4,12,47,49,51] In our own series, the chest tube was removed on the average 8 days after decortication and the children were ready for discharge the following day. The shortened hospitalization and convalescence of decortication patients are obviously beneficial to the patient and family alike.

Although there are no long-term follow-up studies comparing pulmonary function in patients with early decortication versus those treated with tube thoracostomy, delay in either therapy adversely affects the outlook. Hartl[46] has reported a 15-year follow-up study that documented increasing evidence of pleural scarring and obstructive lung disease in those children drained by either method in the later stages of their illness.

Formal decortication requires a standard posterolateral thoracotomy with evacuation of all purulent material and stripping of the empyema rind from the visceral and parietal surfaces. Gentle traction on the inflammatory cortex allows careful separation from the underlying lung (Fig. 24.2A and B). When performed before chronic fibrous ingrowth, decortication does not actually remove the visceral pleura, safely preventing injury to the pulmonary parenchyma, blood loss, and injury to adjacent nerves.

Raffensperger[52] has popularized a technique of minithoracotomy for children with empyema in the fibropurulent stage. A 5-cm minithoracotomy incision is centered over the empyema and the underlying rib resected. After evacuation of the purulent fluid, the adhesions are broken down manually or by suction catheter. The loose

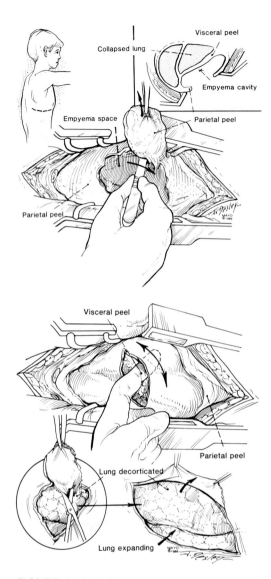

FIGURE 24.2 A. Technique of decortication: through a posterolateral thoracotomy over the empyema cavity the pleural rind is incised and gently elevated. **B.** All of the thick fibrinopurulent cortex is removed, allowing the underlying lung to expand and fill the hemithorax.

solid material is removed from the chest by irrigation or use of blunt forceps, and chest tubes are placed through a separate incision.

Results

In a series of 227 children with postpneumonic empyema reported in 1984,[4] mortality was 8.4%. Most deaths occurred in infants with *Staphylococcus aureus* empyema. Reported fatality rates range from 0% to more than 30%, but recent series have average mortality rates of less than 8%.[4,11,13,22,24,53] The number of infants compared to that of older or immunocompromised patients contributes significantly to fluctuations in these rates.

The prognosis for return of near-normal pulmonary function is good. Pulmonary function studies of 15 children 5–16 years after successful empyema therapy showed no difference when compared to those of normal siblings.[48] Other investigators have found mild restrictive defects in otherwise asymptomatic children.[46,47,54,55] Fears of fibrothorax and chest wall deformity have not been borne out by these studies.

PNEUMATOCELE

Pneumatoceles are thin-walled, air-containing cysts of the lung.[56] Pneumatoceles are seen frequently and characteristically in childhood *Staphylococcal aureus* pneumonia.[4,10,46,51] Their natural history is one of gradual resolution over time.[26,35,57] Surgical intervention for pneumatocele is not necessary unless a pneumatocele is large enough to cause respiratory embarrassment by compression or rupture into the pleural space.[35]

Etiology

Pneumatoceles are seen in 42% to 85% of children during the acute phase of staphylococcal pneumonia.[4,10] In small children with empyemas, pneumatoceles were also seen in 8% of streptococcal pneumonia cases and 5% of *Hemophilus influenzae* pneumonias.[4] Numerous other pathogens have been associated with pneumatoceles.[58–61] An autopsy study of more than 5000 cases with pneumonia identified pneumatoceles secondary to tuberculosis and after measles infection as well as primary staphylococcal pneumonia. The gram-negative aerobes such as *Klebsiella, Escherichia coli,* and *Pseudomonas* have occasionally been implicated as well as anaerobic bacteria.[57] A recent study from Nigeria, where measles is endemic, identified a 9.5% incidence of pneumatoceles in 1341 cases of pneumonia.[46] Over half of the cases of pneumatoceles had evidence of recent measles infection.

Pathology

Pneumatoceles are postulated to arise from necrosis and liquefaction of the lung parenchyma secondary to the inflammatory response to pneumonia.[62] Staphylococcal pneumonia causes a remarkable inflammatory process that is caused in part by the extremely destructive nature of the staphylococcal exotoxins on the infant's pulmonary tissue.[35,63] This results in air leak and potential subpleural dissection to form the typical thin-walled pneumatocele. Recent histopathological evidence has confirmed that an obstructive check-valve phenomenon allows air to enter the pneumatocele but effectively prevents its egress.[64] Although most pneumatoceles gradually decrease in size, an occasional cyst may progress to the point of rupture. Tension pneumothorax, bronchopleural fistula, and empyema may follow.[35]

Diagnosis

Pneumatoceles are diagnosed by chest roentgenogram. Computerized axial tomography (CAT) scanning provides more detailed information[65] but is not practical for the hour-to-hour and day-to-day follow-up observation of an enlarging cyst. The chief concern of diagnosis is differentiation from other pulmonary cysts.[26,66–69] Congenital cysts are true cysts lined by columnar ciliated epithelium. They do not spontaneously disappear but usually remain rather consistent in size and frequently have thicker walls.[35] Posteriorly located basal pneumatoceles may be confused with delayed-onset congenital diaphragmatic hernia, requiring contrast studies of the gastrointestinal tract or imaging of an intact diaphragm to exclude this possibility. The presence of multiple small pneumatoceles can simulate cystic adenomatoid malformation, particularly since both are associated with infection. Again the history of recent staphylococcal pneumonia and the tendency of pneumatoceles to resolve over time differentiates these two processes.

Treatment

Rapidly enlarging pneumatoceles may require urgent catheter cystostomy to decompress the cyst and allow reexpansion of the adjacent lung. Deaths still reported with pneumatoceles are almost exclusively due to respiratory insufficiency associated with large pneumatoceles and an ongoing pneumonic process.[35,46] Patients with large expanding cysts causing respiratory embarrassment cannot tolerate cyst rupture and tension pneumothorax. This surgical emergency is prevented by tube thoracostomy and catheter cystostomy.[35,70] Although as many as one quarter of all pneumatoceles rupture,[10] most are not large and do not cause tension pneumothorax. Prophylactic tube cystostomy is only indicated for those patients with rapidly increasing cysts associated with pulmonary insufficiency.[10,35]

Pyopneumothorax and bronchopleural fistula secondary to cyst rupture are well treated by closed chest drainage and appropriate anti-microbial therapy. The air leak resolves as the inflammation subsides. Open drainage, decortication, or oversewing of the air leak is rarely indicated in the treatment of pneumatoceles.[35]

Prognosis

Once the acute infection subsides, the pneumatoceles gradually decrease in size. The largest recent series of pneumatoceles is in Africa, where measles is still endemic. An analysis of 127 cases reported from Nigeria in 1984[46] showed that 12.6% of pneumatoceles initially increased in size but stabilized by 14 days of treatment. Mortality from pneumatoceles was 2.4%, all with staphyloccocal pneumonia and most with empyema. Complete disappearance of the pneumatocele was seen in 45% of cases after 6 weeks, with the remainder requiring 12 months for reabsorption. The longest time to complete resolution was 18 months.

REFERENCES

1. Andrews NC, Parker EF, Shaw RP: Management of non-tuberculous empyema. *Am Rev Respir Dis* 1962;85:935–936.
2. Adeyemo AO, Adejuyigbe O, Taiwo OO: Pleural empyema in infants and children: Analysis of 298 cases. *J Natl Med Assoc* 1984;76(8):799–805.
3. Clagett OT: Changing aspects of the etiology and treatment of pleural empyema. *Surg Clin North Am* 1973;53:863–866.
4. Freij BJ, Kusmiesz H, Nelson JD, McCracken GH: Parapneumonic effusions and empyema in hospitalized children: A retrospective review of 227 cases. *Pediatr Infect Dis* 1984;3(6):578–591.
5. Grant DR, Finley RJ: Empyema: Analysis of treatment techniques. *Can J Surg* 1985;28(5):449–451.
6. LeBlanc KA, Tucker WY: Empyema of the thorax. *Surg Gynecol Obstet* 1984;158(1):66–70.
7. Hochberg LA, Kramer B: Acute empyema of the chest in children: A review of 300 cases. *Am J Dis Child* 1939;57:1310–1337.
8. Khanna SK: Empyema thoracis in children. *Indian J Pediatr* 1984;51(412):593–601.
9. Kiesewetter WB, Rusnock JR, Girclany BR: Pediatric empyema: A second look at its incidence and importance. *J Pediatr* 1959;54:81–86.
10. Ryckman FC, Rosenkrantz JG: Thoracic surgical problems in infancy and children. *Surg Clin North Am* 1985;65(6):1443–1446.
11. Bechamps GJ, Lynn HB, Wenzl JE: Empyema in children: Review of Mayo Clinic experience. *Mayo Clin Proc* 1970;45(1):43–50.
12. Chonmaitree T, Powell KR: Parapneumonic pleural effusion and empyema in children: Review of a 19-year experience, 1962–1980. *Clin Pediatr (Phila)* 1983;22(6):414–419.
13. Jess P, Brynitz S, Moller AF: Mortality in thoracic empyema. *Scand J Thorac Cardiovasc Surg* 1984;18(1):85–87.
14. Stiles QR, Lindesmith GG, Tucker BL: Pleural empyema in children. *Ann Thorac Surg* 1970;10:37–44.

15. Paget S: Empyema. In: Paget S, ed. *The Surgery of the Chest.* New York: EB Treat, 1897;204–229.

16. Meade RH: Empyema. In: Meade RH, ed. *A History of Thoracic Surgery.* Springfield, Ill: Charles C. Thomas, 1961, 234–256.

17. Estlander JA: Surle résection des côtes dans l'empyème chronique. *Rev Mensuelle* 1879;8:885–888.

18. Eloesser L: An operation for tuberculous empyema. *Surg Gynecol Obstet* 1935;60:1096–1097.

19. Fowler GR: A case of thoracoplasty for the removal of a large cicatrical fibrous growth from the interior of the chest: The result of an old empyema. *Med Rec* 1893;44:838–839.

20. Graham EA, Bell RD: Open pneumothorax: Its relation to the treatment of acute empyema. *Am J Med Sci* 1918;156:839–840.

21. De La Rocha AG: Empyema thoracis. *Surg Gynecol Obstet* 1982;155(12):839–845.

22. Foglia RP, Randolph J: Current indications for decortication in the treatment of empyema in children. *J Pediatr Surg* 1987;22(1):28–33.

23. Hakim M, Milstein BB: Empyema thoracis and infected pneumonectomy space: Case for cyclical irrigation. *Ann Thorac Surg* 1986;41(1):85–88.

24. Kosloske AM: Empyema. In: Welch KJ, Randolf JG, Ravitch MM, O'Neill JA Jr, Rowe MI, eds. *Pediatric Surgery.* Chicago, Ill: Year Book Medical Publishers, 1986;666–669.

25. Abramer EJ, Baptista L, McHendry JA, Conlan AA: The microflora of chronic pleural empyema: An analysis of 89 cases. *S Afr Med J* 1985;68(1):80–82.

26. Avery B: Pleural effusion and empyema. In: Avery B, First LR, eds. *Pediatric Medicine.* Baltimore, Md: Williams & Wilkins, 1989;273–274.

27. Fajardo JE, Chang MJ: Pleural empyema in children: A nationwide retrospective study. *South Med J* 1987;80(5):593–596.

28. Kosloske AM, Cartwright KC: The controversial role of decortication in the management of pediatric empyema. *J Thorac Cardiovasc Surg* 1988;96(1):166–170.

29. Chartrand SA, McCracken GH: Staphylococcal pneumonia in infants and children. *Pediatr Infect Dis* 1982;1:19–23.

30. Ginsberg CM, Howard JB, Nelson JD: Report of 65 cases of *Haemophilus influenzae* B pneumonia. *Pediatrics* 1979;64:283–286.

31. Kevy SV, Lowe BA: Streptococcal pneumonia and empyema in childhood. *N Engl J Med* 1961;264:738–743.

32. Taryle DA, Potts DE, Sahn SA: The incidence and clinical correlate of parapneumonic effusions in pneumococcal pneumonia. *Chest* 1978;74:170–173.

33. DeMeester TR, Lafontaine E: Empyema. In: Sabiston DC, Spencer FC, eds. *Gibbon's Surgery of the Chest.* Philadelphia, Penn: WB Saunders Co, 1983;380–388.

34. Bartlett JG, Finegold SM: Anaerobic pleuropulmonary infections. *Medicine (Baltimore)* 1972;51:413–450.

35. Telander RL: Empyema thoracis in pediatric surgery. In: Holter TM, Ashcraft KW, eds. *Pediatric Surgery.* Philadelphia, Penn: WB Saunders Co, 1980; 213–214.

36. Light RW: Parapneumonic effusions and empyema. *Clin Chest Med* 1985;6(1):55–59.

37. Dines DE: Diagnostic significance of pneumatocele of the lungs. *JAMA* 1969;204:1169–1172.

38. Collins JD, Byrd SE, Bassett LW: Thoracentesis under fluoroscopic control. *JAMA* 1977;237:2751–2752.

39. Gobein RP, Stanley JH, Gobein BS, et al: Percutaneous catheter aspiration and drainage of mediastinal abscess. *Radiology* 1984;151:69–71.

40. Stark DD, Federle MD, Goodman PC: Radiographic assessment of CT and tube thoracostomy. *Am J Radiol* 1983;141:253–258.

41. van Sonnenberg E, Ferrucci JT, Mueller PR, et al: Percutaneous drainage of abscesses and fluid collections: Technique, results, and applications. *Radiology* 1982;142(1):1–10.

42. Ravin CE: Thoracentesis of loculated pleural effusions using grey-scale ultrasonic guidance. *Chest* 1977;71(6):666–668.

43. Nelson JE: Pleural empyema. *Pediatr Infect Dis* 1985;4(suppl 3):531–533.

44. Mayo P: Acute non-tuberculous empyema in children: A 25-year review. *J Ky Med Assoc* 1984; 82(4):163–167.

45. Toomes H, Vogt-Moykopt I, Ahrendt J: Decortication of the lung. *J Thorac Cardiovasc Surg* 1983;31(6):338–341.

46. Oviawe O, Ogundipe O: Pneumatoceles associated with pneumonia: Incidence and clinical course in Nigerian children. *Trop Geogr Med* 1985;37(3):264–269.

47. McLaughlin FJ, Goldmann DA, Rosenbaum DM, et al: Empyema in children: Clinical course and long term follow-up. *Pediatrics* 1984;73(5):587–593.

48. Wise MB, Beaudry DH, Bates DV: Long term follow-up of staphylococcal pneumonia. *Pediatrics* 1966; 38:398–401.

49. Cattaneo SM, Kilman JW: Surgical therapy of empyema in children. *Arch Surg* 1973;106(5):564–567.

50. Hoover EL, Hsu H-K, Ross MJ, et al: Reappraisal of empyema thoracis: Surgical intervention when duration of illness is unknown. *Chest* 1986;90(4):511–515.

50. Murphy D, Lockhart CH, Todd JK: Pneumococcal empyema: Outcome of medical management. *Am J Dis Child* 1980;134:659–662.

51. Ravitch MM, Fein R: The changing picture of pneumonia and empyema in infants and children: A review of the experience at the Harriet Care Home from 1934 to 1958. *JAMA* 1961;175:1039–1044.

52. Raffensperger JG, Luck SR, Shkolnik A, Ricketts RR: Mini-thoracotomy and chest tube insertion for children with empyema. *J Thorac Cardiovasc Surg* 1982;84(4):497–504.

53. Solak H, Yuksek T, Solak N: Methods of treatment of childhood empyema in a Turkish university hospital. *Chest* 1987;92(3):517–519.

56. Tuddenham WJ: Glossary of terms for thoracic radiology: Recommendations of the nomenclature committee of the Fleischner Society. *Am J Radiol* 1984;143:509–517.

57. Amitai I, Mogle P, Godfrey S, Aviad I: Pneumatocele in infants and children: Report of 12 cases. *Clin Pediatr (Phila)* 1983;22(6):420–422.

58. Caglar MK, Yalaz K, Cagler M, Yilgor E: Lobar pneumonia and pneumatocele formation due to *Salmonella paratyphi* B in an infant. *Turk J Pediatr* 1983;28(6):279–283.

59. Mayo P, Saha SP, McElevein RB: Acute empyema in children treated by open thoracostomy and decortication. *Ann Thorac Surg* 1982;34(4):401–407.

60. Stones DK, van Niekerk CH, Cilliers C: Pneumatoceles as a complication of paraffin pneumonia. *S Afr Med J* 1987;72(8):535–537.

61. Thapa BR, Kumar L, Mitra SK: Proteus mirabilis pneumonia with giant pneumatocele. *Indian J Pediatr* 1987;54(4)593–597.

62. Boisset GF: Subpleural emphysema complicating staphylococcal and other pneumonias. *J Pediatr* 1972;81:259–266.

63. O'Driscoll M, Crawford L, Biggar WD: Clinical features and abnormal neutrophil function in disseminated staphylococcal disease. *Pediatr Infect Dis* 1985;4(2):137–141.

64. Quigley MJ, Fraser RS: Pulmonary pneumatocele: Pathology and pathogenesis. *Am J Radiol* 1988;150(6):1275–1277.

66. Burrows PE, Leahy FA, Reed MH: Neonatal pulmonary infarction: A cause of "cystlike" lucencies on the chest roentgenogram. *Am J Dis Child* 1983;137(1):61–64.

67. Godwin JD, Merten DF, Baker ME: Paramediastinal pneumatocele: Alternative explanations to gas in the pulmonary ligament. *Am J Radiol* 1985;145(3):525–530.

68. Wagner RB, Crawford WO, Schimpf PP: Classification of parenchyma injuries of the lung. *Radiology* 1988;167(1):77–82.

69. Woodring JH, Vandiviere HM, Fried AM, et al: Update: The radiographic features of pulmonary tuberculosis. *Am J Radiol* 1986;146(3):497–506.

70. Asplund MW, Beckwith PS, Soltanzadeh H: Successful transthoracic drainage of infected traumatic pneumatocele (letter). *Chest* 1986;90(5):788.

Complications of Lower Respiratory Tract Infection: Empyema Complicating Pneumonia, Pneumatoceles, and Respiratory Embarrassment

Francisco Paris, MD, Santiago Ruiz-Company, MD, Francisco Asensi, MD, Carmen Otero, MD, and Desamparados Perez-Tamarit, MD

The chapter written by Drs Moir and Telander is a well-documented review of pediatric problems in children who have postpneumonic empyemas. Their series is composed of a population that is not comparable to patients seen for the first time in a pediatric hospital. They are working in the Pediatric Surgery Section at the Mayo Foundation, a referral unit that receives selected patients for surgical treatment.

This commentary is based on our experience treating children with postpneumonic empyema at La Fe Hospital during two decades, 1969–1989.[1,2]

Our series is composed of 131 children having this disease, aged less than 15 years (range 1 month–15 years), mean age 6 ± 4. One third of the children were less than 2 years old. Patients with malignancies, immunosuppression, or both were excluded from this study. Pleural empyema was more common in girls (Table D24.1). The clinical interval before hospitalization averaged 17 ± 21 days (range 1–120).

Patients were classified in two groups: (1) children less than 2 years old and (2) children 2–15 years. In the first group (*n* = 44) the most common responsible microorganism was *Staphylococcus*, followed by *Pneumococcus* (Table D24.2). In 16 patients (36%) the microorganisms

© 1991 Elsevier Science Publishing Co., Inc.
655 Avenue of the Americas, New York, NY 10010
Current Topics in General Thoracic Surgery:
An International Series

failed to grow in bacteriological cultures. *Staphylococcus* was present in 15/28 (54%) of the positive cultures, *Pneumococcus* in 5/28 (18%).

In the second group, composed of 87 children older than 2 years, the most common cultured organism was *Pneumococcus*. It was isolated in 16/33 (48%) positive cultures. *Staphylococcus* caused 21% of the empyemas and *Streptococcus* 12%; cultures were sterile in 54 patients and were not obtained for 2 patients.

In our series, 28/131 (21%) children complained of abdominal pain. In the group below 2 years, 11/44 (25%) exhibited abdominal distension; this percentage increased to 40% when *Staphylococcus* was cultured. In the older group 17/87 (13%) children had abdominal symptoms. Seven patients had pseudappendicular symptoms; 3 patients had undergone appendectomy.

Forty-five patients arrived at our unit in very poor condition. The percentage of unfit children was higher in the younger group (61%) and in those with *Staphylococcus*, 13/22 (59%). Fever was present in almost all cases and white cell counts averaged 16.5 ± 8.4 × 1000 (1.9 to 34.4 × 1000).

Radiological studies showed total pleural opacity in 75 children, partial in 27, pyopneumothorax in 18, and encapsulated collections in 11. Of children with staphylococcal empyema, pneumatocele was present in 3, pyopneumothorax in 4, total opacification in 12, and encapsulated collections in 3.

The evacuation of the purulent effusion was

TABLE D24.1 Age and Sex of 131 Children With Postpneumonic Empyema

Sex	Age		
	≤2 years	2–8 years	8–15 years
Male	16	27	16
Female	28	25	19
	44	52	35

achieved by thoracentesis alone in 8 patients and by a closed chest drainage system with suction in 123. We do not agree with Drs Moir and Telander, who state that repeated tube thoracostomy unnecessarily prolongs the disease. In our patients, when the drainage was inadequate the chest tube was removed and a new tube was inserted; repeated thoracostomy drain was needed in 47/131 of the children. A second tube was inserted in 32 children, a third or fourth in 13, and a fifth or sixth in 2. Intrapleural irrigation with physiological saline solution mixed with neomycin was carried out in 48 patients. The mean time of intrapleural drainage was 19 ± 12 days, ranging from 1 to 63 days.

Adequate systemic antibiotic therapy was given, according to the sensitivity tests. Cloxacillin was used for *Staphylococcus.* When the culture was sterile we generally used amplicillin/cephalosporin with or without an aminoglycoside. Corticosteroid therapy was started in almost all patients when the septic period was over.

Pleural empyema was managed by thoracocentesis and/or pleural drainage successfully in 126/129 (98%) of the survivors. The overall mortality rate, 2/131 (1.5%), is lower than in the studies cited by Drs Moir and Telander. The deaths occurred in 2 children, aged 4 and 8

months, with staphylococcal empyema. Clinical evolution before admission occurred in 12 and 23 days, respectively. They showed severe paralytic ileus, advanced toxic syndrome, and leukopenia. Complete right pleural opacity with mediastinal shift was present in both cases. These children died 12 hours and 10 days after admission.

In our series only 3 children (2%) had decortication; their ages were 28 months, 8 years, and 14 years. Clinical evolution before operation was of 30, 47, and 71 days. In one case *Pneumococcus* was isolated, but in the other two the culture was sterile. In one patient six thoracostomy tubes were inserted during 44 days of hospitalization before surgery. The other 2 proceeded directly to surgery after admission. None presented any special perioperative problems.

In our series, the total time of hospitalization was 28 ± 14 days; there were no significant differences between bacteriological types or the patients' ages. When the patients were discharged local infection was controlled and the children were in good condition. Only 15/129 (13%) had radiological sequelae, which resolved after several months of adequate treatment.

The incidence of postpneumonic empyema in children has decreased with the use of antibiotic agents in lower respiratory tract infections. In our hospital, the prevalence of empyema related to pneumonitis was 2.8%. The most com-

TABLE D24.2 Bacteria and Children's Ages: 61 Positive Culture Results*

Bacteria	28 Children ≤2 years	33 Children >2 years
22 (36%) *Staphylococcus*	15 (54%)	7 (21%)
21 (34%) *Pneumococcus*	5 (18%)	16 (48%)
5 (8%) *Streptococcus*	1 (4%)	4 (12%)
3 (5%) Combination of Gram-Positive Organisms	1 (4%)	2 (6%)
9 (15%) Gram-Negative Organisms	5 (18%)	4 (12%)
1 (2%) *Bacteroides*	1 (4%)	—

* Forty-seven percent (47%) of the empyemas.

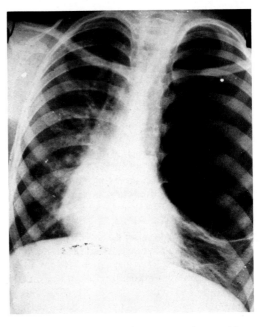

FIGURE D24.1 Large pulmonary tension cyst in a 9-year-old child, after staphylococcal pneumonitis that was surgically removed.

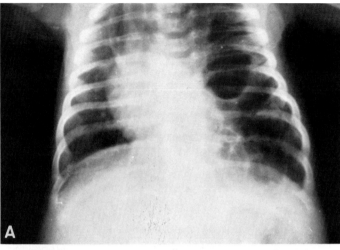

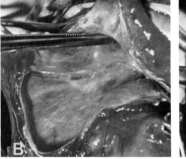
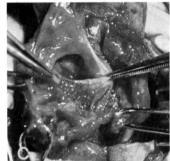

FIGURE D24.2 Cystic adenomatoid malformation in a child aged 1 month with intrathoracic tension phenomena treated by cyst resection. Histological study of the specimen showed cysts with cylindrical epithelium surrounded by adenomatoid parenchyma. **A.** Posterioanterior roentgenograms; **B** and **C.** Surgical views.

mon microorganism causing empyema was *Staphylococcus* followed by *Pneumococcus.* Nevertheless, positive *Staphylococcus* culture findings in the last 35 cases have decreased to 3 (9%), corresponding to 20% of 15 positive cultures.

One third of the children were less than 2 years old; 45 were admitted in very poor condition; 28 complained of abdominal pain or exhibited abdominal distention. These symptoms or signs were most common in patients less than 2 years old, when *Staphylococcus* grew in bacteriological cultures, or under both conditions.

Repeated use of thoracic tubes, or intrapleural irrigations, or both was required in 47/131 (36%) children. Three patients needed thoracotomy and decortication. This 2% decortication rate stands out from the 58% of the series of Moir and Telander, reflecting the differences in population.

Our overall mortality rate, 1.5%, is one of the lowest reported in the literature. The two deaths occurred in infants less than 2 years old who had staphylococcus empyema with toxic syndrome, paralytic ileus, and leukopenia. Radiological sequelae were not frequent and disappeared after several months of appropriate treatment.

Finally, as described by the authors, pneu-

matoceles are thin-walled air cysts of the lung frequently seen after childhood stapylococcal pneumonitis. Surgical intervention is not indicated unless an enlarging cyst under tension compresses the parenchyma, producing mediastinal shift (Fig. D24.1).

Pneumatoceles should be differentiated from other pulmonary cysts with thicker walls that do not vary in size. The presence of small multiple cysts can simulate cystic adenomatoid malformation (Fig. D24.2).

Eighteen patients (14%) had pyopneumothorax caused by the rupture of an infective pulmonary focus. In children with staphylococcal empyema, pneumatocele was present in three cases and pyopneumothorax in another four.

REFERENCES

1. Paris F, Blasco E, Tarazona V, et al: Acute postpneumonic empyema. In: *Proceedings II International on Antibiotics, Valencia, Nov 19–20, 1970.* Beecham, Barcelona, 1970;274–285.
2. Blasco E, Tarazona V, Cantó A, et al: Treatment of pleural pyogenic infections. In: *Proceedings IX Congreso de la Sociedad Española de Patología Respiratoria. Sevilla, Abril, 1976.* Liade, Madrid, 1976;75–89.

Chapter 25

Bronchiectasis and Lung Abscess

Yann Revillon, MD

BRONCHIECTASIS

The incidence of bronchiectasis has been decreasing as the consequence of better prevention of respiratory disease and improvement in physiotherapy. Bronchiectasis is classified as focal or diffuse disease. To date, only focal bronchiectasis can be cured by resection.

Historical Background

Bronchiectasis was first described by Laënnec[1] in 1819. In 1905, Jackson showed that abnormalities of the bronchial wall could be caused by dust particles of bismuth. In 1922, Sicard and Forestier[2] performed the first instillation of radiopaque iodized oil. Churchill and Belsey[3] recommended precise suturing of the different structures of the hilum in 1939. In 1943 Jackson and Huber[4] drew up the first basis for the surgical technique.

Pathology

Bronchiectasis is defined as permanent dilatation of segmental airways. The airways become obstructed by purulent exudate; peripheral airways are inflamed. Bronchomalacia and muscular hypertrophy may develop as a consequence. Intense neovascularization by bronchial arteries is frequent. Pleural adhesions and lymph node hypertrophy are common.

Reid[5] described three types of bronchiectasis: fusiform, cylindrical, and saccular. Bronchiectasis may be localized or diffuse and patchy. The left lower lobe is most frequently affected, perhaps because the left main bronchus is two-thirds the size of the right main bronchus.

Current Topics in General Thoracic Surgery: An International Series

Three theories have been proposed to explain the etiopathogenesis of bronchiectasis: atelectasis, traction, and the middle lobe syndrome. The middle lobar bronchus is long and narrow; this structure results in poor bronchial drainage and repeated bacterial infection. Inflamed lymph nodes may further diminish drainage by compressing the orifice of the bronchus.

The term *reversible bronchiectasis* is applied to bronchial dilatation that may clear within 2 to 3 months of the initial interstitial pneumonia. Only cylindrical dilatations are reversible. The concept of reversibility is important in the context of diagnosis, which requires bronchography, and affects subsequent treatment and outcome.

Etiology

Causes are summarized in Table 25.1. Young children are at high risk for aspiration of foreign bodies such as peanuts or popcorn. An episode of coughing, wheezing, or hemoptysis should raise suspicion of a foreign body. This cause leads to a focal bronchiectasis. Bronchiectasis after foreign body aspiration has an incidence of 3.5% to 16%.[6]

A foreign body may be extracted by endoscopy. However, focal bronchiectasis results from delays in therapy or ineffective treatment. When the aspirated foreign body is vegetable matter, diagnosis is often difficult. Bronchoscopy remains an effective diagnostic tool.

The middle lobe syndrome is an atelectasis persisting more than 2 months. The orifice of the middle bronchus, which is surrounded by lymph nodes, may be compressed by enlarged nodes. Congenital bronchiectasis is very rare and its existence is debatable.

α_1-Antitrypsin deficiency may be associated with bronchiectasis, although this is uncommon in childhood.

TABLE 25.1 Causes of Bronchiectasis

Secondary	Congenital
Pneumonia	Congenital Bronchiectasis
Bronchitis, Measles,	Congenital
Influenza	Hypoglobulinemia
Foreign Body	α_1-Protease Inhibition
Mucus Plug	Deficiency
Bronchogenic Tumor	Cystic Fibrosis
Middle Lobar Syndrome	Pulmonary Sequestration
Tuberculosis	Cardiovascular
Secondary	Malformation
Hypoglobulinemia	Ciliary Dyskinesia
Hypersensitivity	Rheumatic Diseases
Inhalation	
Cigarette Smoking	

Children with cystic fibrosis predominantly have diffuse bronchiectasis. However, focal bronchiectasis may occur more frequently with middle lobe involvement.

Suppurative infections of the respiratory tract develop in children with humoral immunodeficiency (agammaglobulinemia), although use of new therapies has resulted in fewer cases of bronchiectasis.

Kartagener's syndrome (Dextrocardia, sinusitis, bronchiectasis) must be ruled out in all cases.

Symptoms

Fever and cough are the most common symptoms. Production of sputum is seldom noted in children, and hemoptysis resulting from erosion of the bronchial wall is not common. Nutritional disturbance may be associated with severe cases.[7]

Abnormalities of breath sounds occur in 75% of patients, and clubbing of fingers may occur in 25% to 50% (Table 25.2).

Diagnostic Aids

Only focal bronchiectasis is curable with a surgical resection. Therefore, the aim of preoperative assessment is to confirm the diagnosis of bronchiectasis and to determine whether it is focal or diffuse.

The ordinary chest roentgenogram is very helpful. There are areas of circular or polygonal translucency surrounded by dense fibrous bands. Sometimes there is atelectasis. Bronchograms are sufficient for diagnosis.

Bronchoscopy is necessary to find a foreign body, to show the bronchial orifices and mucosa, and to obtain biopsy and sputum samples for culture and pathological evaluation.

In children fiberoptic bronchoscopy has facilitated exclusion of ciliary dyskinesia.

Bronchography is a vital part of the assessment.

Sicard and Forestier in 1922 introduced radiopaque contrast media for visualization of the bronchial tree. Bronchography must be performed by an experienced radiologist and the lung should be free of secretions during the procedure. Therefore, antimicrobial therapy and bronchoscopy may be needed before bronchography. If it is possible, it is better to use local anesthesia than general anesthesia.

Bronchography displays the topography of the lesions. Major alterations are noted and assessed for potential surgical resection. Differences in the size of bronchioles during the respiratory phases are demonstrated[8] and any distention of the collapsed lung can be noted.

Functional assessment can be obtained by spirometry (with bronchodilator) and by arterial blood gas determinations. In children, spirometry often shows a predominantly restrictive impairment.

In children, arterial lung scans delineate defects earlier than ventilation lung scans. Furthermore, in cases of focal lung disease, isotope scanning is very helpful in evaluating the contralateral lung. If the isotope scan finding is normal, bronchography is not necessary.

Computerized angiography[9] is probably the best method to study pulmonary vascularization; it provides information that is more precise than can be obtained from isotope scanning.

Computerized axial tomography (CAT) scan (Figs. 25.1 and 25.2) may reveal thickened and dilated airways. In cases of cystic fibrosis, it permits delineation of bronchiectasis and its topography.

Diseases Associated with Bronchiectasis

Sinusitis

The frequent association of sinusitis with bronchiectasis has been noted by many clinicians.

TABLE 25.2 Symptoms of Bronchiectasis

Symptom	Percentage
Fever	100
Cough	95
Purulent Sputum	59
Hemoptysis	14
Vomiting	4,5
Breath Sound Disturbance	77
Clubbing of the Fingers	27

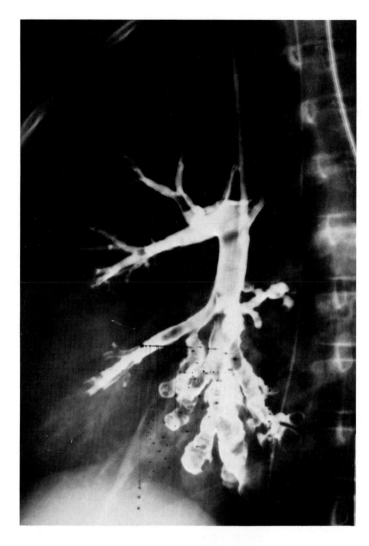

FIGURE 25.1 Definite bronchiectasis of the middle and lower lobes. The upper lobe is not completely normal. Pneumonectomy or bilobectomy?

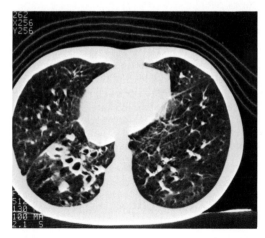

FIGURE 25.2 Computerized axial tomography delineates the topography of the lesions. A bilobectomy is planned.

Roentgenograms of the sinuses are necessary, and sinusitis should be treated to interrupt the cyclical infection between the upper and lower tract.

Asthma

The frequency of asthma in patients with bronchiectasis has been studied. Pulmonary function tests often show obstruction associated with a restrictive impairment.[10]

Treatment

Surgical treatment is often difficult. Pleuropulmonary adhesions, lobar atelectasis, and lymph node hypertrophy may all cause difficult dissection and extensive operative hemorrhage.

The decision to operate requires thorough discussion among chest specialists, pediatricians, anesthesiologists, and surgeons. Only focal lesions are amenable to resectional and curative surgery.

Currently, bronchography and computerized axial tomography can delineate the topography of bronchial lesions. In cases in which focal disease is not clearly defined, differences in size of the bronchi during the respiratory phases and between the normal and affected area are important in the diagnostic evaluation. If the clinical condition is optimal, then surgery can be delayed. However, with hemoptysis and severe infection, resection is necessary. It is always important to appreciate the effectiveness of medical treatment, and sometimes a second assessment is useful.

Medical treatment is difficult and expensive for the child and family. Surgical resection is quicker and often definitive.

Finally, when discussing pulmonary resection in children, one must consider future pulmonary growth.

Preparation for Surgery

Drainage of retained secretions by daily physiotherapy is essential.

Administration of antibiotic agents should be interrupted, although sinusitis and dental infections must be treated.

The quality of the preparation is determined by the culture, quality, and volume of sputum and by the general condition of the child, which includes assessment of nutritional status.

Forty-eight hours before surgery the child is hospitalized for intensive preparation, which includes final bronchial drainage immediately before surgery.

Surgical Treatment

Anesthesia is always difficult. During operation, the child is in the lateral decubitus position, and the incision is posterolateral. Manipulation of the affected lung can lead to flooding of the contralateral lung. Dissection is often difficult and hemorrhagic if large lymph nodes are present and overlying bronchial blood vessels are distended. Bilateral resections have been successfully achieved but require that the more severely damaged area be removed first.

Results

Postoperative complications include atelectasis, pleural effusion, pneumothorax, hemorrhage, and septicemia. However, the incidence of complications has recently been decreasing dramatically. Excellent surgical results are due to improved surgical techniques and control of infections.[11–14]

Relapses, occurring when some segments of diseased lung remain, are usually due to poor preoperative visualization by bronchography.

Among the patients treated in the Hôpital des Enfants Malades in Paris, 85% have had a good result.

Conclusions

Medical treatment is preferred not only for patients with advanced disease but also for those recently diagnosed to permit a determination of the degree to which it can be improved by good medical treatment. Surgical treatment is preferred when the lesion is localized or when there have been repeated hemorrhages or infections. A long observation period is sometimes essential to permit a proper choice of surgical or medical treatment.

LUNG ABSCESS

Lung abscess is a suppurative and necrotic lesion of the pulmonary parenchyma, the frequency of which has decreased in children with progressively more effective treatment of pneumonia.

Etiology

Staphylococcal septicemia has commonly been the cause. A congenital cyst or a sequestered lobe may become infected and lead to the development of an abscess. Bronchopulmonary disease with cystic fibrosis or bronchiectasis can sometimes lead to multiple abscesses. Foreign body aspiration must be considered and a bronchoscopic examination should be performed either to remove or to rule out a foreign body. Congenital hypogammaglobulinemia and other immune deficiencies can predispose to pulmonary abscess.[15]

Diagnosis

The main symptoms are fever, cough, and dyspnea. Roentgenographic examination shows a cavity with or without a fluid level. An inflammatory reaction is often noted. Rupture into the pleural space may lead to a pyopneumothorax.

Treatment

Antimicrobial therapy is the basic treatment, and it is sufficient in cases of consolidation of the lung.

When there is a cavity, drainage under ultrasonography or roentgenographic control permits prompt aspiration and bacteriological study.

If, with conservative treatment, the abscess does not disappear, a lung malformation should be postulated and excised at thoracotomy.

After the pulmonary abscess is treated as outlined, satisfactory resolution is common.

REFERENCES

1. Laënnec RTH: *De l'auscultation médicale, un traité du diagnostic des maladies des poumons et du coeur, fondé principalement sur ce nouveau moyen d'exploration.* Paris: Brosson et Chaude, 1819.
2. Sicard JA, Forestier J: Iodized oil as contrast medium in radioscopy. *Bull Soc Med Hop Paris* 1922;46:463.
3. Churchill ED, Belsey R: Segmental pneumonectomy in bronchiectasis: The lingular segmental of the left upper lobe. *Ann Surg* 1939;109:481.
4. Jackson CL, Huber JF: Correlated applied anatomy of the bronchial tree and lungs with a system of nomenclature. *Dis Chest* 1943;9:319.
5. Reid L: Reduction in bronchial subdivision in bronchiectasis. *Thorax* 1950;5:233.
6. Barker AF, Bardana E: Bronchiectasis: Update of an orphan disease. *Am Rev Respir Dis* 1988;137:969.
7. Nemir RL: Bronchiectasis. In: Kendig EL, ed. *Disorders of the Respiratory Tract in Children.* 3rd ed. Philadelphia, Penn: WB Saunders Co, 1977;446–459.
8. Fraser RG, Mac Klem PT, Brown WG: Airway dynamics in bronchiectasis: A combined cinefluorographic manometry study. *Am J Roentgenol* 1965;93:821.
9. Pariente D, Ernest C, Lacombe P, et al: L'angiographie numérisée: applications pratiques en pédiatrie. *Ann Pediatr* 1983;30(3):175.
10. Varpela E, Laittiner LA, Keskinen H, Korhola O: Asthma allergy and bronchial hyper reactivity to histamine in patients with bronchiectasis. *Clin Allergy* 1978;8(3):273.
11. Glanser EM, Cook CD, Harris GBC: Bronchiectasis: A review of 187 cases in children with follow-up pulmonary function studies in 58. *Acta Paediat Scand* 1966;165:1.
12. Latarjeh M: A propos du traitement chirurgical des dilatations des bronches de l'enfant et de l'adolescent. *Ann Pediatr* 1973;20:49.
13. Sanderson JM, Kennedy MCS, Johnson MF, Manley DCE: Bronchiectasis: Results of surgical and conservative management: A review of 393 cases. *Thorax* 1974;29:407.
14. Wilson JF, Decker AM: The surgical management of childhood bronchiectasis: A review of 96 consecutive pulmonary resections in children with non tuberculosis bronchiectasis. *Ann Surg* 1982;195(3):354.
15. Pulmonary abscess. High AH, Kendig EL: *Disorders of the Respiratory Tract in Children.* 3rd ed. WB Saunders Co, Philadelphia, Penn: 1977;470–474.

Bronchiectasis and Lung Abscess

D. Alex Gillis, MD, BSc, FRCS(C), FACS

Bronchiectasis has largely disappeared as a significant entity from the surgical wards of pediatric hospitals. Predisposing factors are rare. It is unusual for an aspirated foreign body to escape detection. Appropriate immunization and improved medical management have greatly reduced the incidence and seriousness of childhood infections such as pertussis and measles.

The causal relationship of sinusitis to bronchiectasis is controversial. Chronic sinus infection with postnasal drip may result in a repetitive "clearing" cough but is a very uncommon cause of major pulmonary infections. The association of sinusitis, bronchiectasis, and visceral transposition (Kartagener's syndrome) is rare but well recognized.

Chronic right middle lobe atelectasis in children is seen almost exclusively as a complication of asthma. Our experience has been that this is not improved significantly by endoscopic maneuvers, that it has a favorable natural history, and that it does not lead to bronchiectasis.

Although bronchiectasis is almost inevitable in patients with cystic fibrosis, current treatment allows most patients to live well into adulthood. The disease is seldom sufficiently localized to justify selective resection.

Congenital bronchiectasis is rare but is amenable to surgical resection when localized to a lobe or even one entire lung.

Aspiration of regurgitated gastric contents, either repetitively in neurologically damaged children with gastroesophageal reflux or as a complication of anesthesia, may cause significant pulmonary injury but is rarely identified as the sole source of bronchiectasis.

Suppurative pulmonary infections are relatively common in patients with severe immunosuppression, either congenital or related to the chemotherapy of malignant disease or the use of immunosuppressive drugs in patients undergoing organ transplantation. Pulmonary abscesses are typically superficial in relation to the visceral pleura. This has permitted aspiration, surgical drainage, or both without the use of thoracotomy if the process fails to respond to intensive nonsurgical management. Most pulmonary abscesses have a good outcome and seldom require major excisional procedures.

Suppurative pulmonary disease must always raise the suspicion of an underlying congenital abnormality such as sequestration or cystic malformations (eg, cystic adenomatoid disease). This is especially true if the initial inflammatory insult does not resolve completely or leaves the patient with apparent structural changes that are not readily explained.

Bronchography has been almost totally replaced by computerized axial tomography (CAT) scanning as the diagnostic imaging modality of choice in patients with suspected bronchiectasis. The CAT scan has the added advantage of being reproducible for sequential assessments in patients who are being followed or managed nonoperatively. Methods of functional assessment including isotope scanning are useful in making preoperative assessments and in determining operability.

Bronchoscopy is essential to identify foreign bodies or structural abnormalities in the major bronchi properly and to obtain appropriate specimens for cultures. Although rare, endobronchial tumors may obstruct a major orifice in the child.

PART X

Future Challenges

Chapter 26

Transplantation of Thoracic Organs in Children

Pascal R. Vouhé, MD

Replacing the heart, lungs, or both in children with end-stage cardiac or pulmonary disease has long been a surgical dream. This dream is becoming a reality.

In 1967, Kantrowitz transplanted a heart from an anencephalic infant to a 3-week-old infant with tricuspid atresia. In 1968, Cooley performed a combined heart and lung transplantation in an infant with complete atrioventricular canal. Both patients died early, but the surgical feasibility of such procedures in children had been demonstrated. Satisfactory results in adults after heart, and more recently, heart-lung transplantation have prompted worldwide interest in transplantation in the pediatric age group.

However, transplantation in children entails additional concerns along with the general problems encountered in adult programs.

Only a limited number of children are candidates for transplantation of thoracic organs. In France (55 million inhabitants), it has been estimated that every year, 50–100 children below the age of 15 years (1–2 patients/1 million people) need heart or heart-lung transplantation. According to the registry of the International Society for Heart Transplantation, 206 children below the age of 10 years have undergone heart transplantation between 1984 and 1988 all over the world.

Transplantation in children is justifiable only if outstanding results are achieved: complete functional rehabilitation and long-term survival should be obtained.

Before discussing the medical problems associated with transplantation in children, it should be clearly understood that this procedure cannot be undertaken without very strong parental and psychosocial support to deal with the psychological problems that occur during the transition from childhood to adolescence and young adulthood.

Thoracic transplantation includes heart, heart and lung, and lung transplantation. Although many problems are common to these procedures, indications, techniques, and results are different; therefore, they will be discussed separately.

THE IMMUNOLOGICAL BASIS OF TRANSPLANTATION

The Rejection Reaction

The ultimate fate of an allogenic graft is to be destroyed by the adaptive immune system of the host.[1] The rejection reaction involves humoral and cellular events that may take place at any time after the graft.

Hyperacute graft rejection is an explosive reaction that occurs immediately (within minutes) after transplantation and causes loss of the transplanted organ. Hyperacute rejection occurs in recipients already sensitized to the donor's antigens and is caused entirely by cytotoxic antibodies, usually those to class I major histocompatibility complex (MHC) antigens, directed against the donor lymphocytes. This accident can be prevented by obtaining negative white cell crossmatching (donor cells plus recipient serum plus complement) before transplantation.

However, for time-related logistic reasons, it is often impractical to perform a direct crossmatch before every transplantation. Therefore, the serum of any potential recipient is tested against a broad panel of human lymphocytes. If the result of this screening is negative, the risk of presence of cytotoxic antibodies and hyperacute rejection is extremely low and the transplantation can be performed without direct cross-match. However, a minimal risk of hyperacute rejection (perhaps related to antibodies to vascular endothelial cells) remains. On the contrary, in a recipient with preformed cytotoxic antibodies, negative direct cross-matching (recipient serum plus potential donor lymphocytes) is required to allow transplantation.

Acute rejection episodes after allogenic transplantation are presently unpreventable events. They are frequent during the first months after transplant even during adequate immunosuppressive therapy. After the graft has escaped the initial phase of the rejection reactions, cumulative unresponsiveness usually develops, but this is a subtle equilibrium that may be disturbed by many factors, including infection.

Acute rejection reaction is a cellular-mediated event that implies three steps:

1. Antigen presentation and recognition. This mainly involves class I and class II molecules of the MHC present in dendritic cells of the graft with the class II molecules presenting class I. However, minor histocompatibility antigens may also play a significant, although undefined role.

2. Proliferation and differentiation of T lymphocytes. During this phase T-helper (Th) cells play a major role by stimulating T-cytotoxic (Tc) cells and by releasing various lymphokines (tumor necrosis factor α, interleukin 1, interleukin 2, interferon γ).

3. Destruction of the graft by either specific (activated Tc cells) or nonspecific cells (macrophages activated by lymphokines).

Chronic graft rejection may cause late destruction of the graft and appears as accelerated coronary arteriosclerosis after heart transplantation or obliterative bronchiolitis after lung transplantation. The exact mechanism is still unclear. Chronic rejection seems more frequent in patients with major donor/recipient MHC mismatches and probably involves both humoral-mediated and cellular-mediated events. Chronic rejection is presently the major factor in late failure after transplantation, particularly in the pediatric age group.

The Immunosuppressive Treatment

The aim of immunosuppressive treatment is to reduce the frequency and severity of acute graft rejection episodes. Various immunosuppressive agents (including cyclosporine A, corticosteroids, azathioprine, antilymphocyte globulin,

monoclonal antibodies) are currently used to prevent sensitization of preexisting specific mature T cells immediately after the graft, to prevent acute allogeneic reactions afterward, or to treat acute rejection if it occurs. All these measures specifically reduce T cell function but are antigen-nonspecific. They increase the susceptibility to infection and have harmful side effects, particularly in children.

It is possible that in the near future, better solutions will be found for two reasons:

Antigen-specific immunosuppression may be induced by specifically altering the T receptors used by the lymphocytes responsible for rejection. The neonatal period may be a favorable period during which induction of immune tolerance may be possible. This may be due to the persistence during the first few weeks of life of immunosuppressive humoral and cellular factors that play a major role during intrauterine life in inducing tolerance between fetus and mother.

HEART TRANSPLANTATION

Indications

Neonates

Indications for heart transplantation are listed in Table 26.1. Hypoplastic left heart syndrome, untreated, is a lethal condition; death usually occurs within the first 2 weeks of life. There are two options for infants with this common congenital lesion: the Norwood approach and cardiac transplantation. The Norwood approach involves two stages. An initial complex palliative operation is followed by a Fontan-like repair using the right ventricle as the systemic ventricle. The overall mortality is high in most centers. The long-term prognosis with a single right ventricle Fontan circulation is unknown. The Loma Linda experience with cardiac transplantation in neonates with hypoplastic left heart syndrome is very encouraging, yielding a high midterm survival rate and a

TABLE 26.1 Potential Indications for Heart Transplantation in Infants and Children

Neonates
  Hypoplastic Left Heart Syndrome (HLHS)
  Minor Variants of HLHS
  Inoperable Complex Congenital Heart Defects
Infants and Children
  Cardiomyopathies
  Complex Congenital Heart Defects
    Inoperable
    After Failed Palliative or Definitive Surgery
  Multiple Inoperable Cardiac Tumors

low morbidity rate to date.[2] This experience suggests that the immature immunological status of the recipient neonate may be advantageous insofar as problems related to rejection and immunosuppression are less frequent and severe.

Should this finding be confirmed in a large population with a longer follow-up period, the indication for heart transplantation in neonates may be extended to those severe congenital heart defects carrying a poor prognosis with conventional surgical treatment.

However, in our institution, we have presently adopted a more conservative approach and have reserved cardiac transplantation to those infants with minor variants of hypoplastic left heart syndrome (aortic coarctation, valvular aortic stenosis with "hypoplastic" left ventricle, or both) who had survived the neonatal period without surgery or with conventional surgery and who remained in intractable heart failure.

Infants and Children

Children with end-stage cardiac failure, to whom no standard surgical procedures are applicable, are potential candidates for heart transplantation. Questions regarding timing of intervention, particularly in patients with chronic cardiomyopathy, have arisen. On one hand, children with strikingly poor myocardial function may be surprisingly free of symptoms; on the other hand, they may deteriorate very rapidly despite optimal medical management. Furthermore, heart transplantation in a desperately ill patient carries an increased risk. Cardiac replacement should therefore be recommended before an end-stage situation with multiorgan failure occurs.

Various congenital heart defects not amenable to conventional surgical procedures or leading to intractable heart failure after a failed palliative or definitive procedure are potential candidates for cardiac replacement. These patients should be assessed very carefully. They commonly have pulmonary hypertension, which may cause postoperative right heart failure. Pulmonary vascular resistances (PVRs) are determined at cardiac catheterization and provide the major guideline. However, precise measurement of PVR is impossible in the presence of intracardiac shunts, and other factors, such as the anatomy of the malformation, the anatomy of the pulmonary arteries, and the duration of the illness, should be taken into account. If pulmonary hypertension is thought to be of postcapillary origin (systemic ventricle failure or systemic atrioventricular valve dysfunction), standard heart transplantation is indicated although pulmonary vasodilation using isoproterenol and prostaglandin E_1 (PGE_1) or mechanical assistance of the right

TABLE 26.2 Indications for Heart Transplantation in 31 Patients (Laënnec Hospital, 1987–1990)

Variants of HLHS		4
Complex Congenital Heart Defects		9
Inoperable	3	
After Failed Surgery	6	
Cardiomyopathies		18
Idiopathic	14	
Chemotherapy-Induced	3	
Postvalvular Disease	1	

ventricle may be necessary during the early postoperative period. Patients with mild pulmonary vascular damage are candidates for cardiac replacement using an oversized donor heart or the heart from a heart-lung recipient with pulmonary hypertension and a normal cardiac function (domino procedure). Irreversible pulmonary vascular disease is an indication for heart-lung transplantation.

The indications for cardiac transplantation in our series of 31 infants and children below the age of 15 years are listed in Table 26.2.

Besides the presence of fixed pulmonary vascular disease, there are other strict contraindications to heart transplantation, which are summarized in Table 26.3.

The Operation

Selection of the Donor

The usual criteria for acceptable heart donors are shown in Table 26.4. A brain-dead patient should be monitored and treated in the same way as an intensive care unit patient. The donor heart must have excellent function, particularly when a distant procurement is performed. Brain death is known to damage the heart and to lead to a decline in myocardial function. Of utmost importance in evaluating the donor is normal myocardial function, as indicated by echocardiography, immediately before procurement.

A child with end-stage cardiac disease usually has a huge cardiomegaly. Therefore, a heart from a donor significantly larger than the recipient can often be used; this may even be advan-

TABLE 26.3 Contraindications to Heart Transplantation

Irreversible Pulmonary Vascular Disease (See Text)
Irreversible and Severe Hepatic or Renal Dysfunction
Active Systemic Infection
Absence of Adequate Psychosocial Support

TABLE 26.4 Criteria for Acceptable
Heart Donors

Brain Death Declared; Signed Parental Consent
Absence of
   Malignancy (Except Cerebral Malignancy)
   Infection
   Prolonged Cardiac Arrest
Normal Heart
   Minimal Inotropic Requirement
   Normal Function Indicated by Echocardiography
Donor/Recipient Matching
   ABO Blood Group Compatibility
   Size Matching
Anticipated Ischemic time < 5 h

---

tageous to a recipient with borderline elevation of pulmonary vascular resistances.

Procurement and Preservation of the Donor Heart

Harvesting of the heart. The technique of heart procurement may vary, depending on the extent of reconstruction needed by the recipient. Therefore, a clear understanding of the recipient anatomy is fundamental during the process of donor graft procurement. Most of the purely anatomical problems can be bridged successfully if enough donor tissue is obtained through harvesting. According to the anticipated recipient reconstruction, heart harvesting may include the entire aortic arch, the pulmonary arterial bifurcation and main pulmonary arteries, the superior vena cava system, and the pulmonary veins.

Preservation of the graft. An adequate technique of graft preservation must be used to prevent ischemic damage to the heart. At the time of procurement, the coronary arteries are flushed with a cold crystalloid cardioplegic solution. After harvesting, the graft is placed into a cold bath of normal saline solution, wrapped, packed in ice, and transported. At the time of arrival in the transplant room, a cold blood cardioplegic solution is infused and repeated every 20–25 minutes. Just before unclamping the aorta, a warm blood reperfusion solution is administered to prevent reperfusion injury.

Using this protocol, a total ischemic time up to 5 hours is very safe; the acceptable ischemic period may be extended up to 7–8 hours, but the risk of myocardial damage is then significantly increased.

Recipient Operation

The recipient heart excision is carried out at the atrioventricular junction and at the ventriculoarterial junction, thus leaving the maximum length of recipient tissue to allow subsequent reconstruction. The recipient coronary sinus is preserved if it receives an abnormal left superior vena cava.

In a child with cardiomyopathy, the standard technique, as described by Lower and Shumway, is used.[3] A size discrepancy, even if important, between the donor and recipient structures (especially of the atria) is managed by tailoring the donor and/or recipient hearts adequately.

In children with complex congenital diseases, various technical modifications may be necessary. In neonates with hypoplastic left heart syndrome, Bailey's technique is used.[4] The operation is performed under hypothermic circulatory arrest. The donor aortic arch is used to enlarge the hypoplastic aortic arch of the recipient. The presence of transposition of the great arteries is not a major problem. Extensive mobilization of the aortic arch and of the main pulmonary arteries (including division of the ligamentum arteriosum) allows end-to-end anastomosis of the donor and recipient aorta and pulmonary trunk without tension or kinking.

In patients with situs ambiguus, a single atrium receives all the systemic and pulmonary veins. The operation is carried out under hypothermic circulatory arrest to prevent multiple venous cannulations. An intraatrial baffle is constructed, using a prosthetic patch to partition the atrium into a right-sided chamber receiving the systemic veins and a left-sided chamber receiving the pulmonary veins. Standard heart transplantation is then carried out. The problem of managing a recipient with situs inversus is more challenging. The probability of finding a suitable donor with situs inversus is extremely low. Therefore, repositioning the atria should be performed to allow transplantation with a situs solitus donor heart. This can be done by a modification of the Senning procedure. The pulmonary atrium (right-sided) is opened in front of the left pulmonary veins after performance of Sondergaard's maneuver. The interatrial septum is separated from its caudal and cephalad attachments, mobilized, and used to divert the right pulmonary venous blood toward the left-sided opening. Repositioning of the atria is thus obtained.

Previous palliative procedures may need reconstruction. A pulmonary arterial stenosis secondary to a Blalock shunt is repaired by using the donor pulmonary artery. A cavopulmonary shunt is taken down and the superior vena cava and the right pulmonary artery of the donor are used to reconstruct normal venous and pulmonary pathways. Previous complete repair of the malformation leads to pericardial adhesions that increase the difficulty of recipient heart excision. Procedures involving the atria (Senning or Mustard) or the great vessels (arterial switch) must be taken down and may need reconstruction using the donor or recipient tissue or both to allow standard transplantation.

In summary, from a purely technical point of view heart transplantation is always possible although the operative risk is increased if complex reconstructive procedures are needed.[5]

Posttransplant Management

Immunosuppression

Our current protocol of immunosuppression in infants and children is described in Table 26.5. This regimen relies mainly on cyclosporine A therapy. Cyclosporine is begun on the first postoperative day. Whole blood level of cyclosporine is determined daily by monoclonal antibody radioimmunoassay. A high dosage is used during the first month (blood level: 300–400 ng/mL). Cyclosporine dosage is then progressively tapered to a long-term maintenance blood level of 100–150 ng/mL. Long-term use of steroids is avoided; however, in some patients, steroids may be temporarily or permanently necessary because long-term cyclosporine therapy is badly tolerated or unable to ensure adequate immunosuppression.

Diagnosis and Treatment of Rejection

For obvious technical reasons a program of systematic serial endomyocardial biopsies cannot be carried out as it is in adult programs. Cardiac examination is initially performed twice weekly, then weekly after the first month and monthly after 6 months. Routine examination includes physical examination, chest roentgenogram, electrocardiography, and echocardiography to evaluate ventricular function. Some clinical symptoms are particularly suggestive of acute rejection: fever, irritability, poor feeding, unexplained increase in resting heart rate, hepatomegaly, and excessive weight gain. If these findings are associated with echocardiographic evidence of abnormal ventricular systolic or diastolic function or both, rejection is highly probable and immediate rejection treatment may be instituted although confirmation at biopsy is preferable. When rejection is suspected but with a discrepancy between clinical and echocardiographic signs, endomyocardial biopsy is necessary.

Endomyocardial biopsies can be performed even in small infants by using the femoral or the jugular vein with a very low morbidity rate. In our series, 125 endomyocardial biopsies have been performed in 24 children (12 in the same patient) with no mortality and only one serious accident (hemothorax).

If rejection is present at biopsy, it is graded according to Billingham[6] and treatment is instituted with the protocol described in Table 26.6. Acute rejection usually resolves under current treatment (including high-dosage steroids, anti-CD3 monoclonal antibody, or both): this must be

TABLE 26.5 Current Immunosuppressive Regimen in Infants and Children

Postoperative Period
  Cyclosporine A
    IV Infusion 2–6 mg/kg/d
    Adjusted to Maintain Whole Blood Level at 300–400 ng/mL
  Rabbit Antithymocyte Globulin (RATG)
    IV Infusion 5 mg/kg/d
    5- to 7-d Course
  Methylprednisolone
    100 mg/m^2/d for 5 d
    Then Tapering over 5 d
Maintenance Therapy
  Cyclosporine A
    Oral Administration every 8 h or every 12 h
    Adjusted to Maintain Whole Blood Level
      300–400 ng/mL for 1 mo
      150–200 ng/mL for 6 mo
      100–150 ng/mL after 6 mo
  Azathioprine
    Oral Administration every 24 h
    2 mg/kg/d
    To Maintain WBC 4000–6000/m^3
  No Steroids

TABLE 26.6 Treatment Protocol of Acute Rejection

Mild to Moderate Rejection
  Initial Treatment
    Methylprednisolone IV: 1g/1.73 m^2 BSA/d for 3 d
    Control Biopsy at Day 7
  Persistent Rejection
    OKT3: 0.1 mg/kg/d for 10 d
Severe Rejection
  Initial Treatment
    Methylprednisolone IV: 1g/1.73 m^2 BSA/d for 3 d
    OKT3: 0.1 mg/kg/d for 10 d
  Life-Threatening: Extracorporeal Membrane Oxygenation

BSA = Body surface area, OKT3 = Anti-CD3 monoclonal antibody.

confirmed by a control endomyocardial biopsy. Extracorporeal membrane oxygenation may be necessary to control life-threatening rejection episodes.

Prevention of Infection

Prophylactic antibiotics are given during the perioperative period. Cytomegalovirus (CMV) is an extremely common cause of infection in children who have had transplantation. In CMV-seropositive recipients or in patients receiving a CMV-seropositive donor heart, prophylaxis with dihydroxypropoxymethylguanin (DHPG) is used. Routine childhood immunizations use only killed (nonattenuated) vaccine.

Results

Survival

In our series, the actuarial probability of survival was 62% ± 9% at 1 year and 52% ± 11% at 2 years. These results are similar to those obtained in other centers but are less satisfactory than in adult patient series.[7-9]

Causes of Death

Acute graft failure is the main cause (Table 26.7) of early mortality. Early biventricular failure is usually related to primary dysfunction of the graft (decreased myocardial function at the time of procurement, inadequate myocardial preservation with a prolonged ischemic time, or both). Acute right heart failure is frequent in patients with preoperative pulmonary hypertension. Various factors are often associated in the same patient. Inotropic support, pulmonary vasodilation using PGE$_1$, or both are often necessary. Severe failure may be successfully treated by temporary mechanical support (extracorporeal membrane oxygenation or mechanical assist device). In a few cases, urgent retransplantation may be indicated.

Chronic rejection, causing accelerated coronary arteriosclerosis with progressive myocar-

TABLE 26.7 Causes of Death After Heart Transplantation in Children (Laënnec Hospital, 1987–1990)

In-Hospital Deaths		9
Acute Graft Failure	3	
Hyperacute Rejection	2	
Infection	2	
Multiorgan Failure	1	
Late Deaths		4
Chronic Rejection	2	
Sudden Death	1	
Lymphoma	1	

dial dysfunction, seems to be more frequent in the pediatric age group than in the adult population.[10] This may be a major drawback in the long-term prognosis of pediatric recipients.

Rehabilitation, Growth, and Development

Most survivors are leading a normal life with complete rehabilitation and without cardiac medication.

In patients in whom corticosteroids can be completely avoided, normal growth pattern is noted. When prolonged steroid use is necessary, growth retardation is usually observed but catch-up growth can be anticipated once steroids are discontinued.

Complications

Rejection. Acute rejection episodes are very frequent during the first 3 months after transplantation. Of our patients 65% had at least one episode during this early period. The incidence of rejection declines progressively thereafter (only two episodes after 1 year in our series). This rejection pattern is similar to that observed in adult series.

Infection. Infectious complications (including bacterial, viral, fungal, and protozoan infections) are common during the first year after transplantation. They necessitate urgent diagnosis and adequate treatment. Nevertheless, they remain a major cause of mortality.

Immunosuppression-related complications. Systemic hypertension, requiring medical treatment, is very uncommon in our pediatric series (only two cases). This contrasts with the incidence of systemic hypertension noted in adult recipients and may be due to the fact that a virtual single-drug (cyclosporine) regimen is used and that the specific response of children toward long-term cyclosporine therapy differs.

Lymphoproliferative syndrome may develop under immunosuppressive treatment. Early lymphoma (within the first year) usually resolves after reduction in immunotherapy. Late lymphoproliferative disease is a more complex lymphoma, which has a high mortality rate (one in our series).

Renal toxicity is a well-known complication of long-term cyclosporine therapy. Serum creatinine levels usually remain within normal limits. However, we noted a progressive decrease in inulin clearance in some of our patients. Of more concern, 4 patients (in a group of 13) showed moderate to severe tubulointerstitial lesions at kidney biopsy, which was systematically performed 6 to 8 months after grafting. There was no clear relation between the occurrence of renal lesions and the dosage of cyclosporine. This demonstrates the importance of individual factors. The dosage of cyclosporine should be kept as low as possible and strict monitoring of the renal function is mandatory.

HEART AND LUNG TRANSPLANTATION

Indications

Various end-stage cardiac and pulmonary diseases may be indications for heart and lung transplantation in children (Table 26.8). Cystic fibrosis, Eisenmenger's syndrome, and primary pulmonary hypertension are most frequent. Among these patients, some (particularly most cystic fibrosis patients) have normal cardiac function; their hearts may be used as grafts for cardiac recipients with borderline elevation of pulmonary vascular resistances (domino procedure).

Contraindications to heart-lung transplantation are listed in Table 26.9. Normal mechanical properties of the ventilatory system and good nutritional status (particularly in cystic fibrosis patients) are mandatory to allow early postoperative extubation. Uncontrollable intraoperative bleeding remains the major operative risk of heart-lung transplantation. Patients with extensive pleural or mediastinal adhesions secondary to previous thoracic surgery or primary pleural involvement should be excluded. A CAT scan is obtained to assess the severity of pleural lesions. In some patients with unilateral pleural lesions, transplantation of the heart and one lung may be indicated.

The Operation

Selection of the Donor

The importance of careful donor selection cannot be overemphasized. The criteria for acceptable heart-lung donors are shown in Table 26.10. Preserving adequate function of the lungs in brain-dead patients is difficult and necessitates careful

TABLE 26.8 Potential Indications for Heart-Lung Transplantation in Children

Eisenmenger's Syndrome
Congenital Heart Defects With Absent or Hypoplastic
    Pulmonary Arteries
Diffuse Pulmonary Diseases
    Cystic Fibrosis
    Primary Pulmonary Hypertension
    Miscellaneous: Fibrosis, Bronchiectasis, Emphysema

TABLE 26.9 Current Contraindications to Heart-Lung Transplantation

Deterioration of Ventilatory Function
    Phrenic Nerve Palsy
    Kyphoscoliosis
Poor Nutritional Status (Cystic Fibrosis)
Major Pleural Lesions
Previous Thoracic Surgery (Relative)

medical management to prevent lung infection and pulmonary edema. Donor/recipient size matching must be very strict. A graft of the same size as the recipient chest or preferably a little smaller is mandatory. A graft that is larger, even to a slight extent, is discarded because postoperative edema would result in diffuse atelectasis and severe intrapulmonary right-to-left shunting. On the other hand, implantation of small organs in a significantly larger recipient would create space problems with possible prolonged air leak and increased risk of contamination and empyema. The strict enforcement of these various criteria easily explains the scarcity of suitable heart and lung donors.

Procurement and Preservation of the Graft

Harvesting of the graft. The heart and both lungs are removed en bloc.[11] Particular care is taken when detaching the heart-lung bloc from the posterior mediastinum. The mediastinal tissue is carefully ligated on the graft side to prevent postoperative back-bleeding from the graft. The ligatures are placed in contact with the esophagus and the descending aorta to preserve, as much as possible, the bronchial blood supply.

Preservation of the graft. The heart is preserved by the same technique used for isolated

TABLE 26.10 Criteria for Acceptable Heart-Lung Donors

Brain Death Declared; Signed Parental Consent
Absence of Malignancy and Infection
Normal Heart (see Table 26.4)
Normal Lungs
    Normal Gas Exchange
    Clear Lung Fields on Chest Roentgenogram
    Low Ventilation Inflation Pressure
    Short Period of Assisted Ventilation
Donor/Recipient Matching
    ABO Blood Group Compatibility
    Size Matching
Anticipated Ischemic Time < 3–4 h

heart transplantation. The lungs are protected by the Papworth single flush technique.[12] An intravenous prostacyclin infusion (10 ng/kg/min) is begun 5 to 10 minutes before cardiac arrest. After administration of the cardioplegic solution, a protective pulmonary solution (including donor blood, Ringer's lactate solution, salt-poor albumin, mannitol, prostacyclin, and heparin) is infused into the main pulmonary artery under low pressure. The lungs are then immersed in iced saline solution. This current technique provides a safe ischemic time of up to 3 hours; the acceptable ischemic period may probably be extended up to 4 to 5 hours.

Various other techniques (deep hypothermia under cardiopulmonary bypass, crystalloid pneumoplegic solution, pharmacological protection) have been studied experimentally or used with satisfactory clinical results. In the near future, techniques allowing extended safe ischemic time may become available.[13]

Recipient Operation

Under normothermic cardiopulmonary bypass, the heart and each lung are successively removed.[11] The main bronchial stumps and the carina are freed from the surrounding mediastinal tissue. The reimplantation is performed by reanastomosing the trachea, the right atrium, and the ascending aorta.

Heart-lung transplantation is a major thoracic surgical procedure. The thoracic nerves must be carefully preserved. The tracheal blood supply should be preserved to allow satisfactory healing of the airway anastomosis. The intraoperative hemorrhagic risk may be increased by extensive pleural adhesions or a major collateral bronchial circulation.

Posttransplant Management

Management of the Early Postoperative Period

Pulmonary edema is common during the early postoperative course.[14] The best treatment is prevention. Many factors may promote pulmonary edema: suboptimal graft function at the time of procurement, prolonged ischemic time, and loss of the pulmonary lymphatic drainage. Accumulation of fluid in the transplanted lungs is prevented to allow early extubation. Fluids are restricted, diuresis is encouraged, and optimal myocardial function is achieved. A negative fluid balance is obtained for the first 4 to 6 days.

Unsatisfactory healing of the tracheal anastomosis (resulting in early dehiscence or secondary stenosis) may occur. Wrapping of the anastomosis with a pedicule of omentum is no longer done. Preservation of the tracheal blood supply during surgery, maintenance of adequate postoperative cardiac function, early weaning off assisted ventilation and early extubation, and avoidance of corticosteroids during the first 3 weeks (except in cases of acute rejection) permit satisfactory airway healing in most patients.

Prevention of infectious complications is of utmost importance. Prophylactic antibiotics are given for the first week. This includes two major antibiotics unless the recipient, donor, or both have been colonized, in which case antibiotics are chosen according to the intraoperative tracheal cultures. Prophylaxis of CMV infection uses DHPG (between day 15 and day 30) in all patients, except if both donor and recipient are CMV-seronegative. *Pneumocystis carinii* infections may be prevented by prophylactic administration of trimethoprim-sulfamethoxazole (TMP-SMZ).

Management after the Initial Period

During the first 3–6 postoperative months, rejection and infection of the transplanted lungs are very common. These complications have similar clinical and radiological manifestations: fever, shortness of breath, fall in forced expiratory volume in 1 second (FEV_1), lung infiltrates revealed by chest roentgenogram. Accurate diagnosis can be achieved only by transbronchial lung biopsies. In children, at least five to eight biopsy specimens from various lung segments must be obtained. These specimens are taken for histological analysis and immunofluorescence and for viral, bacterial, fungal, and protozoan cultures. Acute rejection or infection or the association of both is thus confirmed and treated adequately. Although less frequent, cardiac rejection may occur independently and require the same management used after isolated heart transplantation.

Late Management

The late results of heart-lung transplantation in children are burdened with a high incidence of obliterative bronchiolitis (OB). There is now increasing evidence that OB is a manifestation of chronic pulmonary rejection.[15] Late rejection may be clinically asymptomatic. Pulmonary function is routinely evaluated very frequently, with particular regard to FEV_1 and forced expiratory flow 25–75 (FEF_{25-75}). Any decrease in one of these measurements, even in the absence of clinical or radiological symptoms, must lead to transbronchial lung biopsies. Rejection, if confirmed at biopsy, is treated with corticosteroids until FEV_1, FEF_{25-75}, or both return to normal values. Ultimately, most heart-lung pediatric recipients require long-term immunosuppression by steroids and cyclosporine.

TABLE 26.11 Heart-Lung Transplantation in Children (Laënnec Hospital, 1988–1990)

Diagnosis	Age (Years)	Follow-up Period (Months)	Outcome Death (n = 4)	Survival (n = 3)	Obliterative Bronchiolitis
Eisenmenger's Syndrome	11	24		FC I	+
Eisenmenger's Syndrome	9	23		FC I tracheal stenosis	0
Primary Pulmonary Hypertension	13	16	OB		+ + +
Primary Pulmonary Hypertension	11	11		FC II	+ +
Bronchiectasis (Congenital Humoral Immune Defect)	11	3	Infection (Tracheal Dehiscence)		
Cystic Fibrosis	15	2	Infection		
Pulmonary Atresia and Ventricular Septal Defect	4	day 1	Malignant Hyperthermia		

Abbreviations: 0 = none, + = mild, + + = moderate, + + + = severe, FC I = functional class I, FC II = functional class II (NYHA).

Results

The results of our own series of heart-lung transplantation in patients below 15 years of age are summarized in Table 26.11. This series, although small, emphasizes the current problems of heart-lung transplantation in children. A 1-year survival rate of 50% to 60% can be anticipated; complete rehabilitation is achieved in survivors, but there is a very high incidence of late obliterative bronchiolitis (OB).

Improvements in the early results should be obtained by very careful selection of both donor and recipient, meticulous attempts to prevent infection, and an aggressive approach in the diagnosis and treatment of early rejection and infection. We hope, on the other hand, that the late incidence of OB will be decreased by our current aggressive protocol for the early diagnosis and treatment of late lung rejection.

LUNG TRANSPLANTATION

Lung transplantation is a rapidly evolving field. The overall worldwide experience remains small, particularly in children, but is expanding very rapidly. From a theoretical point of view, patients with end-stage pulmonary disease and normal cardiac function are potential candidates for lung transplantation. Many patients who are presently considered candidates for heart-lung transplantation may in the future become potential lung recipients.

Single-Lung Transplantation

Single-lung transplantation was the first technique used because it is technically very simple and allows transplantation of two recipients from the same donor.

Surgical Technique

Through a standard lateral thoracotomy and, in most cases, with no need for cardiopulmonary bypass, a pneumonectomy is performed and the donor lung is transplanted by anastomosing, respectively, the bronchus, the pulmonary artery, and a pulmonary venous stump.[16] The left lung is transplanted in preference to the right because the operation is technically simpler, but transplantation is possible on either side according to individual factors. The bronchial anastomosis is wrapped with a pedicle of omentum to promote satisfactory healing.

Indications and Results

Pulmonary fibrosis. Single-lung transplantation is an attractive procedure for patients with severe pulmonary fibrosis since it can be anticipated that most alveolar ventilation and lung perfusion will move preferentially from the native to the transplanted lung, because elastic recoil and vascular resistances are greater in the native fibrotic lung than in the transplanted normal lung.

Current criteria for recipient selection are no evidence of overt right heart failure, possibility of weaning off corticosteroids, adequate nutrition, adequate psychosocial support.

Among 20 adult patients transplanted by the Toronto Lung Transplant Group,[17] there were nine deaths. Most early deaths were related to infectious complications, whereas chronic rejection and obliterative bronchiolitis were the main causes of late death. Late evaluation of the survivors showed significant functional improvement, although exercise capacity was decreased.

The indication for single-lung transplantation is questionable in the pediatric age group since end-stage fibrotic pulmonary disease is rare in children and only incomplete functional re-habilitation is achieved.

Other indications. Recently, single-lung transplantation, in association with repair of the intracardiac defect, has been proposed for patients with Eisenmenger's syndrome.[18] The results remain to be evaluated.

Double-Lung Transplantation

Double-lung transplantation has been designed to obviate the main drawbacks of single-lung transplantation: incomplete rehabilitation and unsuitability for many patients with end-stage pulmonary disease.

Surgical Techniques

Both lungs can be transplanted en bloc.[19] Through a median sternotomy and during cardiopulmonary bypass, both lungs are successively removed and the bronchial stumps are freed from the surrounding mediastinal tissue. The transplanted lungs are connected by a left atrial cuff and the main pulmonary artery. Reimplantation includes bilateral bronchial anastomoses, left atrial anastomosis posterior to the heart, and pulmonary artery anastomosis anteriorly.

Both lungs can also be transplanted sequentially through a bilateral transverse thoracosternotomy. Cardiopulmonary bypass is not indispensable, although it is probably safer for most patients. Cardiac denervation, usually associated with en bloc double-lung transplantation, is thus prevented.[20]

Indications and Results

Double-lung transplantation is an attractive procedure for all patients with end-stage pulmonary disease and normal cardiac function. The potential late cardiac drawbacks of heart-lung transplantation (namely accelerated coronary arteriosclerosis) are avoided. In patients with septic pulmonary disease (cystic fibrosis, bronchiectasis) double-lung transplantation is mandatory since single-lung grafting would lead to contamination of the transplanted lung from the native chronically infected lung left in place. In patients with emphysema, it is anticipated that single-lung transplantation would lead to an increase in intrapulmonary shunting since the overly compliant native lung would receive much of the ventilation and perfusion would preferentially be directed to the transplanted lung; double-lung transplantation is thus theoretically preferable. In all patients with end-stage pulmonary disease, double-lung transplantation is more likely to achieve complete functional rehabilitation.

In the initial experience with double-lung transplantation, there was a high incidence of airway complications at the site of the tracheal anastomosis despite omental wrapping; this was probably related to the suppression of carinal blood supply from the heart. Performing bilateral bronchial anastomoses has significantly reduced the risk of airway complications.[21] Direct revascularization of the bronchial arteries may be an important, although technically demanding, improvement.[22]

Many children may be candidates for double-lung transplantation (particularly cystic fibrosis patients). However, further experience is needed to evaluate the results. The exact incidence of airway complications in patients with small airway conduits remains to be determined. Late results may be burdened with the same risk of obliterative bronchiolitis noted after heart-lung transplantation. Aggressive management of lung rejection is thus necessary.

CONCLUSIONS

Thoracic organ transplantation is a very innovative and exciting field in pediatric surgery. Nevertheless excessive enthusiasm should be tempered by the fact that questions are still unanswered. These concern long-term results, indications in certain conditions, and availability of suitable donors.

As far as the issue of suitable donors is concerned, it has been estimated that the potential pool of pediatric donors can match the number of potential recipients. However, many organs cannot be explanted either because clinical deterioration occurs before procurement or because parental consent is not asked for or obtained.

Many interesting issues are presently under investigation and could widen the horizons of the field of transplantation. The following key questions may find an answer in the next few years:

Does transplant in the neonatal period yield good results as a result of the immature status of the immunological system?

Can the duration of the ischemic time be extended to allow for prospective MCH donor/recipient matching?

Will xenotransplantation be possible with improved techniques of immunological manipulation?

While waiting for all these answers, we believe that in the meantime heart or lung transplantation in children should be reserved for a highly selected group of patients and be performed in a limited number of surgical centers.

A lesson should be learned from the history of heart transplantation in adults.

REFERENCES

1. Welsh K, Male D: Transplantation and rejection. In: Roitt IM, Brostoff J, Male D, eds. *Immunology 1989.* New York: Gower Medical Publishing, 1989.
2. Boucek MM, Kanakriyeh MS, Mathis CM, et al: Cardiac transplantation in infancy: Donors and recipients. *J Pediatr* 1990;116:171–176.
3. Lower RR, Shumway NE: Studies on orthotopic homotransplantation of the canine heart. *Surg Forum* 1960;11:18–20.
4. Bailey LL, Conception W, Shattuck H, Huang L: Method of heart transplantation for treatment of hypoplatic left heart syndrome. *J Thorac Cardiovasc Surg* 1986;92:1–5.
5. Mayer JE, Perry S, O'Brien P, et al: Orthotopic heart transplantation for complex congenital heart disease. *J Thorac Cardiovasc Surg* 1990;99:484–492.
6. Billingham ME: Diagnosis of cardiac rejection by endomyocardial biopsy. *Heart Transplant* 1981;1:25–30.
7. Addonizio LJ, Hsu DT, Fuzesi L, et al: Optimal timing of pediatric heart transplantation. *Circulation* 1989;80(suppl III):84–89.
8. Trento A, Griffith BP, Fricker FJ, et al: Lessons learned in pediatric heart transplantation. *Ann Thorac Surg* 1989;48:617–623.
9. Starnes VA, Bernstein D, Oyer PE, et al: Heart transplantation in children. *J Heart Transplant* 1989;8:20–26.
10. Pahl E, Fricker FJ, Armitage J, et al: Coronary arterio sclerosis in pediatric heart transplant survivors: Limitation of long-term survival. *J Pediatr* 1990;116:177–183.
11. Vouhé PR, Dartevelle PG: Heart lung transplantation: Technical modifications that may improve the early outcome. *J Thorac Cardiovasc Surg* 1989;97:906–910.
12. Hakim M, Higenbottam T, Bethune D, et al: Selection and procurement of combined heart and lung grafts for transplantation. *J Thorac Cardiovasc Surg* 1988;95:474–479.
13. Zenati M, Dowling RD, Armitage JM, et al: Organ procurement for pulmonary transplantation. *Ann Thorac Surg* 1989;48:882–886.
14. Scott JP, Fradet G, Smyth RL, et al: Management following heart and lung transplantation: Five years experience. *Eur J Cardiothorac Surg* 1990;4:197–201.
15. Scott JP, Clelland C, Higgenbottam T, et al: The natural history of obliterative bronchiolatis. *Transplant Proc* 1989;21:2592–2593.
16. Cooper JD, Pearson FG, Patterson GA, et al: Technique of successful lung transplantation in humans. *J Thorac Cardiovasc Surg* 1987;93:173–181.
17. Grossman RF, Frost A, Zamel N, et al: Results of single lung transplantation for bilateral pulmonary fibrosis. *N Engl J Med* 1990;322:727–733.
18. Fremes SE, Patterson GA, Williams WG, et al: Single lung transplantation and closure of patent ductus arteriosus for Eisenmenger's syndrome. *J Thorac Cardiovasc Surg* 1990;100:1–5.
19. Patterson GA, Cooper JD, Goldman B, et al: Technique of successful clinical double lung transplantation. *Ann Thorac Surg* 1988;45:626–633.
20. Pasque MK, Cooper JD, Kaiser CR, et al: Improved technique for bilateral lung transplantation: Rational and initial clinical experience. *Ann Thorac Surg* 1990;49:785–791.
21. Noirclerc MJ, Metras D, Valliant A, et al: Bilateral bronchial anastomoses in double lung and heart lung transplantation. *Eur J Cardiothorac Surg* 1990;4:314–317.
22. Schreinemakers HHJ, Weder W, Miyoshi S, et al: Direct revascularization of bronchial arteries for lung transplantation: An anatomical study. *Ann Thorac Surg* 1990;49:44–54.

Transplantation of Thoracic Organs in Children

G. Alexander Patterson, MD, FRCS(C), FACS

Professor Vouhé has presented a detailed summary of a field that is in its early stages of development. His emphasis on the world's pediatric cardiac experience reflects the size of that experience in comparison to the small experience of combined heart-lung transplantation and almost anecdotal experience of isolated lung transplantation in children. Comments regarding these latter procedures are necessarily influenced by experience with the adult population. Our own program has very limited experience with the pediatric age group.

The reader is given a brief review of the allograft response, an area not familiar to most thoracic surgeons caring for children. Professor Vouhé points out the considerable morbidity and mortality associated with chronic rejection of cardiac and lung allografts in children. This has proved to be the most common cause of late death after combined heart-lung transplantation in children. The problem, of course, is that of making a precise diagnosis of rejection. Bronchoalveolar lavage is useful in excluding opportunistic infection. The Papworth group has clearly shown that transbronchial biopsy is the only reliable method of diagnosing rejection after pulmonary transplantation. The typical clinical parameters of dyspnea, fever, leukocytosis, and pulmonary infiltrate are nonspecific and serve only to indicate the need for transbronchial biopsy. Unfortunately, obtaining adequate-sized biopsy specimens by transbronchial biopsy is a technical challenge in the pediatric age group. The same problem exists after cardiac transplantation, in which repeated endomyocardial biopsy is not practical. A number of clinical, electrocardiographic (ECG), echocardiographic, and computerized axial tomographic parameters

have been proposed to improve the diagnostic accuracy of rejection.

We have relied on triple-drug immunosuppressive therapy using cyclosporin, azathioprine, and corticosteroid. We now use corticosteroid routinely during the early postoperative phase and have observed no detrimental effect on airway healing among isolated lung recipients. Elimination of chronic steroid has obvious attractions. However, we have elected to maintain our patients on chronic steroids because of our concern about the subsequent development of chronic bronchiolitis obliterans. Those pediatric and adult cardiac transplant programs avoiding chronic steroid use have a diminished incidence of infection and systemic hypertension.

Antibiotic prophylaxis is employed routinely. We use broad-spectrum gram-negative and anaerobic coverage in the patients with septic lung disease (cystic fibrosis). In these patients we have also employed inhaled aminoglycoside. Gancyclovir is used routinely for recipients who are (CMV)-positive or who receive a graft from a CMV-positive donor.

RECIPIENT SELECTION

The selection of these young patients must be very careful indeed to maximize the likelihood of success with a very limited donor supply and institutional resource.

Heart

The subject of heart transplantation is covered in detail by Professor Vouhé, and the text reflects his extensive experience. Several groups have discovered that many children with hypoplastic left heart syndrome can survive beyond the neonatal period, improving their chance of obtaining a suitable graft and a successful outcome. The difficulties of cardiac transplantation in the presence of pulmonary hypertension are also well described. Patients with complex congenital abnormalities and associated pulmonary hypertension are likely best treated by combined heart-lung transplantation. However, many patients with Eisenmenger's syndrome would benefit from isolated lung transplantation and simultaneous repair of the cardiac defect, as has been employed in our center[1] and elsewhere.

Isolated Lung Transplantation

Single- and double-lung transplantation have proven to be effective therapeutic modalities for the treatment of end-stage lung disease. Single-lung transplantation has been traditionally employed for fibrotic lung disease.[2] Yet in the past 2 years it has been proved effective in obstructive lung disease,[3] as well as in pulmonary vascular disease.[1] Excellent functional results in these patients have been achieved in an increasing number of transplant centers. In the pediatric age group diaphragmatic hernia and bronchopulmonary dysplasia are two conditions in which single-lung replacement offers a very attractive option.

Double-lung transplantation has been successfully employed for patients with obstructive and septic lung disease (cystic fibrosis, bronchiectasis). However, in most North American centers patients with cystic fibrosis have reached adult life before their disease has become severe enough to warrant consideration of transplantation. Pediatric patients with obstructive lung disease should probably receive bilateral lung grafts since the functional results of bilateral replacement are slightly better than those of single-lung grafts in patients with obstructive lung disease. Early complications associated with donor airway ischemia[4] have been largely overcome by technical innovations (discussed later).

These procedures offer distinct advantages over combined heart-lung transplantation. The recipient heart is left in situ. The donor heart can be used in another recipient, a definite advantage in North America, where the "domino" procedure is not popular among cardiac transplant programs. Functional results are excellent even in patients with severe pretransplantation right ventricular dysfunction.

It should also be pointed out that pleural disease is not a contraindication to pulmonary or combined cardiopulmonary transplantation. Computerized axial tomography (CAT) cannot reliably distinguish visceral and parietal pleural symphysis. Although CAT scanning is of value in the surgical planning for these patients it should not be used to exclude patients from surgical consideration.

Combined Heart-Lung Transplantation

We currently believe that combined heart-lung transplantation has a very limited role in the management of septic, obstructive, or vascular pulmonary disease. These conditions in the main can be effectively managed by isolated lung transplantation. It is our opinion that combined heart-lung transplantation should be employed in those patients with irreparable or end-stage cardiac disease in the presence of primary or secondary pulmonary hypertension.

DONOR SELECTION

Professor Vouhé has outlined the critical importance of rigid donor selection criteria. Ours do not differ significantly. We have identified and successfully employed single-lung donors whose contralateral lung was shown radiographically to be abnormal. Gas exchange with single-lung ventilation and perfusion can be easily determined immediately before harvest.

Satisfactory lung and heart grafts can always be harvested separately from the same donor when both teams approach the harvest in a spirit of cooperation. A variety of pulmonary preservation strategies exist. We employ a pulmonary vasodilator (prostaglandin E_1 [PGE_1], 500 mg, directly into the pulmonary artery) and 4°C modified Euro-Collins flush (500 cc/Kg).

TECHNIQUE

The technical intricacies of pediatric cardiac replacement have been well covered, and I am not in a position to elaborate.

The single-lung technique differs slightly from our original report.[5] We now employ a telescoping bronchial anastomosis, overlapping the recipient and donor bronchus by one cartilaginous ring. We adopted this technique from the San Antonio group[6] along with their recommendation for early routine corticosteroid use. Since making these changes we have not experienced any airway complications among single- or double-lung recipients. We no longer use bronchial omentopexy, preferring to cover the bronchial anastomosis with donor and recipient peribronchial nodal tissue.

The left side offers no technical advantage over the right. Indeed the right is preferable for a number of reasons: it provides easier access for cannulation should cardiopulmonary bypass be required; a much larger circumference bronchial anastomosis is possible at the proximal right main bronchus than at the distal left main bronchus; and among patients with obstructive lung disease receiving single-lung grafts there appears to be a lesser degree of mediastinal shift to the transplanted side if the graft is placed on the right.

The double-lung technique has evolved significantly from our original description.[7] As outlined by the Washington University group[8] we also employ bilateral sequential single-lung transplantation through a transverse incision that provides excellent exposure to both pleural spaces. This permits safe division of all pleural adhesions and control of the augmented bronchial circulation present in many of these patients. Cardiopulmonary bypass can be avoided in most double-lung recipients, particularly those with obstructive lung disease.

FUTURE DIRECTIONS

The critical shortage of donors must be addressed. For cardiac recipients recent, exciting developments in xenograft technology will ultimately prove beneficial. This, of course, may benefit lung recipients as well. However, an immediate alternative is available, particularly for the pediatric group: living related donors. This donor strategy has already been employed successfully in liver transplantation and in a very small number of pulmonary transplants. The ethical considerations are perhaps somewhat fewer in pulmonary transplantation since the risk of pulmonary lobar donation in a young healthy adult would be minimal indeed. However, a much more intriguing question is whether an adult pulmonary lobe would grow after placement in a neonate or child. These questions are being actively pursued in a number of transplant laboratories around the world.

Current immunosuppressive regimens are toxic and provide nonspecific immunosuppression, making the recipient susceptible to a host of infectious agents. Less toxic and more specific immunosuppressive strategies are being actively pursued; some are already at the clinical trial stage. Further advances in this field will provide improved specific graft tolerance and better long-term functional results in an ever-increasing number of children with terminal cardiopulmonary disease.

REFERENCES

1. Fremes SE, Patterson GA, Williams WG, et al: Single lung transplant and closure of patent ductus arteriosus for Eisenmenger's syndrome. *J Thorac Cardiovasc Surg* 1990;100:1–5.
2. Grossman RF, Forst A, Zamel N, et al: Results of single-lung transplantation for bilateral pulmonary fibrosis. *N Engl J Med* 1990;322(11):727–733.
3. Mal H, Andreassian B, Pamela F, et al: Unilateral lung transplantation in end stage pulmonary emphysema. *Am Rev Respir Dis* 1989;140:797–802.
4. Patterson GA, Todd TRT, Cooper JD, et al: Airway complications after double lung transplantation. *J Thorac Cardiovasc Surg* 1990;99:14–21.
5. Cooper JD, Pearson FG, Patterson GA, et al: Technique of successful lung transplantation in humans. *J Thorac Cardiovasc Surg* 1987;93:182–198.
6. Calhoon JH, Grover FL, Gibbons WJ, et al: Single lung transplantation: Alternative indications and technique. *J Thorac Cardiovasc Surg*, in press, 1991.
7. Patterson GA, Cooper JD, Goldman B, et al: Technique of successful clinical double lung transplantation. *Ann Thorac Surg* 1988;45:626–633.
8. Pasque MK, Cooper JD, Kaiser L, et al: Improved technique for bilateral lung transplantation: Rational and initial clinical experience. *Ann Thorac Surg* 1990;49:785–791.

Chapter 27

Fetal Surgery: Practical Considerations and Current Status:
Where Do We Go from Here with Bochdalek Diaphragmatic Hernia?

Kevin C. Pringle, MB, ChB, FRACS

Diaphragmatic hernia has an incidence of 1 in 5000 live births[1,2] and a true mortality of over 60% of babies born alive with diaphragmatic hernia,[1,3] although the precise mortality would be impossible to obtain unless 100% of perinatal deaths had autopsy evaluation. It is interesting to reflect that the mortality from diaphragmatic hernia has not improved significantly since Bowditch reported his first collective review of the literature in 1847.[4,5] (This review included Morgagni's paper, but not Bochdalek's.)

The mortality from diaphragmatic hernia is outlined in Table 27.1. According to the figures in the *World Health Statistics Annual 1988*,[6] if one accepts an incidence of 1 in 5000 live births, then the projected number of babies born with diaphragmatic hernia in 1986 or 1987 is 37 for the Netherlands, 751 for the United States, 155 for the United Kingdom, and 128 for West Germany. If one assumes a conservative 60% mortality from this lesion, then the figures for deaths from diaphragmatic hernia are 22 for the Netherlands, 451 for the United States, 93 for the United Kingdom, and 77 for West Germany. These are of the order of 65% to 75% of the number of deaths from leukemia in the first 14 years of life, and approximately one tenth of the number of the deaths from congenital heart disease in the first year of life. For diaphragmatic hernia, the vast majority

of these deaths occur in the first few hours of life, often even before referral to a pediatric surgeon is possible.[1,7]

Support of selected patients with diaphragmatic hernia using extracorporeal membrane oxygenation (ECMO) has resulted in the salvage of some infants who would otherwise have died.[8-11] However, since approximately half of the babies who die from diaphragmatic hernia do so before they reach a pediatric surgical center,[1,7] ECMO can be expected to make only minimal inroads into the mortality from this lesion.

There are three reasonably clearly defined groups within the clinical spectrum of diaphragmatic hernia.[12,13]

Group 1 patients can never be adequately oxygenated and usually die shortly after birth, regardless of treatment. There is some controversy in the literature as to whether these infants should be offered ECMO. This group supplies the majority of the infants whose lungs have been subjected to morphometric analysis. It is probably the largest group, comprising up to 50% of patients.

Group 2 patients initially do well or occasionally may initially appear to be in group 1 and respond to intubation and ventilation (either before or after repair) but later develop persistent pulmonary hypertension. Collins and co-workers[14] and Geggel and associates[12] have referred to this as the "honeymoon" group. In the past, this group has done poorly, although in many centers most of these babies are now being salvaged by ECMO.

TABLE 27.1 Mortality From Diaphragmatic Hernia

Country (Year)	Total Live Births	Approximate Total DH (1:5000)[a]	Estimated Total Deaths DH (60% Mortality)[b]	Deaths of Various Lesions[c]	
				Congenital Heart Disease 1st Year	Leukemia 0–14 Years
Netherlands (1986)	184,513	37	22	172 (13%)	34 (65%)
United States (1986)	3,756,547	751	451	4921 (9%)	667 (67%)
United Kingdom (1985)	775,617	155	93	657 (14%)	134 (69%)
West Germany (1986)	642,010	128	77	554 (14%)	102 (75%)

DH = diaphragmatic hernia.
[a] Estimate of numbers of liveborn babies with a posterolateral diaphragmatic hernia, assuming an incidence of 1 in 5000 live births.
[b] Estimate of deaths from diaphragmatic hernia, assuming a mortality rate of 60% of live-born babies with a diaphragmatic hernia.
[c] The numbers in parentheses represent the estimated deaths from diaphragmatic hernia expressed as a percentage of the deaths from congenital heart disease in the first year of life or from leukemia in the first 14 years of life.

Group 3 patients have few or no symptoms, and almost all survive. Those seen after the neonatal period tend to have bowel obstruction or gastrointestinal symptoms.[15,16]

Whatever criteria are used to measure lung development, the lungs of infants dying from diaphragmatic hernia are hypoplastic: that is, they are smaller than normal.[12,13,17–19] However, it must be remembered that all the infants whose lungs have been studied by detailed morphometric analysis have died, suggesting that they are at the worst end of the spectrum. Apart from the article by Geggel et al,[12] few studies distinguishing among the three groups have been published. However, with improved techniques, it is possible that most of group 2 and group 3 babies will be able to be salvaged. Further gains in survival, therefore, will only be possible if a significant advance is made in the management of group 1 patients. One possible option for the salvaging of these babies is to repair the diaphragmatic hernia before they are born: that is, a fetal repair.

HISTORY OF FETAL SURGERY

As has been pointed out in a recent review,[20] fetal surgery has a long history, dating back at least to Roman times. Therapeutic fetal surgery has a history recorded from the middle 1960s, when erythroblastosis fetalis was a major problem in obstetrics and neonatology. By 1966, more than 20 cases of open fetal transfusions had been reported.[21–28] These babies were delivered at intervals varying from 1 day to 8 weeks after the surgery. In an era when uteruses were closed with heavy catgut after open procedures, there were no *reported* uterine ruptures or uterine wound dehiscences. It is impossible to ascertain how many of these babies were delivered by vaginal delivery, but it is probable that some had a vaginal delivery shortly after the open fetal surgical procedure.

Open fetal transfusions stopped when percutaneous intraperitoneal transfusions were shown to be much better than open transfusions (in terms of fetal salvage) with the added bonus of having a marked reduction in maternal morbidity.[28] More than anything else, the reduced maternal morbidity associated with percutaneous (needle) transfusions dictated that open transfusions had to be abandoned, and so they were. This leaves the fascinating paradox that, on the one hand, the pioneering work of the late Sir William Liley[29] (who, together with Liggins[30,31] and his other associates perfected percutaneous peritoneal fetal transfusions) made him one of the fathers of fetal therapy and, on the other hand, he was the individual most responsible for our current paucity of knowledge about open fetal surgical procedures in humans. It is fascinating to speculate what might currently be available in the way of open fetal surgical techniques had percutaneous fetal transfusion techniques not been developed.

Experimental Models of Fetal Repair of Diaphragmatic Hernia

The fetal lamb model of diaphragmatic hernia has been most widely used. Olivet and colleagues,[32] de Lorimier and associates,[33,34] and Kent and coworkers[35] developed models of diaphragmatic hernias in fetal lambs, and de Lorimier's group[34] and Kent's group,[35] especially, were able to validate the conclusion that the creation of a diaphragmatic hernia resulted in pulmonary hypoplasia and neonatal physiology strikingly similar to that of human neonates with a diaphragmatic hernia. This group was able to demonstrate the sustained pulmonary hypertension that is seen both in those babies who "honeymoon" and in those who can never be adequately ventilated. Haller and his group were able to simulate a diaphragmatic hernia by placing a silicone rubber (Silastic) balloon in the thorax of the fetal lamb.[36] Harrison and his group expanded on this model by inflating the balloon throughout pregnancy, using a catheter led out through the ewe's abdominal wall.[37] They then simulated repair by deflating the balloon at 120 days gestation.[38] Lambs whose "diaphragmatic hernia" had been "repaired" survived (at least for 2 hours), whereas those whose had not been repaired all died soon after birth, in spite of the fact that the balloon was deflated as soon as the lamb was born, simulating neonatal repair.

Harrison's group then went on to create and repair a diaphragmatic hernia in fetal lambs,[39] and after a few false starts with the fetal repairs realized that an abdominal wall patch would be required during the repair to prevent a rise in intraabdominal pressure that otherwise would effectively occlude umbilical venous return. Again, all of the lambs that had fetal repairs lived for up to 2 hours after birth, whereas none of the lambs born with an unrepaired diaphragmatic hernia survived that long. Pringle's group demanded a more stringent definition of survival for the lambs who had had a fetal repair.[40,41] All but one lived for more than 2 hours, but several died in the first few days of life. Of the lambs who were born with a nonrepaired diaphragmatic hernia, most died soon after birth, sometimes even before a neonatal repair could be completed. However, one lived an amazing 89 hours. There was also a suggestion (not ever reaching statistical significance, because of the small numbers involved) that lambs whose diaphragmatic hernias were repaired at 110 days did better than those whose diaphragmatic hernias were repaired at 120 days.

Examination of the lungs of the lambs with diaphragmatic hernia showed that they were not only small (or hypoplastic) but were indeed dysplastic, with a delay in the development of alveoli and an apparent hyperplasia of the type II (surfactant-producing) cells.[41,42] Fetal repair restored lung structure to normal, with alveoli that were perhaps larger than normal and a marked decrease in the frequency with which type II cells were observed.

For all practical purposes, the fetal lamb model has been taken as far as it is possible to take it. However, there are still several important questions to be answered, especially details of how the fetal lamb lung is repaired after fetal correction of a diaphragmatic hernia. Creation of a diaphragmatic hernia in a fetal lamb of appropriate gestation results in a model that provides striking parallels to the human. Fetal repair of the diaphragmatic hernia at the time that the normal fetal lung is in the late canalicular phase (110 days) or early saccular phase (120 days) of development results in greatly improved survival.[43] The next logical step would be a primate model. However, in spite of repeated applications to the National Institutes of Health, such a study has not been funded. In all probability, it is now likely that the next experiments will be on humans.

Problems with Diagnosis

The diagnosis of a diaphragmatic hernia before birth presents several problems. Antenatal diagnosis of diaphragmatic hernia was reported as early as 1969,[44] but once the use of ultrasound scanning became more widespread, it became apparent that cystic adenomatous malformation of the lung was commonly confused with diaphragmatic hernia and may, in fact, be at least as common as diaphragmatic hernia. Puri and Gorman[7] have also stressed that a significant percentage of babies with diaphragmatic hernia have major associated anomalies. Liveborn babies with diaphragmatic hernia have a relatively low incidence (approximately 15%) of associated major anomalies. However, if all cases with diaphragmatic hernia are considered (including those that are stillborn), the incidence of major anomalies rises considerably. It is, of course, difficult to be sure that a given baby examined at, say, 20 weeks gestation, would or would not proceed safely to term. Puri and Gorman[7] have sounded an appropriate note of caution, stressing that major anomalies must be assiduously sought and that the presence of any major associated anomaly would probably exclude such a baby from consideration for fetal therapy.

Adzick and associates[45] reported a survey of babies born after an antenatal diagnosis. In this survey, 20 fetuses in whom the antenatal diagnosis of diaphragmatic hernia was made were found to have other associated anomalies. Fifteen of these were described as "lethal." Unfortunately, in the survey, only 7 of these lethal associated anomalies were diagnosed before the baby was born.

Another factor that is a very important prognostic indicator in diaphragmatic hernia is whether the liver is in the chest. Babies with the liver in the chest have an extremely poor prognosis, but unfortunately, as Harrison has reported,[46] if the liver is in the chest, then attempts to displace it into the abdomen appear to alter umbilical vein dynamics drastically, causing immediate fetal demise if the liver is suddenly transposed into the fetal abdomen. Moreover, since the sonographic appearance of the liver is very similar to that of the normal fetal lung, it is often extremely difficult to decide whether the fetal liver is, in fact, in the chest or not. Failure to detect an intrathoracic fetal liver may well result in having to abandon the fetal procedure after the mother has been put to all the risks of the procedure, with no possible gain.

Problems with Case Selection

Some of the major problems with case selection have been outlined. It clearly would not be ideal to plan an in utero repair on a fetus with other anomalies or in one with the liver in the chest. On the basis of the survey by Adzick and colleagues,[45] in which babies with polyhydramnios had an 89% mortality, Harrison and co-workers[46] have suggested that it is reasonable to offer fetal repair to mothers with a fetus with a diaphragmatic hernia and polyhydramnios. However, there is a potential flaw in the data presented in the survey. This has never been acknowledged since it was pointed out[47] shortly after the article by Adzick and associates[45] was published. Of the 94 fetuses in that survey, 15 had lethal associated anomalies. We are not told how many of these had polyhydramnios. However, if we assume that all of the fetuses with lethal anomalies had polyhydramnios, then those fetuses should be removed from the group to be potentially offered fetal repair. Under these circumstances, if all of the lethal anomalies could be diagnosed before birth, a fetus with no other anomalies and a diaphragmatic hernia who had polyhydramnios would have an expected mortality of approximately 77%. This means that the fetus with a diaphragmatic hernia and polyhydramnios would have approximately a 20% chance of surviving without fetal repair. In spite of the fact that this was pointed out to the authors of this article, both by means of a letter to the editor[47] and in personal discussion, Harrison has never acknowledged this fact in any of his subsequent writings on this subject.[46,48–50]

The other problem with using polyhydramnios as a prognostic factor to guide selection for fetal repair is the fact that it is a relatively late phenomenon. Benacerraf and Adzick[51] have pointed this out, indicating that it seldom appears until after 26–28 weeks gestation. However, if the fetal lamb model is valid, then fetal repairs would best be made at a stage of gestation when the lung is normally in the canalicular phase of development or the early saccular phase at the latest. This would suggest that the period between 20 and 24 weeks would be the best time for fetal repairs.[43] Certainly, Harrison[46] has suggested that after about 26–28 weeks, it becomes increasingly difficult to prevent premature labor after open fetal surgery.

Clearly, what is needed is a marker that will accurately identify a fetus with no other anomalies who will have at least 95% mortality; that is, one who has at least a 95% probability of dying after a neonatal repair. The mother of such a fetus could be offered a fetal repair. Unfortunately, no such marker has been found, so far.

Attempts have been made to deduce fetal lung volume by measuring chest volume and subtracting cardiac and gut volumes or by determining the ratio of heart volume to hernia volume.[52] These measurements are very difficult to make, and are probably subject to fairly large errors, suggesting that they will not be a reliable prognostic indicator.

The presence or absence of fetal breathing movements does not reliably indicate outcome.[53] The vast majority of babies with diaphragmatic hernia appear to continue to have normal fetal breathing movements throughout gestation, whether they are destined to live or die after birth. It is a reasonable hypothesis that pulmonary blood flow to hypoplastic fetal lungs is lower than pulmonary blood flow to normal fetal lungs at a comparable gestational age. It should be possible to deduce pulmonary blood flow if the flow through the main pulmonary artery and that through the ductus can be measured with sufficient accuracy. At present, this is probably not possible, although some have attempted these measurements. It has proved extremely difficult to assess the outcome for those cases diagnosed antenatally in the various reports in the literature. A reasonably complete compilation of the English language literature is presented in Table 27.2.[44–46,52–54,57–71] In cases where several articles have originated from a given institution, only the most recent report is included in the table on the assumption that it is an update of the data from the previous report(s). There are two exceptions to this rule, where it appears that an isolated case report[54] is followed by a more extensive series[52] that does not appear to include the fetus first reported. It is also probable that some of the patients reported in the San Francisco series of papers[46,55,56] are also included in the survey reported by Adzick and co-workers,[45] but it is impossible to tell how many are doubly reported, and so this factor was ignored. In general, the number of cases reported by the authors is listed in the first column (total number of cases). Where possible, the number of cases reported to have any anomaly (including chromosomal anomalies, but with the single exception of the case of pectus carinatum listed by Adzick and associates in the survey) is noted, as is the number of fetuses whose pregnancy was terminated. This latter figure is somewhat difficult to determine: for ex-

TABLE 27.2 Reported Cases of Antenatal Diagnosis of Diaphragmatic Hernia

Author (Ref)	Total No. of Cases	No. with Anomalies	No. Aborted	No. Available for Possible Repair (PR Group)	Raw Mortality (%)		Mortality for PR Group (%)	
Boyd et al[44]	1	1 (Rh disease)	0	0	1/1	(100)	NA	
Aguero, Zighelborim[57]	1	1	0	1	0/1	(0)	NA	
Griscom[58]	1	1	0	0	1/1	(100)	NA	
Bell, Ternberg[59]	1	0	0	1	1/1	(100)	1/1	(100)
Touloukian, Hobbins[60]	1	NS	NS	1	1/1	(100)	1/1	(100)
Marwood, Davison[61]	1	0	0	1	1/1	(100)	1/1	(100)
Fleischer et al[62]	1	1	0	0	1/1	(100)	0	
Stiller et al[63]	1	1	0	0	1/1	(100)	0	
Adzick et al[45]	94	20	1	74	74/93	(80)	55/74	(74)
Crawford et al[54]	1	0	0	1	0/1	(0)	0/1	(0)
Calisti et al[64]	6	1	0	5	5/6	(83)	4/5	(80)
Kelly et al[65]	1	0	0	1	1/1	(100)	0	
Van den Born– Van den Brook et al[66]	1	0	0	1	0/1		0/1	
Hasegawa et al[67]	8	0	0	8	2/8	(25)	2/8	(25)
Crawford et al[44]	18[a]	3	1	15	9/17	(53)	7/15	(47)
Burge et al[68]	5	1	0	4	5/5	(100)	4/4	(100)
Adzick et al[69]	38	13	4	25	25/34	(74)	16/25	(64)
Harrison[46]	40	11	9[b]	11	22/31	(71)	13/20	(65)
					(77% quoted)			
Thorpe–Beeston[53]	36	18[c]	15	15	11/20	(55)	6/15	(40)
Berk & Grundy[70]	3	1	0	2	1/3	(33)	0	
Hisanga et al[71]	2	1	0	1	2/2	(100)	1/1	(100)
Totals	256	72	30	173	161/225	(71.6)	111/173	(64.2)

NS = not studied, NA = not applicable.
[a] One small anterior diaphragmatic hernia included.
[b] Only seven mentioned in Fig. 27.2.
[c] One survived.

ample, Harrison and colleagues state that nine fetuses were aborted in the San Francisco series but show only seven in Table 27.2.[46] In general, fetuses that were aborted are excluded from the raw mortality data. All cases with any sort of anomaly are excluded from the potential repair (PR) group, since it is unlikely that fetal repair would be offered if any other defect was demonstrated. An attempt is then made to assess the mortality of the fetus with an isolated diaphragmatic hernia (the PR group).

Other factors that have been assessed are the presence of the stomach, liver, or both organs in the chest and a diagnosis at less than 25 weeks of gestational age. The papers in which these factors have been presented are summarized in Table 27.3. For Adzick's two series,[45,69] this was actually less than 24 weeks gestation, and that is also the gestational age cut-off used by Crawford and co-workers.[52] As far as possible (from the information given in the various reports), the mortality figures derived are restricted to cases with isolated diaphragmatic hernia: the PR group.

At least 256 cases of antenatal diagnosis of diaphragmatic hernia have been reported in the English language literature since 1969. The reports of Berk and Grundy[70] and Hisanga et al[71] are included in the table for completeness, but the five fetuses reported are excluded from the analysis, since they report low lecithin/sphingomyelin ratios in the amniotic fluid in association with diaphragmatic hernia, but the diagnosis of diaphragmatic hernia was not made until after birth. Several other reports are excluded from the table because the fetal outcome was not reported. The mortality for cases with fetal diagnosis of diaphragmatic hernia (excluding fetuses of a pregnancy that was terminated, ie, "raw mortality") is 161 of 225 cases (71.6%). The mortality for the group with isolated diaphragmatic hernia (the PR group) was 111 of 173 fetuses (64.2%). For those with isolated diaphragmatic hernia and the stomach in the chest, the mortality was 31 of 58 (53.4%). For fetuses with isolated diaphragmatic hernia and the liver in the chest, the mortality was 90.9% (10 of 11). In those di-

TABLE 27.3 Prognostic Indicators in Antenatal Diagnosis of Diaphragmatic Hernia

Author (Ref)	No. with Stomach in Chest	No. with Liver in Chest	Possible Repair Group Only		No. Diagnosed <25/52	No. <25/52 with Anomalies	PR Mortality (%)
			Mortality with Stomach in Chest	Mortality with Liver in Chest			
Boyd et al[44]	NS	NS	NA	NA	1	1	NA
Bell, Ternberg[59]	NS	1	NA	1/1 (100)	0	0	NA
Adzick et al[45]	NS	NS	NA	NA	4	NS	?3/4 (75)
Crawford et al[54]	1	1	0/1 (0)	0/1 (0)	0	0	0
Calisti et al[64]	2	NS	1/2 (50)	NA	0	0	NA[a]
Kelly et al[65]	1	1	1/1 (100)	1/1 (100)	0	0	NA
Van den Born– Van den Brook et al[66]	1	NS	0/1 (0)	NA	NS	NS	NA
Crawford et al[52]	14	NS	7/14 (50)	NA	7	0	5/7 (71)[c]
Burge et al[68]	4	NS	4/4 (100)[b]	NA	0	0	NA
Adzick et al[69]	NS	NS	NA	NA	14	6	8/8 (100)
Harrison[46]	20	8?	13/20 (65)	8/8 (100)	13[d]	NS	5/8 (62.5)
Thorpe–Beeston[53]	15	NS	6/15 (40)	NA	20	13[e]	
Totals	58	11	31/58 (53.4)	10/11 (90.9)	54	20	23/32 (75)

[a] Two fetuses reported previously by the same group.
[b] ? Includes fetus with heart defect.
[c] One small anterior hernia.
[d] Five aborted.
[e] One survived.
NS = not studied, NA = not applicable.

agnosed before 25 weeks (probably a prerequisite for fetal repair), the mortality was 24 of 32 (75%). This figure is somewhat suspect, however, as neither Adzick and co-workers[45,69] nor Harrison and associates[46] comment on the presence of anomalies in this group. Unfortunately, in only two reports was the presence of the stomach in the chest reported separately in the group diagnosed at less than 24 weeks of age. This was in the report by Crawford and colleagues,[52] and that of Thorpe-Beeston and associates.[53] In this group of fetuses diagnosed before 24 weeks with the stomach in the chest the mortality was 7 of 10 (70%).

From this, it is clear that the presence of the liver in the chest is the only prognostic factor that will predict mortality of greater than 90%. Unfortunately, these data are available from only one series of only eight cases.[46] Given the wide variation of mortality figures for the various parameters reported in the table (which appear to depend on the institution where the babies are treated), this figure is also suspect, especially since the authors did not state whether any of the fetuses with the liver in the chest had any associated anomalies.

The other problem with using the presence of the liver within the chest as a prognostic indicator and a criterion for selection for fetal repair is the extreme technical difficulty reported by Harrison's team in the fetal repair in such cases. It may be that the alternative repair proposed by Ford,[72] with a loose silastic pouch placed above the prolapsed liver via a fetal thoracotomy, may provide the best alternative repair in these cases.

Better prognostic indicators are still needed. Crawford and associates[52] measured a cardiac venticular ratio and a "relative hernia area," comparing the area of the hernia with that of the heart. Although both of these indicators did predict a poor prognostic group, in their small series, neither indicator reliably predicted neonatal death in isolated diaphragmatic hernia. Hasegawa and colleagues[67] used a lung to thoracic area ratio (l/t) in eight fetuses. They defined a normal ratio of 0.52 ± 0.04. Five fetuses had l/t ratios greater than or equal to 0.21. All survived. Of the three fetuses with l/t ratios of 0.11 to 0.19, two died after early repair and ECMO support, and the one fetus with an l/t ratio of 0.11 was salvaged with ECMO. The gestational ages at which these measurements were obtained were not stated. It is possible that any of these three measurements could define a group of fetuses who should *not* be offered fetal repair (ie, those who have a good chance of surviving without fetal repair), but they probably should not be used to select a fetus with a poor prognosis who could be offered fetal repair.

Clearly there is an urgent need for better definition of the contents of the affected hemithorax. Fluid is a wonderful ultrasonic window, and it would, therefore, seem reasonable to inject 5–7 mL of warmed normal saline solution into the fetal abdomen under ultrasonic control. This would provide a degree of ascites, which would almost certainly extend up into the chest. It would clearly define the contents of the chest cavity, including outlining any liver in the chest and clearly defining the lung on the affected side. By providing a reasonable marker for the mediastinum on the left, it should also be possible to define accurately the volume of the right lung. This author, thus, hypothesizes that injection of saline solution into the abdominal cavity would enable the ultrasonographer to measure total lung volume in patients with diaphragmatic hernia accurately. If total lung volume can be accurately determined, then it should be possible to determine the prognosis at term when lung volume is determined by 25 weeks gestation. If this does provide a reliable prognostic indicator, then it may allow selection of possible candidates for fetal repair of diaphragmatic hernia without the risk of performing an unnecessary fetal repair in 20% to 30% of the patients. As soon as a reliable indicator of neonatal outcome is available, fetal repair can ethically be offered to mothers carrying a fetus with a diaphragmatic hernia who appear to be almost certainly (with at least a 95% probability) doomed without fetal repair.

Technical Aspects of Fetal Repair

As Harrison's group demonstrated experimentally[39] and Pringle's group guessed intuitively,[40,41] it is vital to prevent any significant increase in intraabdominal pressure during the fetal repair. Failure to do so results in compression of the intraabdominal umbilical vein, which essentially strangles the fetus. It is also clear from Harrison's report[46] that if the fetal liver is in the chest, then movement of the liver is associated with a most unsatisfactory deterioration in fetal hemodynamics.

Unfortunately, operating on the primate (including the human) uterus is not the same as operating on the quiescent bicornuate ovine (sheep) uterus. Primate models involving fetal surgery were developed in the late 1960s,[73–76] and Michejda's group used a primate model for studying fetal treatment of hydrocephalus.[77,78] Harrison's group have also reported a series of experiments on fetal primates.[79–81] From these papers, it is clear that amniotic fluid volume must be preserved, that the fetus must be kept warm (as must the mother), that the umbilical cord must be kept warm and moist, and that tilting the maternal pelvis to the left prevents caval compression and maintains maternal hemodynamic stability. Halothane appears to be a wonderful uterine relaxant, but some form of preoperative and postoperative tocolysis must be maintained. Indomethacin, as a prostaglandin synthetase inhibitor, appears to be a useful drug when given preoperatively and in the doses used does not appear to cause closure of the fetal ductus arteriosis. It is also vital that the amnion be tightly closed to prevent amniotic leak and oligohydramnios.

In their primate experiments,[79–81] Harrison's group used a GIA stapler to open the uterus. This has the advantage of sealing the amnion to the uterine muscle, facilitating closure. They also used a TIA-90 stapler to close the uterine wall, excising a small segment of uterine muscle. They later found that the stainless steel staples in the uterine wall resulted in a marked reduction in fertility,[81] and so absorbable staples were developed. Harrison appears to have used the same techniques in the 15 experimental human open fetal surgical procedures he has reported.[46,82]

It is clear that an anterior placenta is no particular problem: the uterus is simply tilted forward, and the incision made in the posterior wall. However, it appears best to stay well away from the placenta, or closure may be extremely difficult. Although the lower uterine segment may be an attractive site for the uterine incision, it appears such incisions are more likely to result in postoperative amniotic fluid leak. For the human surgical procedures, Harrison has generally opened the uterus by using the GIA stapler with absorbable staples and closed with absorbable sutures in several layers.[46,82]

Two other points that Harrison emphasizes[46] are the "all or none" approach to fetal surgery (fetuses who prove to have a lesion that cannot be adequately repaired should be evacuated from the uterus) and the importance of close fetal surveillance after open fetal surgery, with aggressive tocolysis for any premature labor.

CONCLUSIONS

As pointed out earlier in this chapter, fetal repair is the only possible chance we have of significantly improving the mortality from diaphragmatic hernia. It will almost certainly have a place in the future. However, patient selection remains a problem, with no clearly defined reliable indicator (present at 25 weeks gestation) of neo-natal demise. (This, after all, was the criterion for patient selection used by Liley for his first four fetal transfusions.) The poor outcome reported by Harrison[46] is not surprising, considering the technical difficulties of a fetal repair and the problems associated with learning to detect an intrathoracic liver. His pioneering efforts in de-fining the technical problems associated with open fetal surgery in humans should be com-mended. However, until adequate patient selec-tion criteria can be defined, fetal repair of dia-phragmatic hernia must remain an experimental procedure. The ethics of offering a procedure that has a definate acute morbidity and potential for major long-term morbidity,[83] when up to 30% to 40% of the fetuses may survive without fetal repair, could be open to question.

REFERENCES

1. Harrison MR, Bjordal RI, Langmark F, Knutrud O: Congenital diaphragmatic hernia: The hidden mor-tality. *J Pediatr Surg* 1978;13:227–230.
2. Ravitch MM, Barton BA: The need for pediatric sur-geons as determined by the volume of work and the mode of delivery of surgical care. *Surgery* 1974;76:754–763.
3. Butler N, Claireaux AE: Congenital diaphragmatic hernia as a cause of perinatal mortality. *Lancet* 1962;1:659–663.
4. Bowditch HI: Diaphragmatic hernia. *Buffalo Med J Month Rev* 1853;9:1–39.
5. Bowditch HI: Diaphragmatic hernia. *Buffalo Med J Month Rev* 1853;9:65–94.
6. *World Health Statistics Annual 1988.* Geneva: World Health Organization, 1988.
7. Puri P, Gorman WA: Natural history of congenital diaphragmatic hernia: Implications for manage-ment. *Pediatr Surg Int* 1987;2:327–330.
8. Hardesty RL, Griffith BP, Debeski RF, et al: Extra-corporeal membrane oxygenation: Successful treat-ment of persistent fetal circulation following repair of congenital diaphragmatic hernia. *J Thorac Car-diovasc Surg* 1981;81:556–563.
9. Stolar CJH, Dillon PW, Altman RP: Management of the infant with congenital diaphragmatic hernia (CDH) and persistent pulmonary hypertension (PPHN). *Jpn J Surg* 1985;15:438–442.
10. Langham MR Jr, Krummel TM, Bartlett RH, et al: Mortality with extracorporeal membrane oxygena-tion following repair of congenital diaphragmatic hernia in 93 infants. *J Pediatr Surg* 1987;22:1150–1154.
11. Heaton JFG, Redmond CR, Graves ED, et al: Con-genital diaphragmatic hernia: Improving survival with extracorporeal membrane oxygenation. *Pe-diatr Surg Int* 1988;3:6–10.
12. Geggel RL, Murphy JD, Langleben D, et al: Congen-ital diaphragmatic hernia: arterial structural changes and persistent pulmonary hypertension after surgical repair. *J Pediatr* 1985;107:457–464.
13. Pringle KC: Lung development in congenital dia-

14. phragmatic hernia. In: Puri P, ed. *Congenital Dia-phragmatic Hernia.* Basel: Karger, 1989;24:28–53.
14. Collins DL, Pomerance JJ, Travis KW, et al: A new approach to congenital posterolateral diaphrag-matic hernia. *J Pediatr Surg* 1977;12:149–156.
15. Woolley MM: Delayed appearance of a left poster-olateral diaphragmatic hernia resulting in signifi-cant small bowel necrosis. *J Pediatr Surg* 1977;12:673–674.
16. Wiseman NE, MacPherson RI: "Acquired" congen-ital diaphragmatic hernia. *J Pediatr Surg* 1977;12:657–665.
17. Areechon W, Reid L: Hypoplasia of lung with con-genital diaphragmatic hernia. *Br Med J* 1963;I:230–233.
18. Kitagawa M, Hislop A, Boyden EA, Reid L: Lung hy-poplasia in congenital diaphragmatic hernia: A quantitative study of airway, artery, and alveolar development. *Br J Surg* 1971;58:342–346.
19. Nguyen L, Guttman FM, de Chadarevian JP, et al: The mortality of congenital diaphragmatic hernia: Is total pulmonary mass inadequate, no matter what? *Ann Surg* 1983;198:766–770.
20. Pringle KC: In utero surgery. In Mannick JA, Cam-eron JC, Jordan GL Jr, et al, eds. *Advances in Sur-gery.* Chicago, Ill: Year Book Medical Publishers, 1986;19:101–138.
21. Freda VJ, Adamsons K: Exchange transfusion in utero: Report of a case. *Am J Obstet Gynecol* 1964;89:817–821.
22. Asensio SH, Figueroa-Longo JG, Pelegrina IA: Intra-uterine exchange transfusion. *Am J Obstet Gynecol* 1966;95:1129–1133.
23. Adamsons K, Freda VJ, James LS, et al: Prenatal treatment of erythroblastosis fetalis following hys-terotomy. *Pediatrics* 1965;35:848–855.
24. Kohorn EI, Wade M, Davies CD: Open intrauterine transfusion. *Proc R Soc Med* 1967;60:42.
25. Asensio SH, Figueroa-Longo JG, Pelegrina IA. Intra-uterine exchange transfusion: A new technique. *Ob-stet Gynecol* 1968;32:350.
26. Seelen J, Van Kessel H, Eskes T, et al: A new method of exchange transfusion in utero: Cannulation of vessels on the fetal side of the human placenta. *Am J Obstet Gynecol* 1966;95:872–876.
27. MacKenzie IZ, MacLean DA, Fry A, et al: Midtrimes-ter intrauterine exchange transfusion of the fetus. *Am J Obstet Gynecol* 1985;143:555.
28. Lucey JF, Butterfield LJ, eds: Intrauterine Transfu-sion and Erythroblastosis Fetalis: Report of the Fifty-Third Ross Conference on Pediatric Research. Aspen, Colorado, March 14–15, 1966. Columbus, Ohio: Ross Laboratories, 1966.
29. Liley AW: Intrauterine transfusion of foetus in hae-molytic disease. *Br Med J* 1963;2:1107–1109.
30. Liggins GC: A self-retaining catheter for fetal peri-toneal transfusion. *Obstet Gynecol* 1966;27:323–326.
31. Liggins GC: Fetal transfusion by the impaling tech-nique. *Obstet Gynecol* 1966;27:617–621.
32. Olivet RT, Rupp WM, Telander RL, Kaye MP: He-modynamics of congenital diaphragmatic hernia in lambs. *J Pediatr Surg* 1978;13:231–235.
33. de Lorimier AA, Tierney DF, Parker HR: Hypoplastic lungs in fetal lambs with surgically produced con-genital diaphragmatic hernia. *Surgery* 1967;62:12–17.
34. Starrett RW, de Lorimier AA: Congenital diaphrag-

matic hernia in lambs: Hemodynamic and ventilatory changes with breathing. *J Pediatr Surg* 1975;10:575–582.

35. Kent GM, Olley PM, Creighton RE, et al: Hemodynamic and pulmonary changes following surgical creation of a diaphragmatic hernia in fetal lambs. *Surgery* 1972;72:427–433.

36. Haller JA, Signer RD, Golladay ES, et al: Pulmonary and ductal hemodynamics in studies of simulated diaphragmatic hernia of fetal and newborn lambs. *J Pediatr Surg* 1976;11:675.

37. Harrison MR, Jester JA, Ross NA: Correction of congenital diaphragmatic hernia in utero: I. The model: Intrathoracic balloon produces fatal pulmonary hypoplasia. *Surgery* 1980;88:174–182.

38. Harrison MR, Bressack MA, Churg AM, de Lorimier AA: Correction of congenital diaphragmatic hernia in utero: II. Simulated correction permits fetal lung growth with survival at birth. *Surgery* 1980;88:260–268.

39. Harrison MR, Ross NA, de Lorimier AA: Correction of congenital diaphragmatic hernia in utero: III. Development of a successful surgical technique using abdominoplasty to avoid compromise of umbilical blood flow. *J Pediatr Surg* 1981;16:934–942.

40. Soper RT, Pringle KC, Scofield JC: Creation and repair of diaphragmatic hernia in the fetal lamb: Techniques and survival. *J Pediatr Surg* 1984;19:33–40.

41. Pringle KC: Fetal lamb and fetal lamb lung growth following creation and repair of a diaphragmatic hernia. In: Nathanielsz PW, ed. *Animal Models in Fetal Medicine.* Ithaca, New York: Perinatology Press, 1984;109–148.

42. Pringle KC, Turner JW, Scofield JC, Soper RT: Creation and repair of diaphragmatic hernia in the fetal lamb: Lung development and morphology. *J Pediatr Surg* 1984;19:131–140.

43. Pringle KC: Human fetal lung development and related animal models. *Clin Obstet Gynecol* 1986;29:502–513.

44. Boyd JJ, Bowman JM, McInnis AC, Kiernan MK: Fetal diaphragmatic hernia detected at intra-uterine transfusion. *Can Med Assoc J* 1969;100:1105–1106.

45. Adzick NS, Harrison MR, Glick DK, et al: Diaphragmatic hernia in the fetus: prenatal diagnosis and outcome in 94 cases. *J Pediatr Surg* 1985;20:357–361.

46. Harrison MR, Langer JC, Adzick NS, et al: Correction of congenital diaphragmatic hernia in utero: V. Initial clinical experience. *J Pediatr Surg* 1990;25:47–57.

47. Pringle KC: Diaphragmatic hernia (letter). *J Pediatr Surg* 1986;21:186.

48. Harrison MR: The fetus with a diaphragmatic hernia. *Pediatr Surg Int* 1988;3:15–22.

49. Harrison MR, Adzick NS, Nakayama DK, de Lorimier AA: Fetal diaphragmatic hernia: Pathophysiology, natural history, and outcome. *Clin Obstet Gynecol* 1986;29:490–501.

50. Harrison MR: Fetal diaphragmatic hernia. In: Puri P, ed. *Congenital Diaphragmatic Hernia.* Basel: Karger, 1989;24:130–142.

51. Benacerraf BR, Adzick NS: Fetal diaphragmatic hernia: Ultrasound diagnosis and clinical outcome in 19 cases. *Am J Obstet Gynecol* 1987;156:573–576.

52. Crawford DC, Wright VM, Drake DP, Allan LD: Fetal diaphragmatic hernia: The value of fetal echocar-

diography in the prediction of postnatal outcome. *Br J Obstet Gynaecol* 1989;96:705–710.

53. Thorpe-Beeston JG, Gosden CM, Nicolaides KH: Prenatal diagnosis of congenital diaphragmatic hernia: Associated malformations and chromosomal defects. *Fetal Ther* 1989;4:21–28.

54. Crawford DC, Drake PP, Kwaitkowski D, et al: Prenatal diagnosis of reversible cardiac hypoplasia associated with congenital diaphragmatic hernia: implications for postnatal management. *J Clin Ultrasound* 1986;14:718.

55. Nakayama DK, Harrison MR, Chinn DH, et al: Prenatal diagnosis and natural history of the fetus with a congenital diaphragmatic hernia: Initial clinical experience. *J Pediatr Surg* 1985;20:118–124.

56. Chinn DH, Filly RA, Cullen PW, et al: Congenital diaphragmatic hernia diagnosed prenatally by ultrasound. *Radiology* 1983;148:119–123.

57. Agüero O, Zighelboim I: Intrauterine diagnosis of fetal diaphragmatic hernia by amniography. *Am J Obstet Gynecol* 1970;107:971–972.

58. Griscom NT: Possible radiologic approaches to fetal diagnosis and therapy. *Clin Perinatol* 1974;1:435–464.

59. Bell MJ, Ternberg JL: Antenatal diagnosis of diaphragmatic hernia. *Pediatrics* 1977;60:738–740.

60. Touloukian RJ, Hobbins JC: Maternal ultrasonography in the antenatal diagnosis of surgically correctable fetal abnormalities. *J Pediatr Surg* 1980;15:373–377.

61. Marwood RP, Davison OW: Antenatal diagnosis of diaphragmatic hernia: Case report. *Br J Obstet Gynaecol* 1981;88:71–72.

62. Fleischer AC, Killam AP, Boehm FH, et al: Hydrops fetalis: Sonographic evaluation and clinical implications. *Radiology* 1981;141:163–168.

63. Stiller RJ, Roberts NS, Weiner S, Vaughn B: Congenital diaphragmatic hernia: Antenatal diagnosis and obstetrical management. *J Clin Ultrasound* 1985;13:212–215.

64. Calisti A, Manzoni C, Pintus C, Perrelli L: Prenatal diagnosis and management of some fetal intrathoracic abnormalities. *Eur J Obstet Gynecol Reprod Biol* 1986;22:61–68.

65. Kelly DR, Grant EG, Zeman RK, et al: In utero diagnosis of congenital diaphragmatic hernia by CT amniography: Case report. *J Comput Assist Tomogr* 1986;10:500–502.

66. Van den Born–van den Broek ME, Box NMA, Van de Vange N, et al: Antenatal ultrasonographic diagnosis of a congenital posterolateral diaphragmatic defect: Case report. *Eur J Obstet Gynecol Reprod Biol* 1987;25:139–144.

67. Hasegawa T, Matsuo Y, Fukuzawa M, et al: Fetal diaphragmatic hernia: Prenatal evaluation of lung hypoplasia and effect of immediate operation. Presented at 22nd Annual Meeting Pacific Association of Pediatric Surgeons, Portland, Oregon, May 21–26, 1989.

68. Burge DM, Atwell JD, Freeman NW: Could the stomach site help predict outcome in babies with left sided congenital diaphragmatic hernia diagnosed antenatally? *J Pediatr Surg* 1989;24:567–569.

69. Adzick NS, Vacanti JP, Lillehei CW, et al: Fetal diaphragmatic hernia: Ultrasound diagnosis and clinical outcome in 38 cases. *J Pediatr Surg* 1989;24:654–658.

70. Berk C, Grundy M: "High risk" lecithin/sphingomyelin ratios associated with neonatal diaphragmatic hernia: Case reports. *Br J Obstet Gynaecol* 1982;89:250–251.

71. Hisanaga S, Shimokawa H, Kashiwabana Y, et al: Unexpectedly low lecithin/sphingomyelin ratio associated with fetal diaphragmatic hernia. *Am J Obstet Gynecol* 1984;149:905–906.

72. Ford WDA: Silastic patch placed via a thoracotomy for fetal repair of diaphragmatic hernia with liver in the chest. Presented at 9th Annual Meeting International Fetal Medicine and Surgery Society, Rotorua, New Zealand, February 23–28, 1990.

73. Chez RA, Smith FG, Hutchinson DL: Renal function in the intra-uterine primate fetus: I. Experimental technique: Rate of formation and chemical composition of urine, *Am J Obstet Gynecol* 1964;90:128–131.

74. Chez RA, Hutchinson DL: The use of experimental surgical techniques in the pregnant *Macaca mulatta. Ann NY Acad Sci* 1969;162:249–253.

75. Parshall CJ, Silverstein AM: Surgical approaches to the study of fetal immunology in primate animals. *Ann NY Acad Sci* 1969;162:254–266.

76. Myers RE: Brain pathology following fetal vascular occlusion: an experimental study. *Invest Ophthalmol Vis Sci* 1969;8:41–50.

77. Michejda M, Hodgen GD: In utero diagnosis and treatment of non-human primate fetal skeletal anomalies: I. Hydrocephalus. *JAMA* 1981;246:1093.

78. Michejda M, Patronus N, de Chiro G, Hodger GD: Fetal hydrocephalus: II. Amelioration of fetal porencephaly by in utero therapy in nonhuman primates. *JAMA* 1984;251:2548–2552.

79. Harrison MR, Anderson MA, Rosen NA, et al: Fetal surgery in the primate: I. Anesthetic, surgical, and tocolytic management to maximize fetal-neonatal survival. *J Pediatr Surg* 1982;17:115–122.

80. Nakayama DK, Harrison MR, Seron-Ferre M, Villa RL: Fetal surgery in the primate: II. Uterine electromyographic response to operative procedures and pharmacologic agents. *J Pediatr Surg* 1984;19:333–339.

81. Adzick NS, Harrison MR, Glick PL, et al: Fetal surgery in the primate: III. Maternal outcome after fetal surgery. *J Pediatr Surg* 1986;21:477–480.

82. Crombleholme TM, Harrison MR, Langer JC, et al: Early experience with open fetal surgery for congenital hydronephrosis. *J Pediatr Surg* 1988;23:1114.

83. Pringle KC: Ethical issues in fetal surgery. In: Puri P, ed. *Modern Problems in Paediatrics,* Basel: Karger, 1986;23:190–201.

Fetal Surgery: Practical Considerations and Current Status: Where Do We Go from Here with Bochdalek Diaphragmatic Hernia?

J. Alex Haller, Jr., MD

Pringle's carefully documented and thoughtful chapter concludes with his position that unless an individual human fetus with a congenital diaphragmatic hernia (CDH) has more than a 90% mortality rate with continuing gestation and delivery, intrauterine repair is not ethically defensible. I agree with his conclusion, especially in a social era when abortion of defective fetuses is legally allowed in the USA and actively encouraged before 24 weeks gestation by most obstetricians. If the CDH is accompanied by other major anomalies, the fetus is surely not an appropriate surgical candidate. If the fetus with CDH has a liver which has herniated into the chest and is accompanied by polyhydramnios, especially before 24 weeks, the mortality rate approaches 95%; these are perhaps the *target* patients for intrauterine surgery. Pringle's suggestion that more sophisticated prenatal testing may lead to earlier diagnosis of CDH with an intrathoracic liver is thought-provoking, as is his proposal that intra-peritoneal injection of saline into the fetus might delineate the liver–diaphragm–thorax anatomy. What say the prenatal diagnosticians?!

A major enigma remains: Why does the presence of liver or, for that matter, intestine and/or spleen *in the chest* above the diaphragm *cause* pulmonary hypoplasia and the devastating accompanying pathophysiology of persistent fetal pulmonary hypertension? The liver, spleen, and intestine are *normally* in the chest in the developing fetus because the lungs are unexpanded and the diaphragm is quite high in the chest and is tightly juxtaposed to the lungs. How does the mere presence of an intact diaphragm muscle act as a physiologic buffer? Or is there another etiology of the pulmonary hypoplasia and hypertension? Therein lies the real continuing challenge! Until better primate models are carefully studied and precise dynamics of pulmonary artery hypertension clarified, I would not want my wife to undergo *two caesarean sections* (one at 22 to 24 weeks and another at 38 to 40 weeks) when the statistical chance of our baby surviving with a CDH is 25 to 30% if left alone. If at 20 to 22 weeks it was discovered that the fetus had the liver placed abnormally in the chest, my wife and I would select transvaginal interruption of pregnancy and try again to have a normal fetus, gestation, and delivery!

We truly need more experimental primate data before more extensive human trials. However, if Harrison's patients give uncoerced informed consent, then his limited and carefully documented *human experiments* may be helpful in further understanding the pathophysiology of congenital diaphragmatic hernia.

© 1991 Elsevier Science Publishing Co., Inc.
655 Avenue of the Americas, New York, NY 10010
Current Topics in General Thoracic Surgery:
An International Series

Chapter 28

Ethical Considerations

Abbyann Lynch, PhD

Attention to "the ethical component" (ie, right action, all things considered) is inseparable from any serious reflection concerning management of clinical practice and pursuit of clinical research. In the following brief discussion, some aspects of the ethical component intrinsic to the practices of pediatric thoracic transplantation and fetal surgery will be examined.

Ethical problems arising in the care of children (including those associated with implementation of the interventions just named) have much in common with those ethical problems related to the care of adults. There is common interest in ensuring that the patients not be harmed, for example. At the same time, on comparison of the two groups in an ethical perspective, there are significant differences. An example of this dissimilarity: ethical decision making for competent adults rests principally on considerations of autonomy; such decision making for children rests principally on considerations of "best interests."

Choosing among the many ethical issues pertaining to the areas first noted, two are identified for comment: the matter of authorization for such interventions and the matter of patient access and subject selection in regard to these interventions.

THERAPEUTIC RESEARCH INTERVENTIONS INVOLVING CHILDREN

The usual model for consideration of therapeutic research interventions for children is that of adult consent. This is recognized as an ethical prerequisite to any medical, research, or educational intervention on the person of another.[1] In ethical

Published 1991 by Elsevier Science Publishing Co., Inc.
655 Avenue of the Americas, New York, NY 10010
Current Topics in General Thoracic Surgery:
An International Series

terms, the primary concern is that the patient or research subject should knowledgeably and freely agree to any proposed intervention on the self. To seek such an agreement is to recognize the inviolability of the individual on whom the intervention is to be practiced; it is to respect that individual's right to self-direction and self-protection.

In functional terms, the ethical concern translates to a fivefold authorization process in which each element is essential to the integrity of the whole: competence of the individual who is to be the subject of the intervention, adequate disclosure of relevant information to that individual, evident understanding by that individual of the information so disclosed, the individual's "freedom" of choice in regard to the proposed intervention, and the individual's continuing competence/understanding/freedom with regard to decision making based on continuing disclosure of relevant information.

In principle, these same criteria should be applied to children. The difficulty is that very young children are not competent to make the necessary choices. The decision to allow medical, research, or educational intervention in this population thus falls to parents or guardians. It then becomes appropriate to speak of authorization or permission for these interventions, rather than to use the term *consent.* This being said, the conditions for consent already outlined apply, albeit analogically.

Given the ethical requisite that individual choice regarding medical and research intervention must prevail, it follows that, with the development of intelligence and psychological awareness of self, including the capacity and responsibility for self-direction, the child who has become an adult will ultimately be the locus for decisions regarding this activity.[2-4] For those children who are neither very young nor yet adult, the ethical process for agreement/disagreement necessarily involves some combination of parental authorization and child assent, on the understanding that the child's knowledgeable dissent will be honored.[5-8]

In light of what has been said, it is evident that the clinician who proposes to offer thoracic transplantation to an older child must be prepared, in principle, to honor that child's ability to understand, and to disclose information suitable to that child's competence. Further, in principle, the clinician must be open to acceptance of the child's knowledgeable disagreement with what is proposed. In practical terms, observance of the ethical principle of respect for person translates here to various suggestions as to appropriate measures to be taken around such disclosure, and to appropriate measures to be taken in the event that child and parent might disagree in this regard. Related to these concerns is that ethical criteria can be made functional only within societal limits, and various civil jurisdictions have different legal requirements dictating such consent (eg, with regard to the recognized age for legal as distinct from the recognized ability for ethical consent to medical intervention). Thus, it might be that the older child could be judged "ethically competent to choose" but apparently barred from so doing in fact, because that child is under the "legal age of majority." In that case, if the child refuses the therapeutic intervention proposed, the clinician who is ethically obliged to honor the child's autonomy and ethically obliged to prevent harm to the child may experience a profound ethical dilemma.

If the ethical standard for allowable medical intervention on the older child is that child's knowledgeable and free choice, what ethical standard applies in the matter of allowable medical intervention on the younger (not ethically competent) child? In popular terms, the recognized guiding principle here is "best interests," usually interpreted to mean that the choice of the parents/legal guardians must ensure that the child come to no harm (minimally, that the child's physical well-being be ensured).

Such a choice may be enforceable under child welfare legislation, should the parents, in terms of their own interest or those of other family members, elect "therapy" that differs from a recognized standard of physical well-being. Thus, for example, should parents refuse a lifesaving procedure on grounds of religious conviction, their decision may be countermanded via legal mechanisms (presuming the court accepts medical consensus that the procedure is, indeed, in the best interests of the child). This being said, parents still have first responsibility in choosing adequate means for meeting the child's best interests. In principle, clinicians must thus be open

to the possibility that there can be legitimate difference of viewpoint between them and parents such that the two parties have quite a different understanding of the child's best interests. In the event that medical consensus may not be clear (eg, clinicians may disagree about the appropriateness of attempting thoracic transplantation in certain cases), the clinician and the parents must be prepared for some kind of ethical negotiation to arrive at agreement about the procedure to be followed.

Currently, the definition of limits of best interest of the child appears to be shifting to include concern for the child's quality of life, as distinguishable from maintenance of the child's physical life only. Within the near future, the best interest focus may well be expanded to include not only consideration of "no harm" as regards the child's physical life and quality of life but also consideration of the best interest of the family as a whole.[10,11]

In summary, there is continuing need to explore the meaning and limits of parental/guardian and clinical responsibility for the development, nurture, well-being, and nonharm of the child and to explore the means for communication and negotiation between these individuals in regard to decisions to be made in the younger child's best interests.

In the matter of involving children in research pursuits or of using the child as a subject for the education of clinical staff, ethical opinion is sharply divided.[12] To some extent, the division rests on the delineation between the goals of therapy, on the one hand, and research and education, on the other. In the former group the goal is clearly the best interests of the patient. In the latter group the primary goal is the benefit of others.

Some thus defend the view that there can be no valid authorization by parents/guardians for research interventions on the child.[13-15] They argue that those whose charge it is to protect children from harm cannot, ethically speaking, expose them to the known or unknown risks of participation in a research or educational activity. Others, for example, the US National Commission,[16-20] argue that so long as there is risk of only minimal harm (a ratio established in comparison with the risk of harms taken by children in everyday life),[21,22] and presuming parents/guardians accept any risk arising in the research enterprise on behalf of the child, then participation of the child in such activity is ethically acceptable. Again, jurisdictional differences make any general statement about the ethical acceptability of these ventures in situ extremely tentative.[13]

Although the conceptual distinction between therapy and research may be clear enough to indicate what the pertinent ethical distinctions in the matter of authorization and consent might be, the delineation of therapy from research in practice is not so easily accomplished. The lack of standard vocabulary used in such discussion makes for real difficulty here, particularly so far as parental decision making is concerned. For example, Harrison speaks of "families who previously accepted the risk and considerable discomfort of an experimental procedure in heroic attempts to help."[23,24] It appears that attempts of this kind should be classified as therapeutically motivated activities that are nonstandard, nonvalidated, innovative. Such attempts can be distinguished from recognized therapy, ie, interventions that are therapeutically motivated, and that are part of the standard, validated activities listed as therapy. Again, both of these groupings are different from research activity, ie, knowledge-oriented comparison of interventions that could involve what appears to be "therapeutic" and what appears to have "therapeutic benefit." In this latter category, consider Harrison's remarks "Now is the time to put fetal surgery to the test of a prospective controlled trial."[23,24]

For the nonclinician, the interventions proposed (whether therapy, research, or innovative therapy) may seem identical. A particular surgical intervention could be identified as therapy, research, or innovative therapy, eg, depending on circumstances. Although it is well recognized that no therapeutic procedure is risk-free, still, in ethical terms, the balance of burdens/benefit to be assumed by a patient receiving standard surgical therapy is quite different from that assumed by a research subject who has surgery in a clinical trial or by the individual who receives nonstandard surgical "therapy." It is evident, then, that those who propose such interventions have an obligation to disclose their nature and intent so that parents/guardians (or child) may make an informed choice concerning participation vis-à-vis the intervention proposed.

If the clinician who is to act as researcher is the clinician who, at the same time, acts as the child's physician, the possibility of conflict of interest arises for that physician, even as it does in the case of the clinician-therapist simultaneously engaged in formal "clinical learning." In both instances, as already noted, the child's parents/child must have this information concerning the clinician's dual role so that their choice regarding participation is ethically informed. If there is parental/guardian/child agreement, but the situation so requires, the clinician must be prepared to set aside the research or the educational venture in terms of protecting the child's best interests.[25]

With reference to the fetus, the matter of authorization of therapy or research represents a most difficult ethical challenge for both the clinician and the mother (or mother/father) of the unborn child. The difficulty arises in part from lack of agreement as to the moral status of the fetus[26,27] and in part from lack of clarity regarding the nature of the interventions proposed,[28,29] a problem to which reference has already been made. Both difficulties are compounded by reason of the fact that any intervention on the fetus will involve intervention on the mother.

In addition to the first two concerns, and considering the fetus only, its moral status will determine ethical obligations in its regard. If seen as "full patient," eg, as a born child would be, then recognized therapy seems indicated and research participation remains questionable. If the fetus is seen as a "lesser moral agent," or lacking in moral status, some will perceive any obligation to therapy here as less stringent or nonexistent, which is not to say that any evidently harmful experimental procedure will be ethically acceptable. Still, if this dilemma of status were resolved, the problem already raised remains: what is the nature of the proposed intervention?[30–32] If its goal is therapy for the fetus, what options are there in the "standard" and "nonstandard" categories, and how are they to be evaluated against the best interests of the fetus (and those of mother/father/family)? What risks are posed; what benefits are anticipated?[33,34]

In addition to the difficulty posed by the question of fetal moral status, there is a further unique ethical concern here. Any intervention involving the fetus can take place safely only with the mother's physical cooperation. Ethically speaking, maternal choice may not be in the interests of the fetus; in such a case, the fetus may be denied what seems therapeutic. In social terms, and in practice, administration of fetal therapy thus becomes a secondary concern, a judgment that poses severe ethical stress for the clinician who attempts to respect fetal best interests as well as maternal autonomy.[35–38] Such uneasiness is exacerbated on consideration of the current double ethical standard regarding fetal well-being: both fetal therapy and termination of pregnancy are acceptable (in certain jurisdictions), at least in principle. Determination of right action in clinical management and clinical research, so far as the fetus is concerned, is thus exceedingly problematic. Can any practicable limit be placed on authorization for interventions in regard to the fetus?

In summary, since no social or ethical consensus regarding the question of the moral status of the fetus is anticipated, the ethical questions arising in care and research involving this "patient"/research subject will remain ever-presenting dilemmas for the individual clinician, the clinician group, and the parents/guardians. It thus appears that attempts at further discussion in this area become ethically obligatory for all concerned.

PATIENT SELECTION

Not all children who might be considered candidates for thoracic transplantation and not all fetuses who might be considered candidates for therapeutic surgery will have an opportunity to receive these services. In some instances, the parents/guardians (or child) may refuse them. In other cases, there may be medical or psychosocial contraindications to provision of these therapeutic interventions. Further, some parents will lack the necessary financial resources to pay for the procedure, or such medical service may not be available because no program exists in their area (eg, there may be a funding problem or shortage of adequately skilled personnel). Finally, it may be that the heart or lung needed by the patient may not be at hand. In each of these instances, the clinician must consider the ethical principles of no harm, beneficence, and justice as they apply to the individual situation. In practical terms, the ethical questions become, What criteria are used to determine "who gets on the list"? Who determines the criteria? How are the criteria to be applied?

Evidently, the matter of "medical selection" of patients to receive thoracic transplantation is a matter calling for astute clinical judgment. According to Vouhé, such "transplantation is justifiable only if outstanding results are achieved: a complete functional rehabilitation and a long-term survival should be obtained." With these as major criteria, the author advises that cardiac replacement, for example, be recommended "before reaching an end-stage situation with multiorgan failure." He lists as well certain medical contraindications to initiation of the transplantation procedure.[39]

There can be no ethical question about medical judgment concerning the severity of a child's illness or of a physician's judgment concerning prognosis. What may be questioned in ethical or social terms is the priority to be given any assigned medical criteria. Thus, some might argue that medical criteria should be quite secondary: those who can pay for service should have such service as they choose. In debating this question, much will depend on the view of medicine

adopted and on the social view of the transplantation endeavor. Certainly, most individuals would agree that donated organs should be distributed to those who can make best use of them, even if such a scheme for allocation causes harm to particular individuals. The very real difficulty, presuming this view is accepted, will be in listing and updating medical criteria and in explaining the reasoning for adoption of such criteria so that public confidence in the process is maintained.

Similar discussion arises with regard to use of psychosocial criteria as a limiting factor in making such transplantation service available. From one perspective, it seems eminently sensible to say that only those patients whose families are able and willing to comply with any required postoperative drug and testing requirement should receive thoracic transplantation. On the other hand, there is serious ethical difficulty in refusing this procedure to a medically suitable child on the grounds that the family is not of an acceptable social configuration or that there are serious concerns about parental compliance. In such a situation, clinicians must be prepared to seek means to remedy the psychosocial problem so as to overcome, as possible, any preventable harm to the child concerned.

A more subtle ethical problem concerns identification of a psychosocial limit in an appropriately nonmedical manner.[40] This calls for use of multidisciplinary skill, for example, a social worker's expertise or a psychologist's. Once the evidence and recommendations are at hand, a further problem will be that of "weighting": how serious a contraindication is parental nonadjustment to the cultural milieu to be, for example? Ought parental illiteracy or inability to communicate easily be nonexceptional impediments to the child's receipt of medical assistance via transplantation?

Lack of financial resources also presents a serious ethical concern. The cost of fetal surgery for diaphragmatic hernia is cited at $15,721 US.[23,24] In jurisdictions in which there is no universal insurance scheme and in which parents have no private insurance or personal resources to cover such costs, individual families whose fetus could benefit must see their fetus suffer and perhaps die because they cannot purchase the medical care needed. Although individual groups might underwrite such costs in particular cases, there is still a question of apparent injustice; it is part of the much larger ethical question regarding distribution of health care resources.

Vouhé points to a serious concern in any attempt to establish a thoracic transplantation program, ie, the availability of suitable organs.[41] Consideration of available alternatives, their risks, and possible benefits thus becomes an ethical imperative, eg, use of the Norwood procedure, attempts to extend ischemic time, use of xenotransplantation, use of the anencephalic infant as donor. Each of these alternatives raises ethical questions in its own right. The ethical controversy surrounding the Baby Fae experience and that surrounding use of "living" anencephalic infants (or maintaining such infants for the benefit of recipients) are examples of current ethical dilemmas that will continue to elicit reasoned discussion as to the "right action" to be chosen. As well, each of these areas will raise the question of availability of thoracic transplantation to a level of social concern, and perhaps to a level of social (and possibly legal) policy. In this perspective, the questions become "public" questions with their resolution not restricted to medical consensus only.[42,43]

What has been said of the ethics of patient access to thoracic transplantation could be said generally of patient access to fetal surgery as well. As to differences, accuracy of selection of patients on medical grounds seems more difficult in the case of the fetus, and that raises many particular and real ethical questions (as Pringle remarks, "The ethics of offering a procedure which has a definite acute morbidity, and the potential for major long-term morbidity, when up to 30–40% of the fetuses may survive without fetal repair, could be open to question").[44] Further, alternatives will differ; for example, extracorporeal membrane oxygenation (ECMO) for affected babies is available, although its use raises ethical concerns.[45]

Overall, the question of patient access to the interventions proposed will raise continuing ethical dilemmas for clinicians, the more so as this becomes a public issue. A particularly troublesome concern arises as the clinician assumes the gatekeeper role in these areas. In that perspective, the physician who is pledged to serve as clinician-advocate for the patient might well find it ethically difficult to serve at one and the same time as that patient's nonadvocate (ie, as the one who must refuse to provide a needed service for the patient in order to render it to someone else).

Along with ethical concern for consent and authorization and no harm in the case of pediatric research is the ethical concern for fair selection of candidates as participants in the research protocol. Since research activity is conducted to increase knowledge for the benefit of the group, it is argued that its burdens should also be shared by the group. As well, there is abiding concern lest those already at risk through physical or mental limitation be unduly burdened by way of the risks implicit in research partici-

pation. Jonas, for example, thus reasons that the first research subjects ought to be those most competent, and only secondarily, those who are weaker.[46] In the interests of justice in research, then, there are two obligations cited: (1) the duty to prevent "overselection," ie, to be fair, as regards population groups chosen as research participants (for example, not all mentally handicapped persons, not all black persons, not all economically disadvantaged persons, unless these are characteristics relevant to the research); (2) the duty to recruit adult or healthy participants before calling on children or those who are infirm.

Historically, public repudiation of the Tuskeegee syphilis study and of the Willowbrook study shows social support for the ethical stances just identified. This approach has been adopted in various government policy statements as well.[47] This is not to argue that pediatric research ought not be done. Questions of consent/authorization and no harm aside, injustice is done to the pediatric group if pediatric research is not pursued. The overall problem raised, ethically speaking, is one of balancing competing interests: the benefit to the group of research done versus the protection required for individuals asked to be research participants. In reference to research activity vis-à-vis thoracic transplantation and fetal surgery, then, and presuming children/fetuses will be involved in such research, right action in selection of these research participants requires that they be chosen equitably, reducing the risk of harm to them as much as possible.

How these ethical concerns are translated into practice will be the responsibility of investigators working in consultation with their own institutional research ethics boards.

CONCLUSION

As scientific knowledge is pursued and developed, as clinical management of patients is practiced and improved, it is axiomatic that ethical challenges will persist and increase. There can be no advance resolution of these challenges; they will differ with different situations, thus requiring varying ethical responses. Nontransient will be the abiding concern for certain human values and for ethical principles in practice, eg, respect for person, no harm, group benefit, and fairness. Clinicians and investigators must be sensitive to such concerns and to the need for reasoned discussion/argument in pursuit of resolution of conflict arising around them. In this contemporary "era of ethics," ethics education for clinical practitioners, early and ongoing, is thus the preferred prophylactic and therapeutic agent. In the future, such education can only be a sine qua non.

REFERENCES

1. President's Commission for the Study of Ethical Problems in Medicine and Biomedical and Behavioral Research: *Making Health Care Decisions: The Ethical and Legal Implications of Informed Consent in the Patient-Practitioner Relationship.* Washington, DC: US Government Printing Office, 1982.
2. Carey S: *Conceptual Change in Childhood.* Cambridge, Mass: MIT Press, 1985.
3. Piaget J, Inhelder B: *The Pscychology of the Child.* New York: Basic Books, 1969.
4. Piaget J: *The Moral Judgment of the Child.* New York: Free Press, 1965.
5. Brock DW: Children's competence for health care decision-making. In: Kopelman LM, Moskop JC, eds. *Children and Health Care: Moral and Social Issues.* London: Kluwer Academic Publishers, 1989, pp. 33–181.
6. Gaylin W, Macklin R, eds: *Who Speaks for the Child?* New York: Plenum Press, 1982.
7. Grisso T, Vierling L: Minors' consent to treatment: a developmental perspective. *Prof Psychol* 1978;9:412–427.
8. Malton GB, Koocher GP, Saks MJ, eds: *Children's Competence to Consent.* New York: Plenum Press, 1983.
9. Weithorn LA, Campbell SB: The competency of children and adolescents to make informed treatment decisions. *Child Dev* 1982;55:1589–1598.
10. Ruddick W: Parents and life prospects. In: O'Neill O, Ruddick W, eds. *Having Children: Philosophical and Legal Reflections on Parenthood.* New York: Oxford University Press, 1979, pp. 123–137.
11. Engelhardt HT Jr: Taking the family seriously: Beyond best interests. In: Kopelman LM, Moskop JC, eds. *Children and Health Care: Moral and Social Issues.* London: Kluwer Academic Publishers, 1989, pp. 231–237.
12. Van Eys J, ed: *Research on Children: Medical Imperatives, Ethical Quandaries and Legal Constraints.* Baltimore, Md: University Park Press, 1978.
13. Medical Research Council (Canada): Ethics in Human Experimentation. Report No. 6, Ottawa. (note p 30, Minority position, P.A. Crepeau.)
14. Ramsey P: The Enforcement of Morals: Nontherapeutic Research on Children. *Hastings Center Report* 1976;6,4:21–30.
15. Ramsey P: "Unconsented touching" and the autonomy absolute. *IRB.* 1980;2,10:9–10.
16. National Commission for the Protection of Human Subjects of Biomedical and Behavioral Research: *Research Involving Children: Report and Recommendations.* Washington, DC: US Government Printing Office, 1977.
17. Nicholson RH, ed: *Medical Research with Children: Ethics, Law, and Practice.* Oxford: Oxford University Press, 1986.
18. Levine RJ: *Ethics and Regulation of Clinical Research.* Baltimore-Munich: Urban and Schwarzenberg, 1981, pp. 155–168.
19. Levine RJ: Children as research subjects. In: Kopelman LM, Moskop JC, eds. *Children and Health Care: Moral and Social Issues.* London: Kluwer Academic Publishers, 1989, pp. 73–87.
20. McCormick RA: Proxy consent in the experimentation situation. *Perspect Biol Med* 1974;18:2–20.
21. Kopelman LM: When is the risk minimal enough for children to be research subjects? In: Kopelman LM, Moskop JC, eds. *Children and Health Care: Moral and Social Issues,* London: Kluwer Academic Publishers, 1989, pp. 89–99.
22. Janofsky J, Starfield B: Assessment of risk in research on children. *J Pediatr* 1981;98(5):842–846.
23. Harrison MR, Adzick NS, Longaker MT, et al: Successful repair in utero of a fetal diaphragmatic hernia after removal of herniated viscera from the left thorax. *N Engl J Med* 1990;322:1582–1584.
24. Newcomer LN: Defining experimental therapy—a third party payer's dilemma. *N Engl J Med* 1990;323,24:1702–1704.
25. Medical Research Council (Canada): Guidelines on Research Involving Human Subjects. Ottawa. Report No. 9.
26. National Commission for the Protection of Human Subjects of Biomedical and Behavioral Research: *Research on the Fetus: Report and Recommendations.* Washington, DC: US Department of Health, Education, and Welfare, 1975.
27. Pringle KC: Ethical issues in fetal surgery. In: Puri P, ed. *Modern Problems in Pediatrics 23.* Basel: Karger, 1986, pp. 190–201.
28. Annas GJ, Elias S: Perspectives on fetal surgery: On the road from experimentation to therapy (and what to do when we arrive). In Milunsky A, Annas GJ, eds. *Genetics and the Law III.* New York: Plenum Press, 1985, pp. 347–363.
29. Macklin R: Ethical implications of surgical experiments. *Am Coll Surgeons Bull* 1985;70,6:2–8.
30. Murray T: Ethical issues in fetal surgery. *Am Coll Surgeons Bull* 1985;70,6:6–10.
31. Walters L: Ethical issues in intrauterine diagnosis and therapy. *Fetal Ther* 1986;1,1:32–37.
32. Jonsen AR: The ethics of fetal surgery. In Milunsky A, Annas GJ, eds. *Genetics and the Law III.* New York: Plenum Press, 1985, pp. 365–368.
33. Bartlett RH, Gazzaniga AB, Toomasin J, et al: Extracorporeal oxygenation (ECMO) in neonatal respiratory failure: 100 cases. *Ann Surg* 1986;204:236–245.
34. Vacanti JP, O'Rourke PP, Lillehei CW, et al. The cardiopulmonary consequences of high-risk congenital diaphragmatic hernia. *Pediatr Surg Int* 1988;3:1–5.
35. Fletcher JC: Drawing moral lines in fetal therapy. *Clin Obstet Gynecol* 1986;29,3:595–602.
36. Engelhardt HT: Current controversies in obstetrics: Wrongful life and forced fetal surgical procedures. *Am J Obstet Gynecol* 1985;151,3:313–318.
37. Ruddick W, Wilcox W: Operating on the fetus. *Hastings Center Report* 1982;12,5:10–14.
38. American Academy of Pediatrics, Committee on Bioethics: Fetal therapy: Ethical considerations. *Pediatrics* 1988;81,6:898–899.
39. Vouhé PR: Transplantation of thoracic organs in children. In *Pediatric Thoracic Surgery.* New York: Elsevier Science Publishing, 1991.
40. Knox RA. Heart transplantation: To pay or not to pay. In Abrams N, Buckner MD, eds. *Medical Ethics* Cambridge, Mass: MIT Press, 1988, pp. 560–564.

41. Evans RW, Manninen DL et al: Donor availability as the primary determinant of the future of heart transplantation. *JAMA* 1986;255(14):1892–1898.

42. Lynch A: Use of the anencephalic infant as organ donor: some "public" questions. *Westminster Affairs* 1988;1(2):3–5.

43. Walters JW, Ashwal S: Organ prolongation in anencephalic infants: Ethical and medical issues. *Hastings Center Report* 1988, pp. 19–27.

44. Pringle KC: Fetal surgery: Practical considerations and current status. In *Pediatric Thoracic Surgery.* New York: Elsevier Science Publishing, 1991.

45. Bartlett RH, Gazzaniga AB, Toomasin J, et al: Extracorporeal oxygen (ECMO) in neonatal respiratory failure: 100 cases. *Ann Surg* 1986;204:236–245.

46. Jonas H: Philosophical reflections on experimenting with human subjects. In Freud PA, ed. *Experimentation with Human Subjects.* New York: American Academy of Arts and Sciences, 1970.

47. National Commission for the Protection of Human Subjects of Biomedical and Behavioral Research: *Research Involving Children: Report and Recommendations.* Washington, DC: US Government Printing Office, 1977.

Index

Page numbers followed by t *represent tables; those followed by* f *represent figures.*

351